# Physical Activity and Health

## A Report of the Surgeon General

D1127985

U.S. DEPARTMENT OF HEALTH AND HUMAN SERVICES
Centers for Disease Control and Prevention
National Center for Chronic Disease Prevention and Health Promotion
The President's Council on Physical Fitness and Sports

Neither the U.S. Public Health Service nor the U.S. Department of Health and Human Services endorses any particular organization or its activities, products or services.


Other Federal Titles from International Medical Publishing
       The Guide to Clinical Preventive Services, 2nd edition
       The Clinician's Handbook of Preventive Services
       First Aid

First edition, 1996.

**Suggested Citation**
U.S. Department of Health and Human Services. *Physical Activity and Health: A Report of the Surgeon General*. Atlanta, GA: U.S. Department of Health and Human Services, Centers for Disease Control and Prevention, National Center for Chronic Disease Prevention and Health Promotion, International Medical Publishing, 1996.


**Physical Activity and Health: A Report of the Surgeon General**

International Medical Publishing, Inc.
P.O. Box 479
McLean, VA 22101-0479
phone 703-519-0807
fax 703-519-0806


Printed in the USA
ISBN: 1-883205-31-X

# Message from Donna E. Shalala
*Secretary of Health and Human Services*

The United States has led the world in understanding and promoting the benefits of physical activity. In the 1950s, we launched the first national effort to encourage young Americans to be physically active, with a strong emphasis on participation in team sports. In the 1970s, we embarked on a national effort to educate Americans about the cardiovascular benefits of vigorous activity, such as running and playing basketball. And in the 1980s and 1990s, we made breakthrough findings about the health benefits of moderate-intensity activities, such as walking, gardening, and dancing.

Now, with the publication of this first Surgeon General's report on physical activity and health, which I commissioned in 1994, we are poised to take another bold step forward. This landmark review of the research on physical activity and health—the most comprehensive ever—has the potential to catalyze a new physical activity and fitness movement in the United States. It is a work of real significance, on par with the Surgeon General's historic first report on smoking and health published in 1964.

This report is a passport to good health for all Americans. Its key finding is that people of all ages can improve the quality of their lives through a lifelong practice of moderate physical activity. You don't have to be training for the Boston Marathon to derive real health benefits from physical activity. A regular, preferably daily regimen of at least 30–45 minutes of brisk walking, bicycling, or even working around the house or yard will reduce your risks of developing coronary heart disease, hypertension, colon cancer, and diabetes. And if you're already doing that, you should consider picking up the pace: this report says that people who are already physically active will benefit even more by increasing the intensity or duration of their activity.

This watershed report comes not a moment too soon. We have found that 60 percent—well over half—of Americans are not regularly active. Worse yet, 25 percent of Americans are not active at all. For young people—the future of our country—physical activity declines dramatically during adolescence. These are dangerous trends. We need to turn them around quickly, for the health of our citizens and our country.

We will do so only with a massive national commitment—beginning now, on the eve of the Centennial Olympic Games, with a true fitness Dream Team drawing on the many forms of leadership that make up our great democratic society. Families need to weave physical activity into the fabric of their daily lives. Health professionals, in addition to being role models for healthy behaviors, need to encourage their patients to get out of their chairs and start fitness programs tailored to their individual needs. Businesses need to learn from what has worked in the past and promote worksite fitness, an easy option for workers. Community leaders need to reexamine whether enough resources have been devoted to the maintenance of parks, playgrounds, community centers, and physical education. Schools and universities need to reintroduce daily, quality physical activity as a key component of a comprehensive education. And the media and entertainment industries need to use their vast creative abilities to show all Americans that physical activity is healthful and fun—in other words, that it is attractive, maybe even glamorous!

We Americans always find the will to change when change is needed. I believe we can team up to create a new physical activity movement in this country. In doing so, we will save precious resources, precious futures, and precious lives. The time for action—and activity—is now.

# Foreword

This first Surgeon General's report on physical activity is being released on the eve of the Centennial Olympic Games—the premiere event showcasing the world's greatest athletes. It is fitting that the games are being held in Atlanta, Georgia, home of the Centers for Disease Control and Prevention (CDC), the lead federal agency in preparing this report. The games' 100-year celebration also coincides with the CDC's landmark 50th year and with the 40th anniversary of the President's Council on Physical Fitness and Sports (PCPFS), the CDC's partner in developing this report. Because physical activity is a widely achievable means to a healthier life, this report directly supports the CDC's mission—to promote health and quality of life by preventing and controlling disease, injury, and disability. Also clear is the link to the PCPFS; originally established as part of a national campaign to help shape up America's younger generation, the Council continues today to promote physical activity, fitness, and sports for Americans of all ages.

The Olympic Games represent the summit of athletic achievement. The Paralympics, an international competition that will occur later this summer in Atlanta, represents the peak of athletic accomplishment for athletes with disabilities. Few of us will approach these levels of performance in our own physical endeavors. The good news in this report is that we do not have to scale Olympian heights to achieve significant health benefits. We can improve the quality of our lives through a lifelong practice of moderate amounts of regular physical activity of moderate or vigorous intensity. An active lifestyle is available to all.

Many Americans may be surprised at the extent and strength of the evidence linking physical activity to numerous health improvements. Most significantly, regular physical activity greatly reduces the risk of dying from coronary heart disease, the leading cause of death in the United States. Physical activity also reduces the risk of developing diabetes, hypertension, and colon cancer; enhances mental health; fosters healthy muscles, bones and joints; and helps maintain function and preserve independence in older adults.

The evidence about what helps people incorporate physical activity into their lives is less clear-cut. We do know that effective strategies and policies have taken place in settings as diverse as physical education classes in schools, health promotion programs at worksites, and one-on-one counseling by health care providers. However, more needs to be learned about what helps individuals change their physical activity habits and how changes in community environments, policies, and social norms might support that process.

Support is greatly needed if physical activity is to be increased in a society as technologically advanced as ours. Most Americans today are spared the burden of excessive physical labor. Indeed, few occupations today require significant physical activity, and most people use motorized transportation to get to work and to perform routine errands and tasks. Even leisure time is increasingly filled with sedentary behaviors, such as watching television, "surfing" the Internet, and playing video games.

Increasing physical activity is a formidable public health challenge that we must hasten to meet. The stakes are high, and the potential rewards are momentous: preventing premature death, unnecessary illness, and disability; controlling health care costs; and maintaining a high quality of life into old age.

David Satcher, M.D., Ph.D.
Director
Centers for Disease Control
and Prevention

Philip R. Lee, M.D.
Assistant Secretary
for Health

Florence Griffith Joyner
Tom McMillen
Co-Chairs
President's Council on
Physical Fitness and Sports

# Preface

*from the Surgeon General*
*U.S. Public Health Service*

I am pleased to present the first report of the Surgeon General on physical activity and health. For more than a century, the Surgeon General of the Public Health Service has focused the nation's attention on important public health issues. Reports from Surgeons General on the adverse health consequences of smoking triggered nationwide efforts to prevent tobacco use. Reports on nutrition, violence, and HIV/AIDS—to name but a few—have heightened America's awareness of important public health issues and have spawned major public health initiatives. This new report, which is a comprehensive review of the available scientific evidence about the relationship between physical activity and health status, follows in this notable tradition.

Scientists and doctors have known for years that substantial benefits can be gained from regular physical activity. The expanding and strengthening evidence on the relationship between physical activity and health necessitates the focus this report brings to this important public health challenge. Although the science of physical activity is a complex and still-developing field, we have today strong evidence to indicate that regular physical activity will provide clear and substantial health gains. In this sense, the report is more than a summary of the science—it is a national call to action.

We must get serious about improving the health of the nation by affirming our commitment to healthy physical activity on all levels: personal, family, community, organizational, and national. Because physical activity is so directly related to preventing disease and premature death and to maintaining a high quality of life, we must accord it the same level of attention that we give other important public health practices that affect the entire nation. Physical activity thus joins the front ranks of essential health objectives, such as sound nutrition, the use of seat belts, and the prevention of adverse health effects of tobacco.

The time for this emphasis is both opportune and pressing. As this report makes clear, current levels of physical activity among Americans remain low, and we are losing ground in some areas. The good news in the report is that people can benefit from even moderate levels of physical activity. The public health implications of this good news are vast: the tremendous health gains that could be realized with even partial success at improving physical activity among the American people compel us to make a commitment and take action. With innovation, dedication, partnering, and a long-term plan, we should be able to improve the health and well-being of our people.

This report is not the final word. More work will need to be done so that we can determine the most effective ways to motivate all Americans to participate in a level of physical activity that can benefit their health and well-being. The challenge that lies ahead is formidable but worthwhile. I strongly encourage all Americans to join us in this effort.

Audrey F. Manley, M.D., M.P.H.
Surgeon General (Acting)

# Acknowledgments

This report was prepared by the Department of Health and Human Services under the direction of the Centers for Disease Control and Prevention, National Center for Chronic Disease Prevention and Health Promotion, in collaboration with the President's Council on Physical Fitness and Sports.

David Satcher, M.D., Ph.D., Director, Centers for Disease Control and Prevention, Atlanta, Georgia.

James S. Marks, M.D., M.P.H., Director, National Center for Chronic Disease Prevention and Health Promotion, Centers for Disease Control and Prevention, Atlanta, Georgia.

Virginia S. Bales, M.P.H., Deputy Director, National Center for Chronic Disease Prevention and Health Promotion, Centers for Disease Control and Prevention, Atlanta, Georgia.

Lisa A. Daily, Assistant Director for Planning, Evaluation, and Legislation, National Center for Chronic Disease Prevention and Health Promotion, Centers for Disease Control and Prevention, Atlanta, Georgia.

Marjorie A. Speers, Ph.D., Behavioral and Social Sciences Coordinator, Office of the Director, (formerly, Director, Division of Chronic Disease Control and Community Intervention, National Center for Chronic Disease Prevention and Health Promotion), Centers for Disease Control and Prevention, Atlanta, Georgia.

Frederick L. Trowbridge, M.D., Director, Division of Nutrition and Physical Activity, National Center for Chronic Disease Prevention and Health Promotion, Centers for Disease Control and Prevention, Atlanta, Georgia.

Florence Griffith Joyner, Co-Chair, President's Council on Physical Fitness and Sports, Washington, D.C.

C. Thomas McMillen, Co-Chair, President's Council on Physical Fitness and Sports, Washington, D.C.

Sandra P. Perlmutter, Executive Director, President's Council on Physical Fitness and Sports, Washington, D.C.

## Editors

Steven N. Blair, P.E.D., Senior Scientific Editor, Director of Research and Director, Epidemiology and Clinical Applications, The Cooper Institute for Aerobics Research, Dallas, Texas.

Adele L. Franks, M.D., Scientific Editor, Assistant Director for Science, National Center for Chronic Disease Prevention and Health Promotion, Centers for Disease Control and Prevention, Atlanta, Georgia.

Dana M. Shelton, M.P.H., Managing Editor, Epidemiologist, Office on Smoking and Health, National Center for Chronic Disease Prevention and Health Promotion, Centers for Disease Control and Prevention, Atlanta, Georgia.

John R. Livengood, M.D., M.Phil., Coordinating Editor, Deputy Director, Epidemiology and Surveillance Division, National Immunization Program, (formerly, Associate Director for Science, Division of Chronic Disease Control and Community Intervention, National Center for Chronic Disease Prevention and Health Promotion), Centers for Disease Control and Prevention, Atlanta, Georgia.

Frederick L. Hull, Ph.D., Technical Editor, Technical Information and Editorial Services Branch, National Center for Chronic Disease Prevention and Health Promotion, Centers for Disease Control and Prevention, Atlanta, Georgia.

Byron Breedlove, M.A., Technical Editor, Technical Information and Editorial Services Branch, National Center for Chronic Disease Prevention and Health Promotion, Centers for Disease Control and Prevention, Atlanta, Georgia.

## Editorial Board

Carl J. Caspersen, Ph.D., Epidemiologist, Division of Nutrition and Physical Activity, National Center for Chronic Disease Prevention and Health Promotion, Centers for Disease Control and Prevention, Atlanta, Georgia.

Aaron R. Folsom, M.D., M.P.H., Professor, Division of Epidemiology, School of Public Health, University of Minnesota, Minneapolis, Minnesota.

William L. Haskell, Ph.D., Professor of Medicine, Stanford University, Palo Alto, California.

Arthur S. Leon, M.D., M.S., Henry L. Taylor Professor and Director of the Laboratory of Physiological Hygiene and Exercise Science, Division of Kinesiology, University of Minnesota, Minneapolis, Minnesota.

James F. Sallis, Jr., Ph.D., Professor, Department of Psychology, San Diego State University, San Diego, California.

Martha L. Slattery, Ph.D., M.P.H., Professor, Department of Oncological Sciences, University of Utah Medical School, Salt Lake City, Utah.

Christine G. Spain, M.A., Director, Research, Planning, and Special Projects, President's Council on Physical Fitness and Sports, Washington, D.C.

Jack H. Wilmore, Ph.D., Professor, Department of Kinesiology and Health Education, University of Texas at Austin, Austin, Texas.

## Planning Board

Terry L. Bazzarre, Ph.D., Science Consultant, American Heart Association, Dallas, Texas.

Steven N. Blair, P.E.D., Senior Scientific Editor, Director of Research and Director, Epidemiology and Clinical Applications, The Cooper Institute for Aerobics Research, Dallas, Texas.

Willis R. Foster, M.D., Office of Disease Prevention and Technology Transfer, National Institute of Diabetes and Digestive and Kidney Diseases, National Institutes of Health, Bethesda, Maryland.

Patty Freedson, Ph.D., Department of Exercise Science, University of Massachusetts, Amherst, Massachusetts. Represented the American Alliance for Health, Physical Education, Recreation and Dance.

William R. Harlan, M.D., Associate Director for Disease Prevention, Office of the Director, National Institutes of Health, Bethesda, Maryland.

James A. Harrell, M.A., Deputy Commissioner, Administration on Children, Youth, and Families, (formerly, Deputy Director, Office of Disease Prevention and Health Promotion, Office of the Assistant Secretary for Health, Department of Health and Human Services), Washington, D.C.

Richard W. Lymn, Ph.D., Muscle Biology Branch, National Institute of Arthritis and Musculoskeletal and Skin Diseases, National Institutes of Health, Bethesda, Maryland.

Russell R. Pate, Ph.D., Chairman, Department of Exercise Science, University of South Carolina, Columbia, South Carolina. Represented the American College of Sports Medicine.

Sandra P. Perlmutter, Executive Director, President's Council on Physical Fitness and Sports, Washington, D.C.

Bruce G. Simons-Morton, Ed.D., M.P.H., Behavioral Scientist, Prevention Research Branch, National Institute of Child Health and Human Development, National Institutes of Health, Bethesda, Maryland.

Denise G. Simons-Morton, M.D., Ph.D., Leader, Prevention Scientific Research Group, DECA, National Heart, Lung, and Blood Institute, National Institutes of Health, Bethesda, Maryland.

## Contributing Authors

Lynda A. Anderson, Ph.D., Public Health Educator, Division of Adult and Community Health, National Center for Chronic Disease Prevention and Health Promotion, Centers for Disease Control and Prevention, Atlanta, Georgia.

Carol C. Ballew, Ph.D., Epidemiologist, Division of Nutrition and Physical Activity, National Center for Chronic Disease Prevention and Health Promotion, Centers for Disease Control and Prevention, Atlanta, Georgia.

Jack W. Berryman, Ph.D., Professor, Department of Medical History and Ethics, School of Medicine, University of Washington, Seattle, Washington.

Lawrence R. Brawley, Ph.D., Professor, University of Waterloo, Ontario, Canada.

David R. Brown, Ph.D., Health Scientist, Division of Nutrition and Physical Activity, National Center for Chronic Disease Prevention and Health Promotion, Centers for Disease Control and Prevention, Atlanta, Georgia.

Lee S. Caplan, M.D., Ph.D., Medical Epidemiologist, Epidemiology and Statistics Branch, Division of Cancer Prevention and Control, National Center for Chronic Disease Prevention and Health Promotion, Centers for Disease Control and Prevention, Atlanta, Georgia.

Ralph J. Coates, Ph.D., Chief, Epidemiology Section, Division of Cancer Prevention and Control, National Center for Chronic Disease Prevention and Health Promotion, Centers for Disease Control and Prevention, Atlanta, Georgia.

Carlos J. Crespo, Dr.P.H., M.S., F.A.C.S.M., Public Health Analyst, National Heart, Lung, and Blood Institute, National Institutes of Health, Bethesda, Maryland.

Loretta DiPietro, Ph.D., M.P.H., Assistant Fellow and Assistant Professor of Epidemiology and Public Health, The John B. Pierce Laboratory and Yale University School of Medicine, New Haven, Connecticut.

Rod K. Dishman, Ph.D., Professor, Department of Exercise Science, University of Georgia, Athens, Georgia.

Michael M. Engelgau, M.D., Chief, Epidemiology and Statistics Branch, Division of Diabetes Translation, National Center for Chronic Disease Prevention and Health Promotion, Centers for Disease Control and Prevention, Atlanta, Georgia.

Walter H. Ettinger, M.D., Professor, Internal Medicine and Public Health Sciences, Bowman Gray School of Medicine, Winston-Salem, North Carolina.

David S. Freedman, Ph.D., Epidemiologist, Division of Nutrition and Physical Activity, National Center for Chronic Disease Prevention and Health Promotion, Centers for Disease Control and Prevention, Atlanta, Georgia.

Frederick Fridinger, Dr.P.H., C.H.E.S., Public Health Educator, Division of Nutrition and Physical Activity, National Center for Chronic Disease Prevention and Health Promotion, Centers for Disease Control and Prevention, Atlanta, Georgia.

Gregory W. Heath, D.Sc., M.P.H., Epidemiologist/ Exercise Physiologist, Division of Adult and Community Health, National Center for Chronic Disease Prevention and Health Promotion, Centers for Disease Control and Prevention, Atlanta, Georgia.

Wendy A. Holmes, M.S., Health Communications Specialist, Division of Nutrition and Physical Activity, National Center for Chronic Disease Prevention and Health Promotion, Centers for Disease Control and Prevention, Atlanta, Georgia.

Elizabeth H. Howze, Sc.D., Associate Director for Health Promotion, Division of Nutrition and Physical Activity, National Center for Chronic Disease Prevention and Health Promotion, Centers for Disease Control and Prevention, Atlanta, Georgia.

Laura K. Kann, Ph.D., Chief, Surveillance Research Section, Division of Adolescent and School Health, National Center for Chronic Disease Prevention and Health Promotion, Centers for Disease Control and Prevention, Atlanta, Georgia.

Abby C. King, Ph.D., Assistant Professor of Health Research and Policy and Medicine, Stanford University School of Medicine, Palo Alto, California.

Harold W. Kohl, III, Ph.D., Director of Research, Baylor College of Medicine, Baylor Sports Medicine Institute, Houston, Texas.

Jeffrey P. Koplan, M.D., M.P.H., President, Prudential Center for Health Care Research, Atlanta, Georgia.

Andrea M. Kriska, Ph.D., M.S., Assistant Professor, Department of Epidemiology, Graduate School of Public Health, University of Pittsburgh, Pittsburgh, Pennsylvania.

Barbara D. Latham, R.D., M.P.H., Public Health Nutritionist, Division of Nutrition and Physical Activity, National Center for Chronic Disease Prevention and Health Promotion, Centers for Disease Control and Prevention, Atlanta, Georgia.

I-Min Lee, M.B.B.S., Sc.D., Assistant Professor of Medicine, Harvard Medical School, Boston, Massachusetts.

Elizabeth Lloyd, M.S., Statistician, Division of Nutrition and Physical Activity, National Center for Chronic Disease Prevention and Health Promotion, Centers for Disease Control and Prevention, Atlanta, Georgia.

Bess H. Marcus, Ph.D., Associate Professor of Psychiatry and Human Behavior, Division of Behavior and Preventive Medicine, Miriam Hospital and Brown University School of Medicine, Providence, Rhode Island.

Dyann Matson-Koffman, Dr.P.H., M.P.H., C.H.E.S., Public Health Educator, Division of Adult and Community Health, National Center for Chronic Disease Prevention and Health Promotion, Centers for Disease Control and Prevention, Atlanta, Georgia.

Marion R. Nadel, Ph.D., Epidemiologist, Epidemiology and Statistics Branch, Division of Cancer Prevention and Control, National Center for Chronic Disease Prevention and Health Promotion, Centers for Disease Control and Prevention, Atlanta, Georgia.

Eva Obarzanek, Ph.D., M.P.H., R.D., Nutritionist, National Heart, Lung, and Blood Institute, National Institutes of Health, Bethesda, Maryland.

Christine M. Plepys, M.S., Health Statistician, Division of Health Promotion Statistics, National Center for Health Statistics, Centers for Disease Control and Prevention, Hyattsville, Maryland.

Michael L. Pollock, Ph.D., Professor of Medicine, Physiology and Health and Human Performance; Director, Center for Exercise Science, University of Florida, Gainesville, Florida.

Michael Pratt, M.D., M.P.H., Medical Epidemiologist, Division of Nutrition and Physical Activity, National Center for Chronic Disease Prevention and Health Promotion, Centers for Disease Control and Prevention, Atlanta, Georgia.

Paul T. Raford, M.D., M.P.H., Special Assistant to the Regional Health Administrator, Environmental Justice Programs, Office of Public Health Science, Region VIII, Department of Health and Human Services, U.S. Public Health Service, Denver, Colorado.

W. Jack Rejeski, Ph.D., Professor, Health and Sports Science, Wake Forest University, Winston-Salem, North Carolina.

Richard B. Rothenberg, M.D., M.P.H., F.A.C.P., Professor and Director, Preventive Medicine Residency Program, Department of Family and Preventive Medicine, Emory University School of Medicine, Atlanta, Georgia.

Mary K. Serdula, M.D., M.P.H., Acting Branch Chief, Chronic Disease Prevention Branch, Division of Nutrition and Physical Activity, National Center for Chronic Disease Prevention and Health Promotion, Centers for Disease Control and Prevention, Atlanta, Georgia.

Charlotte A. Schoenborn, M.P.H., Health Statistician, National Center for Health Statistics, Centers for Disease Control and Prevention, Hyattsville, Maryland.

Denise G. Simons-Morton, M.D., Ph.D., Leader, Prevention Scientific Research Group, DECA, National Heart, Lung, and Blood Institute, National Institutes of Health, Bethesda, Maryland.

Elaine J. Stone, Ph.D., M.P.H., Health Scientist Administrator, Division of Epidemiology and Clinical Applications, National Heart, Lung, and Blood Institute, National Institutes of Health, Bethesda, Maryland.

Marlene K. Tappe, Ph.D., Visiting Behavioral Scientist, Division of Adolescent and School Health, National Center for Chronic Disease Prevention and Health Promotion, Centers for Disease Control and Prevention, Atlanta, Georgia.

Wendell C. Taylor, Ph.D., M.P.H., Assistant Professor of Behavioral Sciences, School of Public Health, University of Texas Health Science Center at Houston, Houston, Texas.

Charles W. Warren, Ph.D., Statistician/Demographer, Division of Adolescent and School Health, National Center for Chronic Disease Prevention and Health Promotion, Centers for Disease Control and Prevention, Atlanta, Georgia.

Deborah R. Young, Ph.D., Assistant Professor of Medicine, Division of Internal Medicine, The Johns Hopkins School of Medicine, Baltimore, Maryland.

## Senior Reviewers

Elizabeth A. Arendt, M.D., Associate Professor of Orthopaedics, University of Minnesota, Minneapolis, Minnesota. Member, President's Council on Physical Fitness and Sports.

Elsworth R. Buskirk, Ph.D., Professor of Applied Physiology, Emeritus, Pennsylvania State University, University Park, Pennsylvania.

B. Don Franks, Ph.D., Professor and Chair, Department of Kinesiology, Louisiana State University, Baton Rouge, Louisiana. Senior Program Advisor, President's Council on Physical Fitness and Sports.

William R. Harlan, M.D., Associate Director for Disease Prevention, Office of the Director, National Institutes of Health, Bethesda, Maryland.

William P. Morgan, Ed.D., Professor, Department of Kinesiology, University of Wisconsin–Madison, Madison, Wisconsin.

Ralph S. Paffenbarger, Jr., M.D., Dr.P.H., Professor of Epidemiology (Retired–Active), Stanford University School of Medicine, Stanford, California.

Russell R. Pate, Ph.D., Chairman, Department of Exercise Science, University of South Carolina, Columbia, South Carolina. Represented the American College of Sports Medicine.

Roy J. Shephard, M.D., Ph.D., D.P.E., F.A.C.S.M., Professor Emeritus of Applied Physiology, University of Toronto, Toronto, Canada.

## Peer Reviewers

Barbara E. Ainsworth, Ph.D., M.P.H., Associate Professor, Department of Epidemiology and Biostatistics, Department of Exercise Science, School of Public Health, University of South Carolina, Columbia, South Carolina.

Tom Baranowski, Ph.D., Professor, Department of Behavioral Science, University of Texas, M. D. Anderson Cancer Center, Houston, Texas.

Oded Bar-Or, M.D., Professor of Pediatrics and Director, Children's Exercise and Nutrition Centre, McMaster University, Chedoke Hospital Division, Hamilton, Ontario, Canada.

Charles B. Corbin, Ph.D., Professor, Department of Exercise Science and Physical Education, Arizona State University, Tempe, Arizona.

Kirk J. Cureton, Ph.D., Professor and Head, Department of Exercise Science, University of Georgia, Athens, Georgia.

Gail P. Dalsky, Ph.D., Assistant Professor of Medicine (in residence), University of Connecticut Health Center, Farmington, Connecticut.

Nicholas A. DiNubile, M.D., Clinical Assistant Professor, Department of Orthopaedic Surgery, Hospital of the University of Pennsylvania; Chief, Orthopaedic Surgery and Sports Medicine, Delaware County Memorial Hospital, Drexel Hill, Pennsylvania.

Barbara L. Drinkwater, Ph.D., Research Physiologist, Pacific Medical Center, Seattle, Washington.

Andrea L. Dunn, Ph.D., Associate Director, Division of Epidemiology and Clinical Applications, The Cooper Institute for Aerobics Research, Dallas, Texas.

Leonard H. Epstein, Ph.D., Professor, Department of Psychology, State University of New York at Buffalo, Buffalo, New York.

Katherine M. Flegal, Ph.D., Senior Research Epidemiologist, National Center for Health Statistics, Centers for Disease Control and Prevention, Hyattsville, Maryland.

Christopher D. Gardner, Ph.D., Research Fellow, Stanford Center for Research in Disease Prevention, Stanford University, Palo Alto, California.

Glen G. Gilbert, Ph.D., Professor and Chairperson, Department of Health Education, University of Maryland, College Park, Maryland.

Andrew P. Goldberg, M.D., Professor of Medicine and Director, Division of Gerontology, University of Maryland School of Medicine, Baltimore, Maryland.

John O. Holloszy, M.D., Professor of Internal Medicine, Washington University School of Medicine, St. Louis, Missouri.

Melbourne F. Hovell, Ph.D., M.P.H., Professor of Health Promotion; Director, Center for Behavioral Epidemiology, Graduate School of Public Health, College of Health and Human Services, San Diego State University, San Diego, California.

Caroline A. Macera, Ph.D., Director, Prevention Center, School of Public Health, University of South Carolina, Columbia, South Carolina.

JoAnn E. Manson, M.D., Dr.P.H., Co-Director of Women's Health, Brigham and Women's Hospital, Harvard Medical School, Boston, Massachusetts.

Jere H. Mitchell, M.D., Professor of Internal Medicine and Physiology; Director, Harry S. Moss Heart Center, University of Texas Southwestern Medical Center, Dallas, Texas.

James R. Morrow, Jr., Ph.D., Professor and Chair, Department of KHPR, University of North Texas, Denton, Texas.

Neville Owen, Ph.D., Professor of Human Movement Science, Deakin University, Melbourne, Australia.

Roberta J. Park, Ph.D., Professor of the Graduate School, University of California, Berkeley, California.

Peter B. Raven, Ph.D., Professor and Chair, Department of Integrative Physiology, University of North Texas Health Science Center, Fort Worth, Texas.

Judith G. Regensteiner, Ph.D., Associate Professor of Medicine, University of Colorado Health Sciences Center, Denver, Colorado.

Bruce G. Simons-Morton, Ed.D., M.P.H., Behavioral Scientist, Prevention Research Branch, National Institute of Child Health and Human Development, National Institutes of Health, Bethesda, Maryland.

Denise G. Simons-Morton, M.D., Ph.D., Leader, Prevention Scientific Research Group, DECA, National Heart, Lung, and Blood Institute, National Institutes of Health, Bethesda, Maryland.

James S. Skinner, Ph.D., Professor, Department of Kinesiology, Indiana University, Bloomington, Indiana.

Thomas Stephens, Ph.D., Principal, Thomas Stephens and Associates, Ottawa, Canada.

Anita Stewart, Ph.D., Associate Professor in Residence, University of California, San Francisco, San Francisco, California.

C. Barr Taylor, M.D., Professor of Psychiatry, Department of Psychiatry and Behavioral Sciences, Stanford University School of Medicine, Stanford, California.

Charles M. Tipton, Ph.D., F.A.C.S.M., Professor of Physiology and Surgery, University of Arizona, Tucson, Arizona.

Zung Vu Tran, Ph.D., Senior Research Scientist, Center for Research in Ambulatory Health Care Administration, Englewood, Colorado.

## Other Contributors

Melissa M. Adams, Ph.D., Assistant Director for Science, Division of Reproductive Health, National Center for Chronic Disease Prevention and Health Promotion, Centers for Disease Control and Prevention, Atlanta, Georgia.

Indu Ahluwalia, M.P.H., Ph.D., EIS Officer, Division of Nutrition and Physical Activity, National Center for Chronic Disease Prevention and Health Promotion, Centers for Disease Control and Prevention, Atlanta, Georgia.

Betty A. Ballinger, Technical Information Specialist, Technical Information and Editorial Services Branch, National Center for Chronic Disease Prevention and Health Promotion, Centers for Disease Control and Prevention, Atlanta, Georgia.

Sandra W. Bart, Policy Coordinator, Office of the Secretary, Executive Secretariat, Department of Health and Human Services, Washington, D.C.

Mary Bedford, Proofreader, Cygnus Corporation, Rockville, Maryland.

Caryn Bern, M.D., Medical Epidemiologist, Division of Nutrition and Physical Activity, National Center for Chronic Disease Prevention and Health Promotion, Centers for Disease Control and Prevention, Atlanta, Georgia.

Karil Bialostosky, M.S., Nutrition Fellow, National Center for Health Statistics, Centers for Disease Control and Prevention, Hyattsville, Maryland.

Thomas E. Blakeney, Program Analyst, National Center for Injury Prevention and Control, Centers for Disease Control and Prevention, Atlanta, Georgia.

Ronette R. Briefel, Dr.P.H., Nutrition Policy Advisor, National Center for Health Statistics, Centers for Disease Control and Prevention, Hyattsville, Maryland.

L. Diane Clark, M.P.H., Public Health Nutritionist, Division of Nutrition and Physical Activity, National Center for Chronic Disease Prevention and Health Promotion, Centers for Disease Control and Prevention, Atlanta, Georgia.

Janet L. Collins, Ph.D., Chief, Surveillance and Evaluation Research Branch, Division of Adolescent and School Health, National Center for Chronic Disease Prevention and Health Promotion, Centers for Disease Control and Prevention, Atlanta, Georgia.

Janet B. Croft, Ph.D., Epidemiogist, Division of Adult and Community Health, National Center for Chronic Disease Prevention and Health Promotion, Centers for Disease Control and Prevention, Atlanta, Georgia.

Ann M. Cronin, Program Analyst, National Institute for Occupational Safety and Health, Centers for Disease Control and Prevention, Atlanta, Georgia.

Gail A. Cruse, M.L.I.S., Technical Information Specialist, Technical Information and Editorial Services Branch, National Center for Chronic Disease Prevention and Health Promotion, Centers for Disease Control and Prevention, Atlanta, Georgia.

John M. Davis, M.P.A., R.D., Public Health Analyst, Division of Nutrition and Physical Activity, National Center for Chronic Disease Prevention and Health Promotion, Centers for Disease Control and Prevention, Atlanta, Georgia.

Earl S. Ford, M.D., M.P.H., Senior Scientist, Division of Nutrition and Physical Activity, National Center for Chronic Disease Prevention and Health Promotion, Centers for Disease Control and Prevention, Atlanta, Georgia.

Christine S. Fralish, M.L.I.S., Chief, Technical Information and Editorial Services Branch, National Center for Chronic Disease Prevention and Health Promotion, Centers for Disease Control and Prevention, Atlanta, Georgia.

Emma L. Frazier, Ph.D., Mathematical Statistician, Division of Diabetes Translation, National Center for Chronic Disease Prevention and Health Promotion, Centers for Disease Control and Prevention, Atlanta, Georgia.

Deborah A. Galuska, M.P.H., Ph.D., EIS Fellow, Division of Nutrition and Physical Activity, National Center for Chronic Disease Prevention and Health Promotion, Centers for Disease Control and Prevention, Atlanta, Georgia.

Dinamarie C. Garcia, M.P.H., C.H.E.S., Intern, Division of Nutrition and Physical Activity, National Center for Chronic Disease Prevention and Health Promotion, Centers for Disease Control and Prevention, Atlanta, Georgia.

Linda S. Geiss, M.A., Health Statistician, Division of Diabetes Translation, National Center for Chronic Disease Prevention and Health Promotion, Centers for Disease Control and Prevention, Atlanta, Georgia.

Wayne H. Giles, M.D., M.S., Epidemiologist, Cardiovascular Health Section, Division of Adult and Community Health, National Center for Chronic Disease Prevention and Health Promotion, Centers for Disease Control and Prevention, Atlanta, Georgia.

Kay Sissions Golan, Public Affairs Specialist, Office of Communication (proposed), Centers for Disease Control and Prevention, Atlanta, Georgia.

Betty H. Haithcock, Editorial Assistant, Technical Information and Editorial Services Branch, National Center for Chronic Disease Prevention and Health Promotion, Centers for Disease Control and Prevention, Atlanta, Georgia.

Helen P. Hankins, Writer-Editor, Technical Information and Editorial Services Branch, National Center for Chronic Disease Prevention and Health Promotion, Centers for Disease Control and Prevention, Atlanta, Georgia.

Rita Harding, Graphic Designer, Cygnus Corporation, Rockville, Maryland.

William A. Harris, M.M., Computer Specialist, Division of Adolescent and School Health, National Center for Chronic Disease Prevention and Health Promotion, Centers for Disease Control and Prevention, Atlanta, Georgia.

Charles G. Helmick, III, M.D., Division of Adult and Community Health, National Center for Chronic Disease Prevention and Health Promotion, Centers for Disease Control and Prevention, Atlanta, Georgia.

Elizabeth L. Hess, Technical Editor, Cygnus Corporation, Rockville, Maryland.

Mary Ann Hill, M.P.P., Director of Communications, President's Council on Physical Fitness and Sports, Washington, D.C.

Thomya L. Hogan, Proofreader, Cygnus Corporation, Rockville, Maryland.

Judy F. Horne, Technical Information Specialist, Technical Information and Editorial Services Branch, National Center for Chronic Disease Prevention and Health Promotion, Centers for Disease Control and Prevention, Atlanta, Georgia.

Catherine A. Hutsell, M.P.H., Public Health Educator, Division of Adult and Community Health, National Center for Chronic Disease Prevention and Health Promotion, Centers for Disease Control and Prevention, Atlanta, Georgia.

Robert Irwin, Special Assistant, Office of the Director, Centers for Disease Control and Prevention, Washington, D.C.

Sandra E. Jewell, M.S., Statistician, Division of Nutrition and Physical Activity, National Center for Chronic Disease Prevention and Health Promotion, Centers for Disease Control and Prevention, Atlanta, Georgia.

Loretta G. Johnson, Secretary, Division of Nutrition and Physical Activity, National Center for Chronic Disease Prevention and Health Promotion, Centers for Disease Control and Prevention, Atlanta, Georgia.

Deborah A. Jones, Ph.D., Epidemiologist, Division of Nutrition and Physical Activity, National Center for Chronic Disease Prevention and Health Promotion, Centers for Disease Control and Prevention, Atlanta, Georgia.

Wanda K. Jones, M.P.H., Dr.P.H., Associate Director for Women's Health, Office of Women's Health, Centers for Disease Control and Prevention, Atlanta, Georgia.

Robert E. Keaton, Consultant, Cygnus Corporation, Rockville, Maryland.

Delle B. Kelley, Technical Information Specialist, Technical Information and Editorial Services Branch, National Center for Chronic Disease Prevention and Health Promotion, Centers for Disease Control and Prevention, Atlanta, Georgia.

Mescal J. Knighton, Writer-Editor, Technical Information and Editorial Services Branch, National Center for Chronic Disease Prevention and Health Promotion, Centers for Disease Control and Prevention, Atlanta, Georgia.

Sarah B. Knowlton, J.D., M.S.W., Attorney Advisor, Office of the General Council, Centers for Disease Control and Prevention, Atlanta, Georgia.

Fred Kroger, Acting Director, Health Communication, Office of Communication (proposed), Centers for Disease Control and Prevention, Atlanta, Georgia.

Sarah A. Kuester, M.P.H., R.D., Public Health Nutritionist, Division of Nutrition and Physical Activity, National Center for Chronic Disease Prevention and Health Promotion, Centers for Disease Control and Prevention, Atlanta, Georgia.

Becky H. Lankenau, M.S., R.D., M.P.H., Dr.P.H., Public Health Nutritionist, Division of Nutrition and Physical Activity, National Center for Chronic Disease Prevention and Health Promotion, Centers for Disease Control and Prevention, Atlanta, Georgia.

Nancy C. Lee, M.D., Associate Director for Science, Division of Cancer Prevention and Control, National Center for Chronic Disease Prevention and Health Promotion, Centers for Disease Control and Prevention, Atlanta, Georgia.

Leandris C. Liburd, M.P.H., Public Health Educator, Division of Diabetes Translation, National Center for Chronic Disease Prevention and Health Promotion, Centers for Disease Control and Prevention, Atlanta, Georgia.

Richard Lowry, M.D., M.S., Medical Epidemiologist, Division of Adolescent and School Health, National Center for Chronic Disease Prevention and Health Promotion, Centers for Disease Control and Prevention, Atlanta, Georgia.

Salvatore J. Lucido, M.P.A., Program Analyst, National Center for Chronic Disease Prevention and Health Promotion, Centers for Disease Control and Prevention, Atlanta, Georgia.

Gene W. Matthews, Esq., Legal Advisor to CDC and ATSDR, Office of the General Council, Centers for Disease Control and Prevention, Atlanta, Georgia.

Brenda W. Mazzocchi, M.S.L.S., Technical Information Specialist, Technical Information and Editorial Services Branch, National Center for Chronic Disease Prevention and Health Promotion, Centers for Disease Control and Prevention, Atlanta, Georgia.

Sharon McDonnell, M.D., M.P.H., Medical Epidemiologist, Division of Nutrition and Physical Activity, National Center for Chronic Disease Prevention and Health Promotion, Centers for Disease Control and Prevention, Atlanta, Georgia.

Michael A. McGeehin, Ph.D., M.S.P.H., Chief, Health Studies Branch, Division of Environmental Hazards and Health Effects, National Center for Environmental Health, Centers for Disease Control and Prevention, Atlanta, Georgia.

Zuguo Mei, M.D., M.P.H. Visiting Scientist, Division of Nutrition and Physical Activity, National Center for Chronic Disease Prevention .and Health Promotion, Centers for Disease Control and Prevention, Atlanta, Georgia.

James M. Mendlein, Ph.D., Epidemiologist, Division of Nutrition and Physical Activity, National Center for Chronic Disease Prevention and Health Promotion, Centers for Disease Control and Prevention, Atlanta, Georgia.

Robert K. Merritt, M.A., Behavioral Scientist, Office on Smoking and Health, National Center for Chronic Disease Prevention and Health Promotion, Centers for Disease Control and Prevention, Atlanta, Georgia.

Gaylon D. Morris, M.P.P., Program Analyst, Office of Program Planning and Evaluation, Centers for Disease Control and Prevention, Atlanta, Georgia.

Melba Morrow, M.A., Division Manager, The Cooper Institute for Aerobics Research, Dallas, Texas.

Marion R. Nadel, Ph.D., Epidemiologist, Division of Cancer Prevention and Control, National Center for Chronic Disease Prevention and Health Promotion, Centers for Disease Control and Prevention, Atlanta, Georgia.

David E. Nelson, M.D., M.P.H., Medical Officer, Division of Adult and Community Health, National Center for Chronic Disease Prevention and Health Promotion, Centers for Disease Control and Prevention, Atlanta, Georgia.

Reba A. Norman, M.L.M., Technical Information Specialist, Technical Information and Editorial Services Branch, National Center for Chronic Disease Prevention and Health Promotion, Centers for Disease Control and Prevention, Atlanta, Georgia.

Ward C. Nyholm, Graphic Designer, Cygnus Corporation, Rockville, Maryland.

Stephen M. Ostroff, M.D., Associate Director for Epidemiologic Science, National Center for Infectious Diseases, Centers for Disease Control and Prevention, Atlanta, Georgia.

Ibrahim Parvanta, M.S., Acting Deputy Chief, Maternal and Child Health Branch, Division of Nutrition and Physical Activity, National Center for Chronic Disease Prevention and Health Promotion, Centers for Disease Control and Prevention, Atlanta, Georgia.

Terry F. Pechacek, Ph.D., Visiting Scientist, Office on Smoking and Health, National Center for Chronic Disease Prevention and Health Promotion, Centers for Disease Control and Prevention, Atlanta, Georgia.

Geraldine S. Perry, Dr.P.H., Epidemiologist, Division of Nutrition and Physical Activity, National Center for Chronic Disease Prevention and Health Promotion, Centers for Disease Control and Prevention, Atlanta, Georgia.

Todd M. Phillips, M.S., Deputy Project Director, Cygnus Corporation, Rockville, Maryland.

Audrey L. Pinto, Writer-Editor, Technical Information and Editorial Services Branch, National Center for Chronic Disease Prevention and Health Promotion, Centers for Disease Control and Prevention, Atlanta, Georgia.

Kenneth E. Powell, M.D., M.P.H., Associate Director for Science, Division of Violence Prevention, National Center for Injury Prevention and Control, Centers for Disease Control and Prevention, Atlanta, Georgia.

Julia H. Pruden, M.Ed., R.D., Public Health Nutritionist, Division of Nutrition and Physical Activity, National Center for Chronic Disease Prevention and Health Promotion, Centers for Disease Control and Prevention, Atlanta, Georgia.

David C. Ramsey, M.P.H., Public Health Educator, Division of Nutrition and Physical Activity, National Center for Chronic Disease Prevention and Health Promotion, Centers for Disease Control and Prevention, Atlanta, Georgia.

Brenda D. Reed, Secretary, Division of Adult and Community Health, National Center for Chronic Disease Prevention and Health Promotion, Centers for Disease Control and Prevention, Atlanta, Georgia.

Susan A. Richardson, Writer-Editor, Cygnus Corporation, Rockville, Maryland.

Christopher Rigaux, Project Director, Cygnus Corporation, Rockville, Maryland.

Angel Roca, Program Analyst, National Center for Chronic Disease Prevention and Health Promotion, Centers for Disease Control and Prevention, Atlanta, Georgia.

Cheryl V. Rose, Computer Specialist, Division of Health Promotion Statistics, National Center for Health Statistics, Centers for Disease Control and Prevention, Hyattsville, Maryland.

Patti Schwartz, Graphic Designer, Cygnus Corporation, Rockville, Maryland.

Bettylou Sherry, Ph.D., Epidemiologist, Maternal and Child Health Branch, Division of Nutrition and Physical Activity, National Center for Chronic Disease Prevention and Health Promotion, Centers for Disease Control and Prevention, Atlanta, Georgia.

Margaret Leavy Small, Behavioral Scientist, Division of Adolescent and School Health, National Center for Chronic Disease Prevention and Health Promotion, Centers for Disease Control and Prevention, Atlanta, Georgia

Joseph B. Smith, Senior Project Officer, Disabilities Prevention Program, National Center for Environmental Health, Centers for Disease Control and Prevention, Atlanta, Georgia.

Terrie D. Sterling, Ph.D., Research Psychologist, Division of Adult and Community Health, National Center for Chronic Disease Prevention and Health Promotion, Centers for Disease Control and Prevention, Atlanta, Georgia.

Emma G. Stupp, M.L.S., Technical Information Specialist, Technical Information and Editorial Services Branch, National Center for Chronic Disease Prevention and Health Promotion, Centers for Disease Control and Prevention, Atlanta, Georgia.

William I. Thomas, M.L.I.S., Technical Information Specialist, Technical Information and Editorial Services Branch, National Center for Chronic Disease Prevention and Health Promotion, Centers for Disease Control and Prevention, Atlanta, Georgia.

Patricia E. Thompson-Reid, M.A.T., M.P.H., Program Development Consultant/Community Interventionist, Division of Diabetes Translation, National Center for Chronic Disease Prevention and Health Promotion, Centers for Disease Control and Prevention, Atlanta, Georgia.

Jenelda Thornton, Staff Specialist, National Center for Chronic Disease Prevention and Health Promotion, Centers for Disease Control and Prevention, Atlanta, Georgia.

Nancy B. Watkins, M.P.H., Health Education Specialist, Division of Adult and Community Health, National Center for Chronic Disease Prevention and Health Promotion, Centers for Disease Control and Prevention, Atlanta, Georgia.

Howell Wechsler, Ed.D., M.P.H., Health Education Research Scientist, Division of Adolescent and School Health, National Center for Chronic Disease Prevention and Health Promotion, Centers for Disease Control and Prevention, Atlanta, Georgia.

Julie C. Will, Ph.D., M.P.H., Epidemiologist, Division of Nutrition and Physical Activity, National Center for Chronic Disease Prevention and Health Promotion, Centers for Disease Control and Prevention, Atlanta, Georgia.

Lynda S. Williams, Program Analyst, National Center for Chronic Disease Prevention and Health Promotion, Centers for Disease Control and Prevention, Atlanta, Georgia.

David F. Williamson, Ph.D., Acting Director, Division of Diabetes Translation, National Center for Chronic Disease Prevention and Health Promotion, Centers for Disease Control and Prevention, Atlanta, Georgia.

Stephen W. Wyatt, D.M.D., M.P.H., Director, Division of Cancer Prevention and Control, National Center for Chronic Disease Prevention and Health Promotion, Centers for Disease Control and Prevention, Atlanta, Georgia.

Matthew M. Zack, M.D., M.P.H., Medical Epidemiologist, Division of Adult and Community Health, National Center for Chronic Disease Prevention and Health Promotion, Centers for Disease Control and Prevention, Atlanta, Georgia.

# PHYSICAL ACTIVITY AND HEALTH

# CHAPTER 1

# INTRODUCTION, SUMMARY, AND CHAPTER CONCLUSIONS

## Contents

## Introduction

This is the first Surgeon General's report to address physical activity and health. The main message of this report is that Americans can substantially improve their health and quality of life by including moderate amounts of physical activity in their daily lives. Health benefits from physical activity are thus achievable for most Americans, including those who may dislike vigorous exercise and those who may have been previously discouraged by the difficulty of adhering to a program of vigorous exercise. For those who are already achieving regular moderate amounts of activity, additional benefits can be gained by further increases in activity level.

This report grew out of an emerging consensus among epidemiologists, experts in exercise science, and health professionals that physical activity need not be of vigorous intensity for it to improve health. Moreover, health benefits appear to be proportional to amount of activity; thus, every increase in activity adds some benefit. Emphasizing the amount rather than the intensity of physical activity offers more options for people to select from in incorporating physical activity into their daily lives. Thus, a moderate amount of activity can be obtained in a 30-minute brisk walk, 30 minutes of lawn mowing or raking leaves, a 15-minute run, or 45 minutes of playing volleyball, and these activities can be varied from day to day. It is hoped that this different emphasis on moderate amounts of activity, and the flexibility to vary activities according to personal preference and life circumstances, will encourage more people to make physical activity a regular and sustainable part of their lives.

The information in this report summarizes a diverse literature from the fields of epidemiology, exercise physiology, medicine, and the behavioral sciences. The report highlights what is known about physical activity and health, as well as what is being learned about promoting physical activity among adults and young people.

### Development of the Report

In July 1994, the Office of the Surgeon General authorized the Centers for Disease Control and Prevention (CDC) to serve as lead agency for preparing the first Surgeon General's report on physical activity and health. The CDC was joined in this effort by the President's Council on Physical Fitness and Sports (PCPFS) as a collaborative partner representing the Office of the Surgeon General. Because of the wide interest in the health effects of physical activity, the report was planned collaboratively with representatives from the Office of the Surgeon General, the Office of Public Health and Science (Office of the Secretary), the Office of Disease Prevention (National Institutes of Health [NIH]), and the following institutes from the NIH: the National Heart, Lung, and Blood Institute; the National Institute of Child Health and Human Development; the National Institute of Diabetes and Digestive and Kidney Diseases; and the National Institute of Arthritis and Musculoskeletal and Skin Diseases. CDC's nonfederal partners—including the American Alliance for Health, Physical Education, Recreation, and Dance; the American College of Sports Medicine; and the American Heart Association—provided consultation throughout the development process.

The major purpose of this report is to summarize the existing literature on the role of physical activity in preventing disease and on the status of interventions to increase physical activity. Any report on a topic this broad must restrict its scope to keep its message clear. This report focuses on disease prevention and therefore does not include the considerable body of evidence on the benefits of physical activity for treatment or rehabilitation after disease has developed. This report concentrates on endurance-type physical activity (activity involving repeated use of large muscles, such as in walking or bicycling) because the health benefits of this type of activity have been extensively studied. The importance of resistance exercise (to increase muscle strength, such as by lifting weights) is increasingly being recognized as a means to preserve and enhance muscular strength and endurance and to prevent falls and improve mobility in the elderly. Some promising findings on resistance exercise are presented here, but a comprehensive review of resistance training is beyond the scope of this report. In addition, a review of the special concerns regarding physical activity for pregnant women and for people with disabilities is not undertaken here, although these important topics deserve more research and attention.

Finally, physical activity is only one of many everyday behaviors that affect health. In particular, nutritional habits are linked to some of the same aspects of health as physical activity, and the two may be related lifestyle characteristics. This report deals solely with physical activity; a Surgeon General's Report on Nutrition and Health was published in 1988.

Chapters 2 through 6 of this report address distinct areas of the current understanding of physical activity and health. Chapter 2 offers a historical perspective: after outlining the history of belief and knowledge about physical activity and health, the chapter reviews the evolution and content of physical activity recommendations. Chapter 3 describes the physiologic responses to physical activity—both the immediate effects of a single episode of activity and the long-term adaptations to a regular pattern of activity. The evidence that physical activity reduces the risk of cardiovascular and other diseases is presented in Chapter 4. Data on patterns and trends of physical activity in the U.S. population are the focus of Chapter 5. Lastly, Chapter 6 examines efforts to increase physical activity and reviews ideas currently being proposed for policy and environmental initiatives.

## Major Conclusions

1. People of all ages, both male and female, benefit from regular physical activity.

2. Significant health benefits can be obtained by including a moderate amount of physical activity (e.g., 30 minutes of brisk walking or raking leaves, 15 minutes of running, or 45 minutes of playing volleyball) on most, if not all, days of the week. Through a modest increase in daily activity, most Americans can improve their health and quality of life.

3. Additional health benefits can be gained through greater amounts of physical activity. People who can maintain a regular regimen of activity that is of longer duration or of more vigorous intensity are likely to derive greater benefit.

4. Physical activity reduces the risk of premature mortality in general, and of coronary heart disease, hypertension, colon cancer, and diabetes mellitus in particular. Physical activity also improves mental health and is important for the health of muscles, bones, and joints.

5. More than 60 percent of American adults are not regularly physically active. In fact, 25 percent of all adults are not active at all.

6. Nearly half of American youths 12–21 years of age are not vigorously active on a regular basis. Moreover, physical activity declines dramatically during adolescence.

7. Daily enrollment in physical education classes has declined among high school students from 42 percent in 1991 to 25 percent in 1995.

8. Research on understanding and promoting physical activity is at an early stage, but some interventions to promote physical activity through schools, worksites, and health care settings have been evaluated and found to be successful.

## Summary

The benefits of physical activity have been extolled throughout western history, but it was not until the second half of this century that scientific evidence supporting these beliefs began to accumulate. By the 1970s, enough information was available about the beneficial effects of vigorous exercise on cardiorespiratory fitness that the American College of Sports Medicine (ACSM), the American Heart Association (AHA), and other national organizations began issuing physical activity recommendations to the public. These recommendations generally focused on cardiorespiratory endurance and specified sustained periods of vigorous physical activity involving large muscle groups and lasting at least 20 minutes on 3 or more days per week. As understanding of the benefits of less vigorous activity grew, recommendations followed suit. During the past few years, the ACSM, the CDC, the AHA, the PCPFS, and the NIH have all recommended regular, moderate-intensity physical activity as an option for those who get little or no exercise. The *Healthy People 2000* goals for the nation's health have recognized the importance of physical activity and have included physical activity goals. The 1995 *Dietary Guidelines for Americans*, the basis of the federal government's nutrition-related programs, included physical activity guidance to maintain and improve weight—30 minutes or more of moderate-intensity physical activity on all, or most, days of the week.

Underpinning such recommendations is a growing understanding of how physical activity affects physiologic function. The body responds to physical activity in ways that have important positive effects on musculoskeletal, cardiovascular, respiratory, and endocrine systems. These changes are consistent with a number of health benefits, including a reduced risk of premature mortality and reduced risks of coronary heart disease, hypertension, colon cancer, and diabetes mellitus. Regular participation in physical activity also appears to reduce depression and anxiety, improve mood, and enhance ability to perform daily tasks throughout the life span.

The risks associated with physical activity must also be considered. The most common health problems that have been associated with physical activity are musculoskeletal injuries, which can occur with excessive amounts of activity or with suddenly beginning an activity for which the body is not conditioned. Much more serious associated health problems (i.e., myocardial infarction, sudden death) are also much rarer, occurring primarily among sedentary people with advanced atherosclerotic disease who engage in strenuous activity to which they are unaccustomed. Sedentary people, especially those with preexisting health conditions, who wish to increase their physical activity should therefore gradually build up to the desired level of activity. Even among people who are regularly active, the risk of myocardial infarction or sudden death is somewhat increased during physical exertion, but their overall risk of these outcomes is lower than that among people who are sedentary.

Research on physical activity continues to evolve. This report includes both well-established findings and newer research results that await replication and amplification. Interest has been developing in ways to differentiate between the various characteristics of physical activity that improve health. It remains to be determined how the interrelated characteristics of amount, intensity, duration, frequency, type, and pattern of physical activity are related to specific health or disease outcomes.

Attention has been drawn recently to findings from three studies showing that cardiorespiratory fitness gains are similar when physical activity occurs in several short sessions (e.g., 10 minutes) as when the same total amount and intensity of activity occurs in one longer session (e.g., 30 minutes). Although, strictly speaking, the health benefits of such intermittent activity have not yet been demonstrated, it is reasonable to expect them to be similar to those of continuous activity. Moreover, for people who are unable to set aside 30 minutes for physical activity, shorter episodes are clearly better than none. Indeed, one study has shown greater adherence to a walking program among those walking several times per day than among those walking once per day, when the total amount of walking time was kept the same. Accumulating physical activity over the course of the day has been included in recent recommendations from the CDC and ACSM, as well as from the NIH Consensus Development Conference on Physical Activity and Cardiovascular Health.

Despite common knowledge that exercise is healthful, more than 60 percent of American adults are not regularly active, and 25 percent of the adult population are not active at all. Moreover, although many people have enthusiastically embarked on vigorous exercise programs at one time or another, most do not sustain their participation. Clearly, the processes of developing and maintaining healthier habits are as important to study as the health effects of these habits.

The effort to understand how to promote more active lifestyles is of great importance to the health of this nation. Although the study of physical activity determinants and interventions is at an early stage, effective programs to increase physical activity have been carried out in a variety of settings, such as schools, physicians' offices, and worksites. Determining the most effective and cost-effective intervention approaches is a challenge for the future. Fortunately, the United States has skilled leadership and institutions to support efforts to encourage and assist Americans to become more physically active. Schools, community agencies, parks, recreational facilities, and health clubs are available in most communities and can be more effectively used in these efforts.

School-based interventions for youth are particularly promising, not only for their potential scope—almost all young people between the ages of 6 and 16 years attend school—but also for their potential impact. Nearly half of young people 12–21 years of age are not vigorously active; moreover, physical activity sharply declines during adolescence. Childhood and adolescence may thus be pivotal times for preventing sedentary behavior among adults by maintaining the habit of physical activity throughout the school years. School-based interventions have been shown to be successful in increasing physical activity levels. With evidence that success in this arena is possible, every effort should be made to encourage schools to require daily physical education in each grade and to promote physical activities that can be enjoyed throughout life.

Outside the school, physical activity programs and initiatives face the challenge of a highly technological society that makes it increasingly convenient to remain sedentary and that discourages physical activity in both obvious and subtle ways. To increase physical activity in the general population, it may be necessary to go beyond traditional efforts. This report highlights some concepts from community initiatives that are being implemented around the country. It is hoped that these examples will spark new public policies and programs in other places as well. Special efforts will also be required to meet the needs of special populations, such as people with disabilities, racial and ethnic minorities, people with low income, and the elderly. Much more information about these important groups will be necessary to develop a truly comprehensive national initiative for better health through physical activity. Challenges for the future include identifying key determinants of physically active lifestyles among the diverse populations that characterize the United States (including special populations, women, and young people) and using this information to design and disseminate effective programs.

## Chapter Conclusions

### Chapter 2: Historical Background and Evolution of Physical Activity Recommendations

1. Physical activity for better health and well-being has been an important theme throughout much of western history.

2. Public health recommendations have evolved from emphasizing vigorous activity for cardio-respiratory fitness to including the option of moderate levels of activity for numerous health benefits.

3. Recommendations from experts agree that for better health, physical activity should be performed regularly. The most recent recommendations advise people of all ages to include a minimum of 30 minutes of physical activity of moderate intensity (such as brisk walking) on most, if not all, days of the week. It is also acknowledged that for most people, greater health benefits can be obtained by engaging in physical activity of more vigorous intensity or of longer duration.

4. Experts advise previously sedentary people embarking on a physical activity program to start with short durations of moderate-intensity activity and gradually increase the duration or intensity until the goal is reached.

5. Experts advise consulting with a physician before beginning a new physical activity program for people with chronic diseases, such as cardiovascular disease and diabetes mellitus, or for those who are at high risk for these diseases. Experts also advise men over age 40 and women over age 50 to consult a physician before they begin a vigorous activity program.

6. Recent recommendations from experts also suggest that cardiorespiratory endurance activity should be supplemented with strength-developing exercises at least twice per week for adults, in order to improve musculoskeletal health, maintain independence in performing the activities of daily life, and reduce the risk of falling.

## Chapter 3: Physiologic Responses and Long-Term Adaptations to Exercise

1. Physical activity has numerous beneficial physiologic effects. Most widely appreciated are its effects on the cardiovascular and musculoskeletal systems, but benefits on the functioning of metabolic, endocrine, and immune systems are also considerable.

2. Many of the beneficial effects of exercise training—from both endurance and resistance activities—diminish within 2 weeks if physical activity is substantially reduced, and effects disappear within 2 to 8 months if physical activity is not resumed.

3. People of all ages, both male and female, undergo beneficial physiologic adaptations to physical activity.

## Chapter 4: The Effects of Physical Activity on Health and Disease

### Overall Mortality

1. Higher levels of regular physical activity are associated with lower mortality rates for both older and younger adults.

2. Even those who are moderately active on a regular basis have lower mortality rates than those who are least active.

### Cardiovascular Diseases

1. Regular physical activity or cardiorespiratory fitness decreases the risk of cardiovascular disease mortality in general and of coronary heart disease mortality in particular. Existing data are not conclusive regarding a relationship between physical activity and stroke.

2. The level of decreased risk of coronary heart disease attributable to regular physical activity is similar to that of other lifestyle factors, such as keeping free from cigarette smoking.

3. Regular physical activity prevents or delays the development of high blood pressure, and exercise reduces blood pressure in people with hypertension.

### Cancer

1. Regular physical activity is associated with a decreased risk of colon cancer.

2. There is no association between physical activity and rectal cancer. Data are too sparse to draw conclusions regarding a relationship between physical activity and endometrial, ovarian, or testicular cancers.

3. Despite numerous studies on the subject, existing data are inconsistent regarding an association between physical activity and breast or prostate cancers.

### Non–Insulin-Dependent Diabetes Mellitus

1.) Regular physical activity lowers the risk of developing non–insulin-dependent diabetes mellitus.

### Osteoarthritis

1. Regular physical activity is necessary for maintaining normal muscle strength, joint structure, and joint function. In the range recommended for health, physical activity is not associated with joint damage or development of osteoarthritis and may be beneficial for many people with arthritis.

2. Competitive athletics may be associated with the development of osteoarthritis later in life, but sports-related injuries are the likely cause.

### Osteoporosis

1. Weight-bearing physical activity is essential for normal skeletal development during childhood and adolescence and for achieving and maintaining peak bone mass in young adults.

2. It is unclear whether resistance- or endurance-type physical activity can reduce the accelerated rate of bone loss in postmenopausal women in the absence of estrogen replacement therapy.

### Falling

1. There is promising evidence that strength training and other forms of exercise in older adults preserve the ability to maintain independent living status and reduce the risk of falling.

### Obesity

1. Low levels of activity, resulting in fewer kilocalories used than consumed, contribute to the high prevalence of obesity in the United States.

2. Physical activity may favorably affect body fat distribution.

## Physical Activity and Health

### Mental Health
1. Physical activity appears to relieve symptoms of depression and anxiety and improve mood.
2. Regular physical activity may reduce the risk of developing depression, although further research is needed on this topic.

### Health-Related Quality of Life
1. Physical activity appears to improve health-related quality of life by enhancing psychological well-being and by improving physical functioning in persons compromised by poor health.

### Adverse Effects
1. Most musculoskeletal injuries related to physical activity are believed to be preventable by gradually working up to a desired level of activity and by avoiding excessive amounts of activity.
2. Serious cardiovascular events can occur with physical exertion, but the net effect of regular physical activity is a lower risk of mortality from cardiovascular disease.

## Chapter 5: Patterns and Trends in Physical Activity

### Adults
1. Approximately 15 percent of U.S. adults engage regularly (3 times a week for at least 20 minutes) in vigorous physical activity during leisure time.
2. Approximately 22 percent of adults engage regularly (5 times a week for at least 30 minutes) in sustained physical activity of any intensity during leisure time.
3. About 25 percent of adults report no physical activity at all in their leisure time.
4. Physical inactivity is more prevalent among women than men, among blacks and Hispanics than whites, among older than younger adults, and among the less affluent than the more affluent.
5. The most popular leisure-time physical activities among adults are walking and gardening or yard work.

### Adolescents and Young Adults
1. Only about one-half of U.S. young people (ages 12–21 years) regularly participate in vigorous physical activity. One-fourth report no vigorous physical activity.

2. Approximately one-fourth of young people walk or bicycle (i.e., engage in light to moderate activity) nearly every day.
3. About 14 percent of young people report no recent vigorous or light-to-moderate physical activity. This indicator of inactivity is higher among females than males and among black females than white females.
4. Males are more likely than females to participate in vigorous physical activity, strengthening activities, and walking or bicycling.
5. Participation in all types of physical activity declines strikingly as age or grade in school increases.
6. Among high school students, enrollment in physical education remained unchanged during the first half of the 1990s. However, daily attendance in physical education declined from approximately 42 percent to 25 percent.
7. The percentage of high school students who were enrolled in physical education and who reported being physically active for at least 20 minutes in physical education classes declined from approximately 81 percent to 70 percent during the first half of this decade.
8. Only 19 percent of all high school students report being physically active for 20 minutes or more in daily physical education classes.

## Chapter 6: Understanding and Promoting Physical Activity
1. Consistent influences on physical activity patterns among adults and young people include confidence in one's ability to engage in regular physical activity (e.g., self-efficacy), enjoyment of physical activity, support from others, positive beliefs concerning the benefits of physical activity, and lack of perceived barriers to being physically active.
2. For adults, some interventions have been successful in increasing physical activity in communities, worksites, and health care settings, and at home.
3. Interventions targeting physical education in elementary school can substantially increase the amount of time students spend being physically active in physical education class.

# HISTORICAL BACKGROUND, TERMINOLOGY, EVOLUTION OF RECOMMENDATIONS, AND MEASUREMENT

## Contents

**Contents,** *continued*

# CHAPTER 2
# HISTORICAL BACKGROUND, TERMINOLOGY, EVOLUTION OF RECOMMENDATIONS, AND MEASUREMENT

## Introduction

*The exercise boom is not just a fad; it is a return to 'natural' activity—the kind for which our bodies are engineered and which facilitates the proper function of our biochemistry and physiology. Viewed through the perspective of evolutionary time, sedentary existence, possible for great numbers of people only during the last century, represents a transient, unnatural aberration.* (Eaton, Shostak, Konner 1988, p. 168)

This chapter examines the historical development of physical activity promotion as a means to improve health among entire populations. The chapter focuses on Western (i.e., Greco-Roman) history, because of the near-linear development of physical activity promotion across those times and cultures leading to current American attitudes and guidelines regarding physical activity. These guidelines are discussed in detail in the last half of the chapter. To flesh out this narrow focus on Western traditions, as well as to provide a background for the promotional emphasis of the chapter, this chapter begins by briefly outlining both anthropological and historical evidence of the central, "natural" role of physical activity in prehistoric cultures. Mention is also made of the historical prominence of physical activity in non-Greco-Roman cultures, including those of China, India, Africa, and precolonial America.

Archaeologists working in conjunction with medical anthropologists have established that our ancestors up through the beginning of the Industrial Revolution incorporated strenuous physical activity as a normal part of their daily lives—and not only for the daily, subsistence requirements of their "work" lives. Investigations of preindustrial societies still intact today confirm that physical capability was not just a grim necessity for success at gathering food and providing shelter and safety (Eaton, Shostak, Konner 1988). Physical activity was enjoyed throughout everyday prehistoric life, as an integral component of religious, social, and cultural expression. Food supplies for the most part were plentiful, allowing ample time for both rest and recreational physical endeavors.

Eaton, Shostak, and Konner (1988) describe a "Paleolithic rhythm" (p. 32) observed among contemporary hunters and gatherers that seems to mirror the medical recommendations for physical activity in this report. This natural cycle of regularly intermittent activity was likely the norm for most of human existence. Sustenance preoccupations typically were broken into 1- or 2-day periods of intense and strenuous exertion, followed by 1- or 2-day periods of rest and celebration. During these rest days, however, less intense but still strenuous exertion accompanied 6- to 20-mile round-trip visits to other villages to see relatives and friends and to trade with other clans or communities. There or at home, dancing and cultural play took place.

As the neolithic Agricultural Revolution allowed more people to live in larger group settings and cities, and as the specialization of occupations reduced the amount and intensity of work-related physical activities, various healers and philosophers began to stress that long life and health depended on preventing illnesses through proper diet, nutrition, and physical activity. Such broad prescriptions for health, including exercise recommendations, long predate the increasingly specific guidelines of classical Greek philosophy and medicine, which are the predominant historical focus of this chapter.

In ancient China as early as 3000 to 1000 B.C., the classic *Yellow Emperor's Book of Internal Medicine* (Huang Ti 1949) first described the principle that human harmony with the world was the key to prevention and that prevention was the key to long life (Shampo and Kyle 1989). These principles grew into concepts that became central to the 6th century Chinese philosophy Taoism, where longevity through simple living attained the status of a philosophy that has guided Chinese culture through the present day. tai chi chuan, an exercise system that teaches graceful movements, began as early as 200 B.C. with Hua T'o and has recently been shown to decrease the incidence of falls in elderly Americans (Huard and Wong 1968; see Chapter 4).

In India, too, proper diet and physical activity were known to be essential principles of daily living. The *Ajur Veda,* a collection of health and medical concepts verbally transmitted as early as 3000 B.C., developed into Yoga, a philosophy that included a comprehensively elaborated series of stretching and flexibility postures. The principles were first codified in 600 B.C. in the *Upanishads* and later in the *Yoga Sutras* by Patanjali sometime between 200 B.C. and 200 A.D. Yoga philosophies also asserted that physical suppleness, proper breathing, and diet were essential to control the mind and emotions and were prerequisites for religious experience. In both India and China during this period, the linking of exercise and health may have led to the development of a medical subspecialty that today would find its equivalent in sports medicine (Snook 1984).

Though less directly concerned with physical health than with social and religious attainment, physical activity played a key role in other ancient non-Greco-Roman cultures. In Africa, systems of flexibility, agility, and endurance training not only represented the essence of martial arts capability but also served as an integral component of religious ritual and daily life. The Samburu and the Masai of Kenya still feature running as a virtue of the greatest prowess, linked to manhood and social stature.

Similarly, in American Indian cultures, running was a prominent feature of all major aspects of life (Nabokov 1981). Long before the Europeans invaded, Indians ran to communicate, to fight, and to hunt. Running was also a means for diverse American Indian cultures to enact their myths and thereby construct a tangible link between themselves and both the physical and metaphysical worlds. Among the Indian peoples Nabokov cites are the Mesquakie of Iowa, the Chemeheuvi of California, the Inca of Peru, the Zuni and other Pueblo peoples of the American Southwest, and the Iroquois of the American East, who also developed the precursor of modern-day lacrosse. Even today, the Tarahumarahe of northern Mexico play a version of kickball that involves entire villages for days at a time (Nabokov 1981; Eaton, Shostak, Konner 1988).

## Western Historical Perspective

Besides affecting the practice of preventive hygiene (as is discussed throughout this section), the ancient Greek ideals of exercise and health have influenced the attitudes of modern western culture toward physical activity. The Greeks viewed great athletic achievement as representing both spiritual and physical strength rivaling that of the gods (Jaeger 1965). In the classical-era Olympic Games, the Greeks viewed the winners as men who had the character and physical prowess to accomplish feats beyond the capability of most mortals. Although participants in the modern Olympic Games no longer compete with the gods, today's athletes inspire others to be physically active and to realize their potential—an inspiration as important for modern peoples as it was for the ancient Greeks.

### Early Promotion of
### Physical Activity for Health

Throughout much of recorded western history, philosophers, scientists, physicians, and educators have promoted the idea that being physically active contributes to better health, improved physical functioning, and increased longevity. Although some of these claims were based on personal opinions or clinical judgment, others were the result of systematic observation.

Among the ancient Greeks, the recognition that proper amounts of physical activity are necessary for healthy living dates back to at least the 5th century B.C. (Berryman 1992). The lessons found in the "laws of health" taught during the ancient period sound familiar to us today: to breathe fresh air, eat proper foods, drink the right beverages, take plenty of exercise, get the proper amount of sleep, and include our emotions when analyzing our overall well-being.

Western historians agree that the close connection between exercise and medicine dates back to three Greek physicians—Herodicus (ca. 480 B.C.), Hippocrates (ca. 460–ca. 377 B.C.), and Galen (A.D. 129–ca. 199). The first to study therapeutic gymnastics—or gymnastic medicine, as it was often called—was the Greek physician and former exercise instructor, Herodicus. His dual expertise united the gymnastic with the medical art, thereby preparing the way for subsequent Greek study of the health benefits of physical activity.

Although Hippocrates is generally known as the father of preventive medicine, most historians credit Herodicus as the influence behind Hippocrates' interest in the hygienic uses of exercise and diet (Cyriax 1914; Precope 1952; Licht 1984; Olivova 1985). *Regimen*, the longer of Hippocrates' two works dealing with hygiene, was probably written sometime around 400 B.C. In Book l, he writes:

> Eating alone will not keep a man well; he must also take exercise. For food and exercise, while possessing opposite qualities, yet work together to produce health. For it is the nature of exercise to use up material, but of food and drink to make good deficiencies. And it is necessary, as it appears, to discern the power of various exercises, both natural exercises and artificial, to know which of them tends to increase flesh and which to lessen it; and not only this, but also to proportion exercise to bulk of food, to the constitution of the patient, to the age of the individual, to the season of the year, to the changes in the winds, to the situation of the region in which the patient resides, and to the constitution of the year. (1953 reprint, p. 229)

Hippocrates was a major influence on the career of Claudius Galenus, or Galen, the Greek physician who wrote numerous works of great importance to medical history during the second century. Of these works, his book entitled *On Hygiene* contains the most information on the healthfulness of exercise.

Whether by sailing, riding on horseback, or driving, or via cradles, swings, and arms, everyone, even infants, Galen said, needed exercise (Green 1951 trans., p. 25). He further stated:

> The uses of exercise, I think, are twofold, one for the evacuation of the excrements, the other for the production of good condition of the firm parts of the body. For since vigorous motion is exercise, it must needs be that only these three things result from it in the exercising body— hardness of the organs from mutual attrition, increase of the intrinsic warmth, and accelerated movement of respiration. These are followed by all the other individual benefits which accrue to the body from exercise; from hardness of the organs, both insensitivity and strength for function; from warmth, both strong attraction for things to be eliminated, readier metabolism, and better nutrition and diffusion of all substances, whereby it results that solids are softened, liquids diluted, and ducts dilated. And from the vigorous movement of respiration the ducts must be purged and the excrements evacuated. (p. 54)

The classical notion that one could improve one's health through one's own actions—for example, through eating right and getting enough sleep and exercise—proved to be a powerful influence on medical theory as it developed over the centuries. Classical medicine had made it clear to physicians and the lay public alike that responsibility for disease and health was not the province of the gods. Each person, either independently or in counsel with his or her physician, had a moral duty to attain and preserve health. When the Middle Ages gave way to the Renaissance, with its individualistic perspective and its recovery of classical humanistic influences, this notion of personal responsibility acquired even greater emphasis. Early vestiges of a "self-help" movement arose in western Europe in the 16th century. As that century progressed, "laws of bodily health were expressed as value prescriptions" (Burns 1976, p. 208).

More specifically, "orthodox Greek hygiene," as Smith (1985, p. 257) called it, flourished as part of the revival of Galenic medicine as early as the 13th century. The leading medical schools of the world—Italy's Salerno, Padua, and Bologna—taught hygiene to their students as part of general instruction in the theory and practice of medicine . The works of Hippocrates and Galen dominated a system whereby "the ultimate goal was to be able to practise medicine in the manner of the ancient physicians" (Bylebyl 1979, p. 341).

Hippocrates' *Regimen* also became important during the Renaissance in a literature that Gruman (1961) identified as "prolongevity hygiene" and defined as "the attempt to attain a markedly increased longevity by means of reforms in one's way of life" (p. 221). Central to this literature was the belief that persons who decided to live a temperate life, especially by reforming habits of diet and exercise, could significantly extend their longevity. Beginning with the writings of Luigi Cornaro in 1558, the classic Greek preventive hygiene tradition achieved increasing attention from those wishing to live longer and healthier lives.

Christobal Mendez, who received his medical training at the University of Salamanca, was the author of the first printed book devoted to exercise, *Book of Bodily Exercise* (1553). His novel and comprehensive ideas preceded developments in exercise physiology and sports medicine often thought to be unique to the early 20th century. The book consists of four treatises that cover such topics as the effects of exercise on the body and on the mind. Mendez believed, as the humoral theorists did, that the physician had to clear away excess moisture in the body. Then, after explaining the ill effects of vomiting, bloodletting, purging, sweating, and urination, he noted that "exercise was invented and used to clean the body when it was too full of harmful things. It cleans without any of the above-mentioned inconvenience and is accompanied by pleasure and joy (as we will say). If we use exercise under the conditions which we will describe, it deserves lofty praise as a blessed medicine that must be kept in high esteem" (1960 reprint, p. 22).

In 1569, Hieronymus Mercurialis' *The Art of Gymnastics Among the Ancients* was published in Venice. Mercurialis quoted Galen extensivly and provided a descriptive compilation of ancient material from nearly 200 works by Greek and Roman authors. In general, Mercurialis established the following exercise principles: people who are ill should

not be given exercise that might aggravate existing conditions; special exercises should be prescribed on an individual basis for convalescent, weak, and older patients; people who lead sedentary lives need exercise urgently; each exercise should preserve the existing healthy state; exercise should not disturb the harmony among the principal humors; exercise should be suited to each part of the body; and all healthy people should exercise regularly.

Although Galenism and the humoral theory of medicine were displaced by new ideas, particularly through the study of anatomy and physiology, the Greek principles of hygiene and regimen continued to flourish in 18th century Europe. For some 18th century physicians, such nonintervention tactics were practical alternatives to traditional medical therapies that employed bloodletting and heavy dosing with compounds of mercury and drugs—"heroic" medicine (Warner 1986), in which the "cure" was often worse than the disease.

George Cheyne's *An Essay of Health and Long Life* was published in London in 1724. By 1745, it had gone through 10 editions and various translations. Cheyne recommended walking as the "most natural" and "most useful" exercise but considered riding on horseback as the "most manly" and "most healthy" (1734 reprint, p. 94). He also advocated exercises in the open air, such as tennis and dancing, and recommended cold baths and the use of the "flesh brush" to promote perspiration and improve circulation.

John Wesley's *Primitive Physic*, first published in 1747, was influenced to a large degree by George Cheyne. In his preface, Wesley noted that "the power of exercise, both to preserve and restore health, is greater than can well be conceived; especially in those who add temperance thereto" (1793 reprint, p. iv). William Buchan's classic *Domestic Medicine*, written in 1769, prescribed proper regimen for improving individual and family health. The book contained rules for the healthy and the sick and stressed the importance of exercise for good health in both children and adults.

During the 19th century, both the classical Greek tradition and the general hygiene movement were finding their way into the United States through American editions of western European medical treatises or through books on hygiene written by American physicians. The "self-help" era was also in full bloom during antebellum America. Early vestiges of a self-help movement had arisen in western Europe in the 16th century. As that century progressed, "laws of bodily health were expressed as value prescriptions" (Burns 1976, p. 208). Classical Greek preventive hygiene was part of formal medical training through the 18th century and continued on in the American health reform literature for most of the 19th century. During the latter period, an effort was made to popularize the Greek laws of health, to make each person responsible for the maintenance and balance of his or her health. Individual reform writers thus wrote about self-improvement, self-regulation, the responsibility for personal health, and self-management (Reiser 1985). If people ate too much, slept too long, or did not get enough exercise, they could only blame themselves for illness. By the same token, they could also determine their own good health (Cassedy 1977; Numbers 1977; Verbrugge 1981; Morantz 1984).

A.F.M. Willich's *Lectures on Diet and Regimen* (1801) emphasized the necessity of exercise within the bounds of moderation. He included information on specific exercises, the time for exercise, and the duration of exercise. The essential advantages of exercise included increased bodily strength, improved circulation of the blood and all other bodily fluids, aid in necessary secretions and excretions, help in clearing and refining the blood, and removal of obstructions.

John Gunn's classic *Domestic Medicine, Or Poor Man's Friend*, was first published in 1830. His section entitled "Exercise" recommended temperance, exercise, and rest and valued nature's way over traditional medical treatment. He also recommended exercise for women and claimed that all of the "diseases of delicate women" like "hysterics and hypochondria, arise from want of due exercise in the open, mild, and pure air" (1986 reprint, p. 109). Finally, in an interesting statement for the 1830s if not the 1990s, Gunn recommended a training system for all: "The advantages of the training systems are not confined to pedestrians or walkers—or to pugilists or boxers alone; or to horses which are trained for the chase and the race track; they extend to man in all conditions; and were training introduced into the United States, and made use of by physicians in many cases instead of medical drugs,

the beneficial consequences in the cure of many diseases would be very great indeed" (p. 113).

## Associating Physical Inactivity with Disease

Throughout history, numerous health professionals have observed that sedentary people appear to suffer from more maladies than active people. An early example is found in the writings of English physician Thomas Cogan, author of *The Haven of Health* (1584); he recommended his book to students who, because of their sedentary ways, were believed to be most susceptible to sickness.

In his 1713 book *Diseases of Workers*, Bernardino Ramazzini, an Italian physician considered the father of occupational medicine, offered his views on the association between chronic inactivity and poor health. In the chapter entitled "Sedentary Workers and Their Diseases," Ramazzini noted that "those who sit at their work and are therefore called 'chair-workers,' such as cobblers and tailors, suffer from their own particular diseases." He concluded that "these workers . . . suffer from general ill-health and an excessive accumulation of unwholesome humors caused by their sedentary life," and he urged them to at least exercise on holidays "so to some extent counteract the harm done by many days of sedentary life" (1964 trans., pp. 281–285).

Shadrach Ricketson, a New York physician, wrote the first American text on hygiene and preventive medicine (Rogers 1965). In his 1806 book *Means of Preserving Health and Preventing Diseases*, Ricketson explained that "a certain proportion of exercise is not much less essential to a healthy or vigorous constitution, than drink, food, and sleep; for we see that people, whose inclination, situation, or employment does not admit of exercise, soon become pale, feeble, and disordered." He also noted that "exercise promotes the circulation of the blood, assists digestion, and encourages perspiration" (pp. 152–153).

Since the 1860s, physicians and others had been attempting to assess the longevity of runners and rowers. From the late 1920s (Dublin 1932; Montoye 1992) to the landmark paper by Morris and colleagues (1953), observations that premature mortality is lower among more active persons than sedentary persons began to emerge and were later replicated in a variety of settings (Rook 1954;

Brown et al. 1957; Pomeroy and White 1958; Zukel et al. 1959). The hypothesis that a sedentary lifestyle leads to increased mortality from coronary heart disease, as well as the later hypothesis that inactivity leads to the development of some other chronic diseases, has been the subject of numerous studies that provide the major source of data supporting the health benefits of exercise (see Chapter 4).

## Health, Physical Education, and Fitness

The hygiene movement found further expression in 19th century America through a new literature devoted to "physical education." In the early part of the century, many physicians began using the term in journal articles, speeches, and book titles to describe the task of teaching children the ancient Greek "laws of health." As Willich explained in his *Lectures on Diet and Regimen* (1801), "by *physical education* is meant the bodily treatment of children; the term *physical* being applied in opposition to *moral*" (p. 60). In his section entitled "On the Physical Education of Children," he continued to discuss stomach ailments, bathing, fresh air, exercise, dress, and diseases of the skin, among other topics. Physical education, then, implied not merely exercising the body but also becoming educated about one's body.

These authors were joined by a number of early 19th century educators. For example, an article entitled "Progress of Physical Education" (1826), which appeared in the first issue of *American Journal of Education,* declared that "the time we hope is near, when there will be no literary institution unprovided with the proper means to healthful exercise and innocent recreation, and when literary men shall cease to be distinguished by a pallid countenance and a wasted body" (pp. 19–20). Both William Russell, who was the journal's editor, and Boston educator William Fowler believed that girls as well as boys should have ample outdoor exercise. Knowledge about one's body also was deemed crucial to a well-educated and healthy individual by several physicians who, as Whorton has suggested, "dedicated their careers to birthing the modern physical education movement" (p. 282).

Charles Caldwell held a prominent position in Lexington, Kentucky's, Transylvania University Medical Department. Although he wrote on a variety of medical topics, his *Thoughts on Physical Education*

in 1834 gained him national recognition. Caldwell defined physical education as "that scheme of training, which contributes most effectually to the development, health, and perfection of living matter. As applied to man, it is that scheme which raises his whole system to its summit of perfection.... Physical education, then, in its philosophy and practice, is of great compass. If complete, it would be tantamount to an entire system of Hygeiene. It would embrace every thing, that, by bearing in any way on the human body, might injure or benefit it in its health, vigor, and fitness for action" (pp. 28–29).

During the first half of the 19th century, systems of gymnastic and calisthenic exercise that had been developed abroad were brought to the United States. The most influential were exercises advanced by Per Henrik Ling in Sweden in the early 1800s and the "German system" of gymnastic and apparatus exercises that was based on the work of Johan Christoph GutsMuths and Friedrich Ludwig Jahn. Also, Americans like Catharine Beecher (1856) and Dioclesian Lewis (1883) devised their own extensive systems of calisthenic exercises intended to benefit both women and men. By the 1870s, American physicians and educators frequently discussed exercise and health. For example, physical training in relation to health was a regular topic in the *Boston Medical and Surgical Journal* from the 1880s to the early 1900s.

Testing of physical fitness in physical education began with the extensive anthropometric documentation by Edward Hitchcock in 1861 at Amherst College. By the 1880s, Dudley Sargent at Harvard University was also recording the bodily measurements of college students and promoting strength testing (Leonard and Affleck 1947). During the early 1900s, the focus on measuring body parts shifted to tests of vital working capacity. These tests included measures of blood pressure (McCurdy 1901; McKenzie 1913), pulse rate (Foster 1914), and fatigue (Storey 1903). As early as 1905, C. Ward Crampton, former director of physical training and hygiene in New York City, published the article "A Test of Condition" in *Medical News*. Attempts to assess physical fitness had constituted a significant aspect of the work of turn-of-the-century physical educators, many of whom were physicians.

Allegations that American conscripts during World War I were inadequately fit to serve their country helped shift the emphasis of physical education from health-related exercise to performance outcomes. Public concern stimulated legislation to make physical education a required subject in schools. But the financial austerities of the Great Depression had a negative effect on education in general, including physical education (Rogers 1934). At the same time, the combination of increased leisure time for many Americans and a growing national interest in college and high school sports shifted the emphasis on physical education away from the earlier aim of enhancing performance and health to a new focus on sports-related skills and the worthy use of leisure time.

Physical efficiency was a term widely used in the literature of the 1930s. Another term, physical condition, also found its way into research reports. In 1936, Arthur Steinhaus published one of the earliest articles on "physical fitness" in the *Journal of Health, Physical Education, and Recreation*; in 1938, C. H. McCloy's article "Physical Fitness and Citizenship" appeared in the same journal.

As the United States entered World War II, the federal government showed increasing interest in physical education, especially toward physical fitness testing and preparedness. In October 1940, President Franklin Roosevelt named John Kelly, a former Olympic rower, to the new position of national director of physical training. The following year, Fiorella La Guardia, the Mayor of New York City and the director of civilian defense for the Federal Security Agency, appointed Kelly as assistant in charge of physical fitness; tennis star Alice Marble was also chosen to promote physical fitness among girls and women (Park 1989; Berryman 1995).

In 1943, Arthur Steinhaus chaired a committee appointed by the Board of Directors of the American Medical Association to review the nature and role of exercise in physical fitness (Steinhaus et al. 1943), and C. Ward Crampton chaired a committee on physical fitness under the direction of the Federal Security Agency. Crampton and his 73-member advisory council were charged with developing physical fitness in the civilian population (Crampton 1941; Park 1989).

In 1941, Morris Fishbein, editor of the *Journal of the American Medical Association*, stated that "from the point of view on physical fitness we are a far

better nation now than we were in 1917," but he cautioned Americans not to believe "we have attained an optimum in physical fitness" (p. 54). He realized the magnitude of the fitness problem when he noted that the poor results of physical examinations reported by the Selective Service Boards were "a challenge to the medical profession, to the social scientists, the physical educators, the public health officials, and all those concerned in the United States with the physical improvement of our population" (p. 55). The goals most frequently cited for physical education between 1941 and 1945 were resistance to disease, muscular strength and endurance, cardiorespiratory endurance, muscular growth, flexibility, speed, agility, balance, and accuracy (Larson and Yocom 1951).

After World War II concluded, a continuing interest in physical fitness convinced other key members of the medical profession and the American Medical Association to continue studying exercise. Much of this interest can be attributed to the pioneering work of Thomas K. Cureton, Jr., and his Physical Fitness Research Laboratory at the University of Illinois (Shea 1993). Cardiologists, health education specialists, and physicians in preventive medicine were becoming aware of the contributions of exercise to the overall health and efficiency of the heart and circulatory system. In 1946, the American Medical Association's Bureau of Health Education designed and organized the Health and Fitness Program to provide "assistance to local organizations throughout the nation in the development of satisfactory health education programs" (Fishbein 1947, p. 1009). The program became an important link among physical educators, physicians, and physiologists.

The event that attracted the most public attention to physical fitness, including that of President Dwight D. Eisenhower, was the publication of the article "Muscular Fitness and Health" in the December 1953 issue of the *Journal of Health, Physical Education, and Recreation*. The authors, Hans Kraus and Ruth Hirschland of the Institute of Physical Medicine and Rehabilitation at the New York University Bellevue Medical Center, stated that 56.6 percent of the American schoolchildren tested "failed to meet even a minimum standard required for health" (p. 17). When this rate was compared with the 8.3 percent failure rate for European children, a

17

call for reform went out. Kraus and Hirschland labeled the lack of sufficient exercise "a serious deficiency comparable with vitamin deficiency" and declared "an urgent need" for its remedy (pp. 17–19). John Kelly, the former national director of physical fitness during World War II, notified Pennsylvania Senator James Duff of these startling test results. Duff, in turn, brought the research to the attention of President Eisenhower, who invited several athletes and exercise experts to a meeting in 1955 to examine this issue in more depth. A President's Conference on Fitness of American Youth, held in June 1956, was attended by 150 leaders from government, physical education, medical, public health, sports, civic, and recreational organizations. This meeting eventually led to the establishment of the President's Council on Youth Fitness and the President's Citizens Advisory Committee on the Fitness of American Youth (Hackensmith 1966; Van Dalen and Bennett 1971).

When John Kennedy became president in 1961, one of his first actions was to call a conference on physical fitness and young people. In 1963, the President's Council on Youth Fitness was renamed the President's Council on Physical Fitness. In 1968, the word "sports" was added to the name, making it the President's Council on Physical Fitness and Sports (PCPFS). The PCPFS was charged with promoting physical activity, fitness, and sports for Americans of all ages.

During the 1960s, a number of educational and public health organizations published articles and statements on the importance of fitness for children and youths. The American Association for Health, Physical Education, and Recreation (AAHPER) expanded its physical fitness testing program to include college-aged men and women. The association developed new norms from data collected from more than 11,000 boys and girls 10–17 years old. The AAHPER also joined with the President's Council on Physical Fitness to conduct the AAHPER Youth Fitness Test, which had motivational awards. In 1966, President Lyndon Johnson's newly created Presidential Physical Fitness Award was incorporated into the program.

In the mid-1970s, the need to promote the health—rather than exclusively the performance—benefits of exercise and physical fitness began to reappear. In 1975, AAHPER stated it was time to differentiate physical fitness related to health from performance related to athletic ability (Blair, Falls, Pate 1983). Accordingly, AAHPER commissioned the development of the Health Related Physical Fitness Test. This move in youth fitness paralleled the adoption of the aerobic concept, which promoted endurance-type exercise among the public (Cooper 1968).

## Exercise Physiology Research and Health

The study of the physiology of exercise in a modern sense began in Paris, France, when Antoine Lavoisier in 1777 and Lavoisier and Pierre de Laplace in 1780 developed techniques to measure oxygen uptake and carbon dioxide production at rest and during exercise. During the 1800s, European scientists used and advanced these procedures to study the metabolic responses to exercise (Scharling 1843; Smith 1857; Katzenstein 1891; Speck 1889; Allen and Pepys 1809). The first major application of this research to humans—Edward Smith's study of the effects of "assignment to hard labor" by prisoners in London in 1857—was to determine if hard manual labor negatively affected the health and welfare of the prisoners and whether it should be considered cruel and unusual punishment.

William Byford published "On the Physiology of Exercise" in the *American Journal of Medical Sciences* in 1855, and Edward Mussey Hartwell, a leading physical educator, wrote a two-part article, "On the Physiology of Exercise," for the *Boston Medical and Surgical Journal* in 1887. The first important book on the subject, George Kolb's *Beitrage zur Physiologie Maximaler Muskelarbeit Besonders des Modernen Sports*, was published in 1887 (trans. *Physiology of Sport*, 1893) (cited in Langenfeld 1988 and Park 1992). The following year, Fernand Lagrange's *Physiology of Bodily Exercise* was published in France.

From the early 1900s to the early 1920s, several works on exercise physiology began to appear. George Fitz, who had established a physiology of exercise laboratory during the early 1890s, published his *Principles of Physiology and Hygiene* in 1908. R. Tait McKenzie's *Exercise in Education and Medicine* (1909) was followed by such works as Francis Benedict and Edward Cathcart's *Muscular Work, A Metabolic Study with Special Reference to the Efficiency of the Human Body as a Machine* (1913). The next year, a professor of physiology at the University of London, F.A. Bainbridge, published a second edition of *Physiology of Muscular Exercise* (Park 1981).

In 1923, the year Archibald Hill was appointed Joddrell Professor of Physiology at University College, London, the physiology of exercise acquired one of its most respected researchers and staunchest supporters, for Hill had won the Nobel Prize in Medicine and Physiology the year before. Hill's 1925 presidential address on "The Physiological Basis of Athletic Records" to the British Association for the Advancement of Science appeared in *The Lancet* (1925a) and *Scientific Monthly* (1925b), and in 1926 he published his landmark book *Muscular Activity*. The following year, Hill published *Living Machinery*, which was based largely on his lectures before audiences at the Lowell Institute in Boston and the Baker Laboratory of Chemistry in Ithaca, New York.

Several leading physiologists besides Hill were interested in the human body's response to exercise and environmental stressors, especially activities involving endurance, strength, altitude, heat, and cold. Consequently, they studied soldiers, athletes, aviators, and mountain climbers as the best models for acquiring data. In the United States, such research was centered in the Boston area, first at the Carnegie Nutrition Laboratory in the 1910s and later at the Harvard Fatigue Laboratory, which was established under the leadership of Lawrence Henderson in 1927 (Chapman and Mitchell 1965; Dill 1967; Horvath and Horvath 1973). That year, Henderson and colleagues first demonstrated that endurance exercise training improved the efficiency of the cardiovascular system by increasing stroke volume and decreasing heart rate at rest. Two years later, Schneider and Ring (1929) published the results of a 12-week endurance training program on one person, demonstrating a 24-percent increase in "crest load of oxygen" (maximal oxygen uptake). Over the next 15 years, a limited number of exercise training studies were published that evaluated the response of maximal oxygen uptake or endurance performance capacity to exercise training. These included noteworthy reports by Gemmill and colleagues (1931), Robinson and Harmon (1941), and Knehr, Dill, and Neufeld (1942) on endurance training responses by male college students. However, none of those early studies compared the effects of different types, intensities, durations, or frequencies of exercise on performance capacity or health-related outcomes.

Activities surrounding World War II greatly influenced the research in exercise physiology, and several laboratories, including the Harvard Fatigue Laboratory, began directing their efforts toward topics of importance to the military. The other national concern that created much interest among physiologists was the fear (discussed earlier in this chapter), that American children were less fit than their European counterparts. Research was directed toward the concept of fitness in growth and development, ways to measure fitness, and the various components of fitness (Berryman 1995). Major advances were also made in the 1940s and 1950s in developing the components of physical fitness (Cureton 1947) and in determining the effects of endurance and strength training on measures of performance and physiologic function, especially adaptations of the cardiovascular and metabolic systems. Also investigated were the effects of exercise training on health-related outcomes, such as cholesterol metabolism (Taylor, Anderson, Keys 1957; Montoye et al. 1959).

Starting in the late 1950s and continuing through the 1970s, a rapidly increasing number of published studies evaluated or compared different components of endurance-oriented exercise training regimens. For example, Reindell, Roskamm, and Gerschler (1962) in Germany, Christensen (1960) in Denmark, and Yakovlev and colleagues (1961) in Russia compared—and disagreed—about the relative benefits of interval versus continuous exercise training in increasing cardiac stroke volume and endurance capacity. Other investigators began to evaluate the effects of different modes (Sloan and Keen 1959) and durations (Sinasalo and Juurtola 1957) of endurance-type training on physiologic and performance measures.

Karvonen and colleagues' (1957) landmark paper that introduced using "percent maximal heart rate reserve" to calculate or express exercise training intensity was one of the first studies designed to compare the effects of two different exercise intensities on cardiorespiratory responses during exercise. Over the next 20 years, numerous investigators documented the effects of different exercise training regimens on a variety of health-related outcomes among healthy men and women and among persons under medical care (Bouchard, Shephard, Stephens 1994). Many of these studies evaluated the effects of endurance or aerobic exercise training on cardiorespiratory capacity and were initially summarized by Pollock (1973). The American College of Sports Medicine (ACSM) (1975, 1978) and the American Heart Association (AHA) (1975) further refined the results of this research (see the section on "Evolution of Physical Activity Recommendations," later in this chapter).

Over the past two decades, experts from numerous disciplines have determined that exercise training substantially enhances physical performance and have begun to establish the characteristics of the exercise required to produce specific health benefits (Bouchard, Shephard, Stephens 1994). Also, behavioral scientists have begun to evaluate what determines physical activity habits among different segments of the population and are developing strategies to increase physical activity among sedentary persons (Dishman 1988). The results of much of this research are cited in the other chapters of this report and were the focus of the various conferences, reports, and guidelines summarized later in this chapter.

As the literature of exercise science has matured and recommendations have evolved, certain widely agreed-on terms have emerged. Because a number of these occur throughout the rest of this chapter and report, they are presented and briefly defined in the following section.

## Terminology of Physical Activity, Physical Fitness, and Health

This section discusses four broad terms used frequently in this report: physical activity, exercise (or exercise training), physical fitness, and health. Also included is a glossary (Table 2-1) of more specific terms and concepts crucial to understanding the material presented in later parts of this chapter and report.

**Physical activity.** Physical activity is defined as bodily movement produced by the contraction of skeletal muscle that increases energy expenditure above the basal level. Physical activity can be categorized in various ways, including type, intensity, and purpose.

Because muscle contraction has both mechanical and metabolic properties, it can be classified by either property. This situation has caused some confusion. Typically, mechanical classification stresses whether the muscle contraction produces movement of the limb: isometric (same length) or static exercise if there is no movement of the limb, or isotonic (same tension) or dynamic exercise if there is movement of the limb. Metabolic classification involves the availability of oxygen for the contraction process and includes aerobic (oxygen available) or anaerobic (oxygen unavailable) processes. Whether an activity is aerobic or anaerobic depends primarily on its intensity. Most activities involve both static and dynamic contractions and aerobic and anaerobic metabolism. Thus, activities tend to be classified according to their dominant features.

The physical activity of a person or group is frequently categorized by the context in which it occurs. Common categories include occupational, household, leisure time, or transportation. Leisure-time activity can be further subdivided into categories such as competitive sports, recreational activities (e.g., hiking, cycling), and exercise training.

**Exercise (or exercise training).** Exercise and physical activity have been used synonymously in the past, but more recently, exercise has been used to denote a subcategory of physical activity: "physical activity that is planned, structured, repetitive, and purposive in the sense that improvement or maintenance of one or more components of physical fitness is the objective" (Caspersen, Powell, Christensen 1985). Exercise training also has denoted physical activity performed for the sole purpose of enhancing physical fitness.

**Physical fitness.** Physical fitness has been defined in many ways (Park 1989). A generally accepted approach is to define physical fitness as the ability to carry out daily tasks with vigor and alertness, without undue fatigue, and with ample energy to enjoy leisure-time pursuits and to meet unforeseen emergencies. Physical fitness thus includes cardiorespiratory endurance, skeletal muscular endurance, skeletal muscular strength, skeletal muscular power, speed, flexibility, agility, balance, reaction time, and body composition. Because these attributes differ in their importance to athletic performance versus health, a distinction has been made between performance-related fitness and health-related fitness (Pate 1983; Caspersen, Powell, Christensen 1985). Health-related fitness has been

## Table 2-1. Glossary of terms

**Aerobic training**—Training that improves the efficiency of the aerobic energy-producing systems and that can improve cardiorespiratory endurance.[*]

**Agility**—A skill-related component of physical fitness that relates to the ability to rapidly change the position of the entire body in space with speed and accuracy.[†]

**Anaerobic training**—Training that improves the efficiency of the anaerobic energy-producing systems and that can increase muscular strength and tolerance for acid-base imbalances during high-intensity effort.[*]

**Balance**—A skill-related component of physical fitness that relates to the maintenance of equilibrium while stationary or moving.[†]

**Body composition**—A health-related component of physical fitness that relates to the relative amounts of muscle, fat, bone, and other vital parts of the body.[†]

**Calorimetry**—Methods used to calculate the rate and quantity of energy expenditure when the body is at rest and during exercise.[*]

    **Direct calorimetry**—A method that gauges the body's rate and quantity of energy production by direct measurement of the body's heat production; the method uses a calorimeter, which is a chamber that measures the heat expended by the body.[*]

    **Indirect calorimetry**—A method of estimating energy expenditure by measuring respiratory gases. Given that the amount of $O_2$ and $CO_2$ exchanged in the lungs normally equals that used and released by body tissues, caloric expenditure can be measured by $CO_2$ production and $O_2$ consumption.[*]

**Cardiorespiratory endurance (cardiorespiratory fitness)**—A health-related component of physical fitness that relates to the ability of the circulatory and respiratory systems to supply oxygen during sustained physical activity.[†]

**Coordination**—A skill-related component of physical fitness that relates to the ability to use the senses, such as sight and hearing, together with body parts in performing motor tasks smoothly and accurately.[†]

**Detraining**—Changes the body undergoes in response to a reduction or cessation of regular physical training.[*]

**Endurance training/endurance activities**—Repetitive, aerobic use of large muscles (e.g., walking, bicycling, swimming).[‡]

**Exercise** (exercise training)—Planned, structured, and repetitive bodily movement done to improve or maintain one or more components of physical fitness.

**Flexibility**—A health-related component of physical fitness that relates to the range of motion available at a joint.[*]

**Kilocalorie (kcal)**—A measurement of energy. 1 kilocalorie = 1 Calorie = 4,184 joules = 4.184 kilojoules.

**Kilojoule (kjoule)**—A measurement of energy. 4.184 kilojoules = 4,184 joules = 1 Calorie = 1 kilocalorie.

**Maximal heart rate reserve**—The difference between maximum heart rate and resting heart rate.[*]

**Maximal oxygen uptake ($\dot{V}O_2$ max )**—The maximal capacity for oxygen consumption by the body during maximal exertion. It is also known as aerobic power, maximal oxygen consumption, and cardiorespiratory endurance capacity.[*]

**Maximal heart rate (HR max)**—The highest heart rate value attainable during an all-out effort to the point of exhaustion.[*]

**Metabolic equivalent (MET)**—A unit used to estimate the metabolic cost (oxygen consumption) of physical activity. One MET equals the resting metabolic rate of approximately 3.5 ml $O_2 \cdot kg^{-1} \cdot min^{-1}$.[*]

**Muscle fiber**—An individual muscle cell.[*]

**Muscular endurance**—The ability of the muscle to continue to perform without fatigue.[*]

**Overtraining**—The attempt to do more work than can be physically tolerated.[*]

**Physical activity**—Bodily movement that is produced by the contraction of skeletal muscle and that substantially increases energy expenditure.

**Physical fitness**—A set of attributes that people have or achieve that relates to the ability to perform physical activity.

**Power**—A skill-related component of physical fitness that relates to the rate at which one can perform work.

**Relative perceived exertion (RPE)**—A person's subjective assessment of how hard he or she is working. The Borg scale is a numerical scale for rating perceived exertion.[*]

**Reaction time**—A skill-related component of physical fitness that relates to the time elapsed between stimulation and the beginning of the reaction to it.[†]

**Resistance training**—Training designed to increase strength, power, and muscle endurance.[*]

**Resting heart rate**—The heart rate at rest, averaging 60 to 80 beats per minute.[*]

**Retraining**—Recovery of conditioning after a period of inactivity.[*]

**Speed**—A skill-related component of physical fitness that relates to the ability to perform a movement within a short period of time.[†]

**Strength**—The ability of the muscle to exert force.[*]

**Training heart rate (THR)**—A heart rate goal established by using the heart rate equivalent to a selected training level (percentage of $\dot{V}O_2$ max ). For example, if a training level of 75 percent $\dot{V}O_2$ max is desired, the $\dot{V}O_2$ at 75 percent is determined and the heart rate corresponding to this $VO_2$ is selected as the THR.[*]

[*]From Wilmore JH, Costill DL. *Physiology of sport and exercise*. Champaign, IL: Human Kinetics, 1994.
[†] From Corbin CB, Lindsey R. *Concepts in physical education with laboratories*. 8th ed. Dubuque, IA: Times Mirror Higher Education Group, 1994.
[‡]Adapted from Corbin CB, Lindsey R, 1994, and Wilmore JH, Costill DL, 1994.

said to include cardiorespiratory fitness, muscular strength and endurance, body composition, and flexibility. The relative importance of any one attribute depends on the particular performance or health goal.

**Health.** The 1988 International Consensus Conference on Physical Activity, Physical Fitness, and Health (Bouchard et al. 1990) defined health as "a human condition with physical, social, and psychological dimensions, each characterized on a continuum with positive and negative poles. Positive health is associated with a capacity to enjoy life and to withstand challenges; it is not merely the absence of disease. Negative health is associated with morbidity and, in the extreme, with premature mortality." Thus, when considering the role of physical activity in promoting health, one must acknowledge the importance of psychological well-being, as well as physical health.

## Evolution of Physical Activity Recommendations

In the middle of the 20th century, recommendations for physical activity to achieve fitness and health benefits were based on systematic comparisons of effects from different profiles of exercise training (Cureton 1947; Karvonen, Kentala, Mustala 1957; Christensen 1960; Yakolav et al. 1961; Reindell, Roskamm, Gerschler 1962). In the 1960s and 1970s, expert panels and committees, operating under the auspices of health- or fitness-oriented organizations, began to recommend specific physical activity programs or exercise prescriptions for improving physical performance capacity or health (President's Council on Physical Fitness 1965; AHA 1972, 1975; ACSM 1975). These recommendations were based on substantial clinical experience and on scientific data available at that time.

Pollock's 1973 review of what type of exercise was needed to improve aerobic power and body composition subsequently formed the basis for a 1978 position statement by the ACSM titled "The Recommended Quantity and Quality of Exercise for Developing and Maintaining Fitness in Healthy Adults." This statement outlined the exercise that healthy adults would need to develop and maintain cardiorespiratory fitness and healthy body composition. These guidelines recommended a frequency of

exercise training of 3–5 days per week, an intensity of training of 60–90 percent of maximal heart rate (equivalent to 50–85 percent of maximal oxygen uptake or heart rate reserve), a duration of 15–60 minutes per training session, and the rhythmical and aerobic use of large muscle groups through such activities as running or jogging, walking or hiking, swimming, skating, bicycling, rowing, cross-country skiing, rope skipping, and various endurance games or sports (Table 2-2).

Between 1978 and 1990, most exercise recommendations made to the general public were based on this 1978 position statement, even though it addressed only cardiorespiratory fitness and body composition. By providing clear recommendations, these guidelines proved invaluable for promoting cardiorespiratory endurance, although many people overinterpreted them as guidelines for promoting overall health. Over time, interest developed in potential health benefits of more moderate forms of physical activity, and attention began to shift to alternative physical activity regimens (Haskell 1984; Blair, Kohl, Gordon 1992; Blair 1993).

In 1990, the ACSM updated its 1978 position statement by adding the development of muscular strength and endurance as a major objective (ACSM 1990). The recommended frequency, intensity, and mode of exercise remained similar, but the duration was slightly increased from 15–60 minutes to 20–60 minutes per session, and moderate-intensity resistance training (one set of 8–12 repetitions of 8–10 different exercises at least 2 times per week) was suggested to develop and maintain muscular strength and endurance (Table 2-2). These 1990 recommendations also recognized that activities of moderate intensity may have health benefits independent of cardiorespiratory fitness:

> Since the original position statement was published in 1978, an important distinction has been made between physical activity as it relates to health versus fitness. It has been pointed out that the quantity and quality of exercise needed to obtain health-related benefits may differ from what is recommended for fitness benefits. It is now clear that lower levels of physical activity than recommended by this position statement may reduce the risk for certain chronic degenerative diseases

22

*and yet may not be of sufficient quantity or quality to improve [maximal oxygen uptake]. ACSM recognizes the potential health benefits of regular exercise performed more frequently and for longer duration, but at lower intensities than prescribed in this position statement.*

In conjunction with a program to certify exercise professionals at various levels of experience and competence, the ACSM has published five editions of *Guidelines for Exercise Testing and Prescription* (ACSM 1975, 1980, 1986, 1991, 1995b) that describe the components of the exercise prescription and explain how to initiate and complete a proper exercise training program (Table 2-2). The ACSM has also published recommendations on the role of exercise for preventing and managing hypertension (1993) and for patients with coronary heart disease (1994) and has published a position stand on osteoporosis (1995a). For the most part, newer recommendations that focus on specific health outcomes are consistent with the ACSM's 1978 and 1990 position statements, but they generally expand the range of recommended activities to include moderate-intensity exercise.

Between the 1960s and 1990s, other U.S. health and fitness organizations published recommendations for physical activity. Because these organizations used the same scientific data as the ACSM, their position statements and guidelines are similar. A notable example is *Healthy People 2000* (USDHHS 1990), the landmark publication of the U.S. Public Health Service that lists various health objectives for the nation. (The objectives for physical activity and fitness, as revised in 1995 [USDHHS 1995], are included as Appendix A of this chapter.) Other recommendations include specific exercise programs developed for men and women by the President's Council on Physical Fitness (1965) and the YMCA (National Council YMCA 1989). The AHA (1972, 1975, 1992, 1993, 1994, 1995) has published for both health professionals and the public a series of physical activity recommendations and position statements directed at CHD prevention and cardiac rehabilitation. In 1992, the AHA published a statement identifying physical inactivity as a fourth major risk factor for CHD, along with smoking, high blood pressure, and high blood cholesterol (Fletcher et al. 1992). The American Association of Cardiovascular

and Pulmonary Rehabilitation has also published guidelines for using physical activity for cardiac (1991, 1995) and pulmonary (1993) rehabilitation. Some of these recommendations provide substantial advice to ensure that exercise programs are safe for people at increased risk for heart disease or for patients with established disease.

Between the 1970s and the mid-1990s, exercise training studies conducted on middle-aged and older persons and on patients with lower functional capacity demonstrated that significant cardiorespiratory performance and health-related benefits can be obtained at more moderate levels of activity intensity than previously realized. In addition, population-based epidemiologic studies demonstrated dose-response gradients between physical activity and health outcomes. As a result of these findings, the most recent CDC-ACSM guidelines recommend that all adults perform 30 or more minutes of moderate-intensity physical activity on most, and preferably all, days—either in a single session or "accumulated" in multiple bouts, each lasting at least 8–10 minutes (Pate et al. 1995). This guideline thus significantly differs from the earlier ones on three points: it reduces the minimum starting exercise intensity from 60 percent of maximal oxygen uptake to 50 percent in healthy adults and to 40 percent in patients or persons with very low fitness; it increases the frequency of exercise sessions from 3 days per week to 5–7 days per week, depending on intensity and session duration; and it includes the option of accumulating the minimum of 30 minutes per day in multiple sessions lasting at least 8–10 minutes (Pate et al. 1995). This modification in advice acknowledges that people who are sedentary and who do not enjoy, or are otherwise not able to maintain, a regimen of regular, vigorous activity can still derive substantial benefit from more moderate physical activity as long as it is done regularly.

The NIH Consensus Development Conference Statement on Physical Activity and Cardiovascular Health identifies physical inactivity as a major public health problem in the United States and issues a call to action to increase physical activity levels among persons in all population groups. (See Appendix B for full text of the recommendations.) The core recommendations, similar to those jointly made by the CDC and the ACSM (Pate et al. 1995), call for

Physical Activity and Health

Table 2-2.  Selected physical activity recommendations in the United States (1965–1996)

| Source | Objective | Type/mode |
|---|---|---|
| PCPF (1965) | Physical fitness | General fitness |
| AHA Recommendations (1972) | CHD prevention | Endurance |
| YMCA (1973) | General health and fitness | Endurance, strength, flexibility |
| ACSM Guidelines (1975) | Cardiorespiratory fitness | Endurance, strength, flexibility |
| AHA Recommendations (1975) | Secondary prevention in patients with heart disease | Endurance |
| ACSM Position Statement (1978) | Cardiorespiratory fitness and body composition | Endurance |
| USDHEW–Healthy People (1979) | Disease prevention/ health promotion | Endurance |
| ACSM Guidelines (1980) | Cardiorespiratory fitness | Endurance, strength, flexibility |
| ACSM Guidelines (1986) | Cardiorespiratory fitness | Endurance, strength, flexibility |
| USDHHS–Surgeon General's Report on Nutrition and Health (1988) | Weight control | Endurance |
| USPSTF (1989) | Primary prevention in clinical practice | Not specified, implied endurance |
| ACSM Position Stand (1990) | Cardiorespiratory and muscular fitness | Endurance, strength |
| ACSM Guidelines (1991) | Cardiorespiratory fitness | Endurance, strength, flexibility |
| USHHS/USDA Dietary Guidelines (1990) | Health promotion/disease prevention, weight maintenance | Not specified |
| AACVPR (1991) | Cardiac rehabilitation | Endurance, strength |
| DHHS-Healthy People 2000 (1991)* | Disease prevention/health promotion | Endurance, strength, flexibility |
| AHA Position Statement (1992) | CVD prevention and rehabilitation | Endurance |
| AHA Standards (1992 and 1995) | CHD prevention and rehabilitation | Endurance, strength |
| AACVPR (1993) | Pulmonary rehabilitation | Endurance |
| ACSM Position Statement (1993) | Prevention and treatment of hypertension | Endurance, strength |

| Endurance | | | Resistance training |
|---|---|---|---|
| Intensity | Frequency | Duration | |
| Five levels | 5 x week | Approximately 30 minutes | Selected calisthenics |
| 70–85% MHR | 3–7 x week | 15–20 minutes | Not addressed |
| 80% $\dot{V}O_2$ max | 3 x week | 40–45 minutes | Not specified |
| 60–90% $\dot{V}O_2$ max<br>60–90% HRR | 3 x week | 20–30 minutes | Not specified |
| 70–85% MHR | 3–4 x week | 20–60 minutes | Not addressed |
| 50–85% $\dot{V}O_2$ max<br>50–85% HRR<br>60–90% MHR | 3–5 x week | 15–60 minutes | Not addressed |
| Moderate/hard | 3 x week | 15–30 minutes | Not addressed |
| 50–85% $\dot{V}O_2$ max/HRR<br>60–90% MHR | 3–5 x week | 15–60 minutes | Not specified |
| 50–85% $\dot{V}O_2$ max/HRR<br>60–90% MHR | 3–5 x week | 15–60 minutes | Not specified |
| Not specified | ≥ 3 x week | ≥ 20 minutes | Not addressed |
| At least moderate | Not specified | Not specified | Not addressed |
| 50–85% $\dot{V}O_2$ max<br>50–85% HRR<br>60–90% MHR | 3–5 x week | 20–60 minutes | 1 set, 8–12 repetitions<br>8–10 exercises<br>2 days x week |
| 40–85% $\dot{V}O_2$ max<br>55–90% MHR<br>RPE = 12–16 | 3–5 x week | 15–60 minutes | Not specified |
| Not specified | Not specified | Not specified | Not addressed |
| Exercise following ACSM (1986) and AHA (1983) recommendations | 3–5 x week | 15–60 minutes | 1–3 sets, 12–15 repetitions<br>major muscle groups<br>2–3 days x week |
| Light/moderate/vigorous | 3–5 x week | 20–30 minutes | Not specified |
| > 50% $\dot{V}O_2$ max | 3–4 x week | 30–60 minutes | Not addressed |
| 50–60% $\dot{V}O_2$ max<br>50–60% HR reserve | ≥ 3 x week | ≥ 30 minutes | 1 set, 10–15 repetitions<br>8–10 exercises,<br>2–3 days x week |
| 60% HR reserve | 3 x week | 20–30 minutes | Not addressed |
| 40–70% $\dot{V}O_2$ max | 3–5 x week | 20–60 minutes | Not specified |

25

**Table 2-2.** *Continued*

| Source | Objective | Type/mode |
|---|---|---|
| AHA Position Statement (1993) | CVD prevention and rehabilitation | Moderate intensity (i.e., brisk walking) integrated into daily routine |
| ACSM Position Stand (1994) | Secondary prevention in patients with coronary heart disease | Endurance, strength |
| AHA Position Statement (1994) | Cardiac rehabilitation | Endurance and strength training of moderate intensity following other guidelines |
| Physical Activity Guidelines for Adolescents (1994)[†] | Lifetime health promotion for adolescents | Endurance |
| AACVPR (1995) | Cardiac rehabilitation | Endurance, strength |
| ACSM Guidelines (1995) | Cardiorespiratory fitness and muscular fitness | Endurance, strength |
| ACSM Position Stand (1995) | Prevention of osteoporosis | Strength, flexibility, coordination, cardiorespiratory fitness |
| AHCPR (1995) | Cardiac rehabilitation | Endurance, strength |
| AMA Guidelines for Adolescent Preventive Services (GAPS) (1994) | Health promotion/ physical fitness | Endurance |
| CDC/ACSM (1995)[‡] | Health promotion | Endurance |
| USHHS/USDA Dietary Guidelines (1995) | Health promotion/disease prevention, weight maintenance | Endurance |
| NHLBI Consensus Conference (1996) | CVD prevention for adults and children and cardiac rehabilitation | Endurance |
| USPSTF (1996) | Primary prevention in clinical practice | Endurance, strength, flexibility |

| | Endurance | | Resistance training |
|---|---|---|---|
| Intensity | Frequency | Duration | |
| Not specified | Not specified | Not specified | Not addressed |
| 40–85% $\dot{V}O_2$ max<br>40–85% HRR<br>55–90% MHR | 3 x week,<br>nonconsecutive days | 20–40 minutes | Not specified |
| Not specified | Not specified | Not specified | Not specified |
| Moderate/vigorous | 3 x week, vigorous<br>daily, moderate | ≥ 20 minutes, vigorous<br>not specified, moderate | Not addressed |
| > 50% $\dot{V}O_2$ max<br>RPE 12–14 | 3–5 x week | 30–45 minutes, 200–300<br>kcal per session or<br>1,000–1,500 kcal per week | 1 set, 10–15 repetitions,<br>major muscle groups<br>2–3 days x week |
| 40–85% $\dot{V}O_2$ max/HRR<br>RPE 12–16 | 3-5 x week | 12–15 minutes initially:<br>20–30 minutes for<br>conditioning and<br>maintaining | 1 set, 8–12 repetitions<br>8–10 exercises<br>2 days x week |
| Not specified | Not specified | Not specified | Not specified |
| 70–85% MHR | 3 x week | 20–40 minutes | Not specified |
| Moderate | ≥ 3 x week | 20–30 minutes | Not addressed |
| Moderate/hard | All or most days | ≥ 30 minutes per day<br>in bouts of at least 8–10<br>minutes | Not specified |
| Moderate | All or most days | ≥ 30 minutes per day | Not addressed |
| Moderate/hard | All or most days | ≥ 30 minutes per day | Not addressed |
| Moderate | Most days | 30 minutes | Not specified |

*See Appendix B for listing of objectives.   †See Sallis and Patrick, 1994.   ‡See Pate et al., 1995.

Key to associations: AACVPR = American Association for Cardiovascular and Pulmonary Rehabilitation; ACSM = American College of Sports Medicine; AHA = American Heart Association; AHCPR = Agency for Health Care Policy and Research; CDC = Centers for Disease Control and Prevention; NHLBI = National Heart, Lung, and Blood Institute; PCPF = President's Council on Physical Fitness; USDA = United States Department of Agriculture; USDHEW = United States Department of Health, Education, and Welfare; USDHHS = United States Department of Health and Human Services; USPSTF = United States Preventive Services Task Force; YMCA = Young Men's Christian Association.

Key to abbreviations: CHD = coronary heart disease; CVD = cardiovascular disease; HRR = heart rate reserve; MHR = maximal heart rate; RPE = rating of perceived exertion; $\dot{V}O_2$ max = maximal oxygen uptake.

Not addressed = not included in recommendations. Not specified = recommended but not quantified.

all children and adults to accumulate at least 30 minutes per day of moderate-intensity physical activity. The recommendations also acknowledge that persons already achieving this minimum could experience greater benefits by increasing either the duration or the intensity of activity. In addition, the statement recommends more widespread use of cardiac rehabilitation programs that include physical activity.

The consensus statement from the 1993 International Consensus Conference on Physical Activity Guidelines for Adolescents (Sallis and Patrick 1994) emphasizes that adolescents should be physically active every day as part of general lifestyle activities and that they should engage in 3 or more 20-minute sessions of moderate to vigorous exercise each week. The American Academy of Pediatrics has issued several statements encouraging active play in preschool children, assessment of children's activity levels, and evaluation of physical fitness (1992, 1994). Both the consensus statement and the American Academy of Pediatrics' statements emphasize active play, parental involvement, and generally active lifestyles rather than specific vigorous exercise training. They also acknowledge the need for appropriate school physical education curricula.

Recognizing the important interrelationship of nutrition and physical activity in achieving a balance between energy consumed and energy expended, the 1988 Surgeon General's Report on Nutrition and Health (USDHHS 1988) recommended physical activities such as walking, jogging, and bicycling for at least 20 minutes, 3 times per week. The 1995 *Dietary Guidelines for Americans* greatly expanded physical activity guidance to maintain and improve weight. The bulletin recommends that all Americans engage in 30 minutes of moderate-intensity physical activity on all, or most, days of the week (USDA/USDHHS 1995).

The U.S. Preventive Services Task Force (USPSTF) has recommended that health care providers counsel all patients on the importance of incorporating physical activities into their daily routines to prevent coronary heart disease, hypertension, obesity, and diabetes (Harris et al. 1989; USPSTF 1989, 1996). Similarly, the American

Medical Association's *Guidelines for Adolescent Preventive Services (GAPS)* (AMA 1994) recommends that physicians provide annual physical activity counseling to all adolescents.

## Summary of Recent Physical Activity Recommendations

Sedentary persons can increase their physical activity in many ways. The traditional, structured approach originally described by the ACSM and others involved rather specific recommendations regarding type, frequency, intensity, and duration of activity. Recommended activities typically included fast walking, running, cycling, swimming, or aerobics classes. More recently, physical activity recommendations have adopted a lifestyle approach to increasing activity (Pate et al. 1995). This method involves common activities, such as brisk walking, climbing stairs (rather than taking the elevator), doing more house and yard work, and engaging in active recreational pursuits. Recent physical activity recommendations thus acknowledge both the structured and lifestyle approaches to increasing physical activity. Either approach can be beneficial for a sedentary person, and individual interests and opportunities should determine which is used. The most recent recommendations cited agree on several points:

- All people over the age of 2 years should accumulate at least 30 minutes of endurance-type physical activity, of at least moderate intensity, on most—preferably all—days of the week.

- Additional health and functional benefits of physical activity can be achieved by adding more time in moderate-intensity activity, or by substituting more vigorous activity.

- Persons with symptomatic CVD, diabetes, or other chronic health problems who would like to increase their physical activity should be evaluated by a physician and provided an exercise program appropriate for their clinical status.

- Previously inactive men over age 40, women over age 50, and people at high risk for CVD should first consult a physician before embarking on a program of vigorous physical activity to which they are unaccustomed.
- Strength-developing activities (resistance training) should be performed at least twice per week. At least 8–10 strength-developing exercises that use the major muscle groups of the legs, trunk, arms, and shoulders should be performed at each session, with one or two sets of 8–12 repetitions of each exercise.

## Measurement of Physical Activity, Fitness, and Intensity

The ability to relate physical activity to health depends on accurate, precise, and reproducible measures (Wilson et al. 1986; National Center for Health Statistics 1989). Measurement techniques have evolved considerably over the years (Park 1989), creating a shifting pattern of strength and weakness in the evidence supporting the assertion that physical activity improves health (Ainsworth et al. 1994). The complexity is heightened by the different health implications of measuring activity, gauging intensity, and assessing fitness. The tools currently in use (Table 2-3) must be evaluated not only for their efficacy in measuring an individual's status, but also for their applicability as instruments in larger-scale epidemiologic research. These tools vary considerably in the age groups to which they can be applied, as well as in their cost, in their likelihood of affecting the behavior they try to measure, and in their acceptability. For example, many of the tools that are appropriate for young and middle-aged persons are less so for the elderly and may have no relevance at all for children. A brief review of these approaches provides some insight into the current constellation of strengths and weaknesses on which epidemiologic conclusions rest.

### Measuring Physical Activity

#### Measures Based on Self-Report

Physical activity is a complex set of behaviors most commonly assessed in epidemiologic studies by asking people to classify their level of physical activity (LaPorte, Montoye, Caspersen 1985; Caspersen 1989). Techniques used to gather this self-reported information include diaries, logs, recall surveys, retrospective quantitative histories, and global self-reports (Kannel, Wilson, Blair 1985; Wilson et al. 1986; Powell et al. 1987; Caspersen 1989). Surveys are practical for assessing physical activity in large populations because they are not costly, are relatively easy to administer, and are generally acceptable to study participants (Montoye and Taylor 1984; LaPorte, Montoye, Caspersen 1985; Caspersen 1989). Information obtained from self-report instruments has often been converted into estimates of energy expenditure (i.e., kilocalories or kilojoules; metabolic equivalents [METs]) or some other summary measure that can be used to categorize or rank persons by their physical activity level. This technique has also been used to convert job classifications into summary measures.

*Diaries* can detail virtually all physical activity performed during a specified (usually short) period. A summary index can be derived from a diary by 1) summing the total duration of time spent in a given activity multiplied by an estimated rate of energy expenditure for that activity, or 2) listing accumulated time across all activities or time accrued within specific classes of activities. Comparisons with indirect calorimetry or with caloric intake have shown that diaries are accurate indices of daily energy expenditure (Acheson et al. 1980). Because diaries are commonly limited to spans of 1–3 days, they may not represent long-term physical activity patterns (LaPorte, Montoye, Caspersen 1985). Diaries require intensive effort by the participant, and their use may itself produce changes in the physical activities the participant does during the monitoring period (LaPorte, Montoye, Caspersen 1985; Caspersen 1989).

*Logs* are similar to diaries but provide a record of participation in specific types of physical activity rather than in all activites (King et al. 1991). The time that activity was started and stopped may be recorded, either soon after participation or at the end of the day. Logs can be useful for recording participation in an exercise training program. But as with diaries, they can be inconvenient for the participant, and their use may itself influence the participant's behavior.

Table 2-3. Assessment procedures and their potential use in epidemiologic research

| Measurement tool | Applicable age groups | Use in large scale studies | Low $ cost | Low time cost | Low subject time cost | Low subject effort cost | Likely to influence behavior | Acceptable to persons | Socially acceptable | Activity specific |
|---|---|---|---|---|---|---|---|---|---|---|
| **Surveying** | | | | | | | | | | |
| Task specific diary | adult, elderly | yes | yes | yes | no | no | yes | ? | yes | yes |
| Recall questionnaire | adult, elderly | yes | yes | yes | yes | yes | no | yes | yes | yes |
| Quantitative history | adult, elderly | yes | yes | no | no | no | no | yes | yes | yes |
| Global self-report | adult, elderly | yes | yes | yes | yes | yes | no | yes | yes | no |
| **Monitoring** | | | | | | | | | | |
| Behavioral observation | adult, elderly | no | no | no | no | yes | yes | ? | ? | yes |
| Job classification | adult | yes | yes | yes | yes | yes | no | yes | yes | yes |
| Heart rate monitor | all | no | no | no | yes | yes | no | yes | yes | no |
| Heart rate and motion sensor | all | no | no | no | yes | yes | no | yes | yes | no |
| Electronic motion sensor | adult, elderly | yes | no | yes | yes | yes | no | yes | yes | no |
| Pedometer | adult, elderly | yes | yes | yes | yes | yes | no | yes | yes | no |
| Gait assessment | child, adult, elderly | no | no | yes | yes | yes | no | yes | yes | no |
| Accelerometers | all | yes | yes | yes | yes | yes | no | yes | yes | no |
| Horizontal time monitor | child, adult, elderly | no | no | yes | yes | yes | no | yes | yes | no |
| Stabilometers | infant | no | no | yes | yes | yes | no | yes | yes | no |
| Direct calorimetry | all | no | no | no | no | no | yes | no | no | yes |
| Indirect calorimetry | adult, elderly | no | no | no | no | no | yes | no | no | yes |
| Doubly labeled water | child, adult, elderly | yes | no | no | yes | yes | no | yes | yes | no |

Modified from LaPorte, Montoye, Caspersen. *Public Health Reports*, 1985.

Note that most tests that are applicable for adults can be used in adolescents as well. Few tests can be applied to the pediatric age groups; among infants, only direct calorimetry, accelerometers, heart rate monitoring, and stabilometers can be used with accuracy.

*Recall surveys* are less likely to influence behavior and generally require less effort by the respondent than either diaries or logs, although some participants have trouble remembering details of past participation in physical activity (Baranowski 1985). Recall surveys of physical activity generally have been used for time frames of from 1 week to a lifetime (Kriska et al. 1988; Blair et al. 1991). They can ascertain either precise details about physical activity or more general estimates of usual or typical participation. The recall survey is the method used for the national and state-based information systems providing data for Chapter 5 of this report.

The *retrospective quantitative history*—the most comprehensive form of physical activity recall survey —generally requires specific detail for time frames of up to 1 year (LaPorte, Montoye, Caspersen 1985). If the time frame is long enough, the quantitative history can adequately represent year-round physical activity. For example, the Minnesota Leisure-Time Physical Activity Questionnaire and the Tecumseh questionnaire obtained information on the average frequency and duration of participation for a specific list of physical activities performed over the previous year (Montoye and Taylor 1984; Taylor et al. 1978). Unfortunately, obtaining this abundance of data is a heavy demand on the respondent's memory, and the complexity of the survey generates additional expense (LaPorte, Montoye, Caspersen 1985).

*Global self-reports*, another type of recall survey, ask individuals to rate their physical activity relative to other people's in general or to that of a similar age and sex group. This easy-to-use approach, which was employed for the National Health Interview Survey (NCHS, Bloom 1982), tends to best represent participation in vigorous physical activity (Washburn, Adams, Haile 1987; Caspersen and Pollard 1988; Jacobs et al. 1993). A weakness of this approach is that persons reporting the same rating may have different actual physical activity profiles (Washburn, Adams, Haile 1987; Caspersen and Pollard 1988).

Although survey approaches generally apply to adults, adolescents, and the elderly, survey instruments must often be tailored to the specific demographic requirements of the group under study. Recently, some researchers have suggested developing special survey instruments for older persons (Voorrips et al. 1991; Dipietro et al. 1993; Washburn et al. 1993) and adolescents or children (Noland et al. 1990; Sallis et al. 1993).

### Measures Based on Direct Monitoring

The major alternative to surveys is to directly measure physical activity through behavioral observation, mechanical or electronic devices, or physiologic measurements (Table 2-3). Such approaches eliminate the problems of poor memory and biased self-reporting but are themselves limited by high cost and the burden on participants and staff. Consequently, these measures have been used primarily in small-scale studies, though they have been used recently in some large-scale studies (Lakka, Nyyssonen, Salonen 1994).

Behavioral observation is the straightforward process of watching and recording what a person does. Using general guidelines for caloric expenditure associated with specific activities, a summary estimate of caloric output can be obtained from such observation. An important subtype of this approach is the classification of work based on the amount of physical activity it requires. These approaches can be labor-intensive (hence prohibitively expensive for large-scale studies) but are usually well accepted by study participants.

In the category of mechanical or electronic measurement, various instruments have been used to monitor heart rate and thus provide a continuous recording of a physiologic process that reflects both the duration and intensity of physical activity. Heart rate is typically used to estimate daily energy expenditure (i.e., oxygen uptake) on physical activity; the underlying assumption is that a linear relationship exists between heart rate and oxygen uptake. A major disadvantage of heart rate monitoring is the need to calibrate the heart rate–energy expenditure curve for each individual. Another limitation is that the relationship between heart rate and energy expenditure is variable for low-intensity physical activities. Most monitors have to be worn for extended periods by the participant, and they pose some discomfort and inconvenience.

Other approaches for using heart rate to measure physical activity include using the percentage of time spent during daily activities in various ranges of heart rate (Gilliam et al. 1981), using the difference between mean daily heart rate and resting heart rate (Sallis et al. 1990), and using the integration of the area under a heart rate versus time curve adjusted for resting heart rate (Freedson 1989). Heart rate alone may not be a suitable surrogate for determining the level of physical activity, given that other factors, such as psychological stress or changes in body temperature, can significantly influence heart rate throughout the day.

A variety of sensors have been developed to measure physical activity by detecting motion. Pedometers, perhaps the earliest motion sensors, were designed to count steps and thus measure the distance walked or run. However, not all pedometers are reliable enough for estimating physical activity in either laboratory or field research (Kashiwazaki et al. 1986; Washburn, Janney, Fenster 1990). Electronic motion sensors tend to perform better than their mechanical counterparts (Wong et al. 1981; Taylor et al. 1982; LaPorte et al. 1983). Their output has been significantly correlated with energy expenditure assessed with indirect calorimetry in controlled laboratory conditions using graded treadmill exercise (Balogun, Amusa, Onyewadume 1988; Haskell et al. 1993; Montoye et al. 1996), under short-term controlled activity (e.g., walking or cycling over a measured course) for heart rate during laboratory and daily activities, and for observed behavior in a controlled setting (Klesges and Klesges 1987; Rogers et al. 1987; Freedson 1989; Sallis et al. 1990; Washburn, Janney, Fenster 1990). Direct validation has shown reasonable correlation with physical activity records completed over a year (Richardson et al. 1995). Recording simultaneously both the heart rate and the motion from sensors on several parts of the body and then calibrating each individual's heart rate and motion sensor output versus oxygen uptake for various activities can accurately estimate the energy expended from physical activity (Haskell et al. 1993). Several other devices (e.g., accelerometers, stabilometers) are of lesser value for large-scale studies, and their use is limited to small physiologic investigations.

Methods for physiologically monitoring energy expenditure include direct calorimetry (requiring the participant to remain in a metabolic chamber) and indirect calorimetry (requiring the participant to wear a mask and to carry equipment for analyzing expired air). Both methods are too expensive and complicated for use in large-scale studies. Another physiologic measurement, the use of doubly labeled water, offers researchers special opportunities to assess energy expenditure. By using two stable isotopes ($^2H_2O$ and $H_2 {}^{18}O$) measured every few days or weeks in the urine, researchers can calculate the rate of carbon dioxide production—a reflection of the rate of energy production in humans over time. According to their body weight, study participants drink a specified amount of these isotopes. A mass spectrometer is used to track the amount of unmetabolized isotope in the urine. Although this technique obtains objective data with little effort on the part of participants, two disadvantages are its relatively high cost and its inability to distinguish between types of activities performed. The technique has been proven accurate when compared with indirect calorimetry (Klein et al. 1984; Westerterp et al. 1988; Edwards et al. 1990).

### Measuring Intensity of Physical Activity

Common terms used to characterize the intensity of physical activity include light or low, moderate or mild, hard or vigorous, and very hard or strenuous (Table 2-4). A frequent approach to classifying intensity has been to express it relatively—that is, in relation to a person's capacity for a specific type of activity. For example, the intensity prescribed for aerobic exercise training usually is expressed in relation to the person's measured cardiorespiratory fitness (ACSM 1990). Because heart rate during aerobic exercise is highly associated with the increase in oxygen uptake, the percentage of maximal heart rate is often used as a surrogate for estimating the percentage of maximal oxygen uptake (ACSM 1990). Exercise intensity can also be expressed in absolute terms, such as a specific type of activity with an assigned intensity (for example, walking at 4 miles per hour or jogging at 6 miles per hour). Such quanta of work can also be described in absolute terms as METs, where one MET is about $3.5 \, ml \, O_2 \cdot kg^{-1} \cdot min^{-1}$, corresponding to the body at rest. The workloads in the just-quoted example are equivalent to 4 and 10 METs, respectively. The number of METs associated with a wide range of specific activities can be estimated from aggregated laboratory and field measurements (Ainsworth, Montoye, Leon 1994).

The process of aging illustrates an important relationship between absolute and specific measures. As people age, their maximal oxygen uptake decreases. Activity of a given MET value (an absolute intensity) therefore requires a greater percentage of their maximal oxygen uptake (a relative intensity). The aforementioned walk at 4 miles per hour (4 METs) may be light exercise for a 20-year-old, moderate for a 60-year-old, and vigorous for an 80-year-old.

Most exercise training studies have used relative intensity to evaluate specific exercise training regimens. On the other hand, observational studies relating physical activity to morbidity or mortality usually report absolute intensity or total amount of physical activity estimated from composite measures that include intensity, frequency, and duration. It is thus difficult to compare the intensity of activity that improves physiologic markers with the intensity of activity that may reduce morbidity and mortality.

**Table 2-4.** Classification of physical activity intensity, based on physical activity lasting up to 60 minutes

| | Endurance-type activity | | | | | | | | Strength-type exercise |
|---|---|---|---|---|---|---|---|---|---|
| | Relative intensity | | | Absolute intensity (METs) in healthy adults (age in years) | | | | | Relative intensity* |
| Intensity | $\dot{V}O_2$ max (%) heart rate reserve (%) | Maximal heart rate (%) | RPE† | Young (20–39) | Middle-aged (40–64) | Old (65–79) | Very old (80+) | RPE | Maximal voluntary contraction (%) |
| Very light | <25 | <30 | <9 | <3.0 | <2.5 | <2.0 | ≤1.25 | <10 | <30 |
| Light | 25–44 | 30–49 | 9–10 | 3.0–4.7 | 2.5–4.4 | 2.0–3.5 | 1.26–2.2 | 10–11 | 30–49 |
| Moderate | 45–59 | 50–69 | 11–12 | 4.8–7.1 | 4.5–5.9 | 3.6–4.7 | 2.3–2.95 | 12–13 | 50–69 |
| Hard | 60–84 | 70–89 | 13–16 | 7.2–10.1 | 6.0–8.4 | 4.8–6.7 | 3.0–4.25 | 14–16 | 70–84 |
| Very hard | ≥85 | ≥90 | >16 | ≥10.2 | ≥8.5 | ≥6.8 | ≥4.25 | 17–19 | >85 |
| Maximal‡ | 100 | 100 | 20 | 12.0 | 10.0 | 8.0 | 5.0 | 20 | 100 |

Table 2-4 provided courtesy of Haskell and Pollock.
*Based on 8–12 repetitions for persons under age 50 years and 10–15 repetitions for persons aged 50 years and older.
†Borg rating of Relative Perceived Exertion 6–20 scale (Borg 1982).
‡Maximal values are mean values achieved during maximal exercise by healthy adults. Absolute intensity (METs) values are approximate mean values for men. Mean values for women are approximately 1–2 METs lower than those for men.

Recent public health guidelines and research reports have used absolute intensity to define appropriate levels of physical activity, but the term "absolute" may convey a misplaced sense of precision. For example, the CDC-ACSM guidelines (Pate et al. 1995) use absolute intensity to classify brisk walking as moderate physical activity. In contrast, *Healthy People 2000* objective 1.3 defines brisk walking as "light to moderate" intensity and takes into account the age- and sex-related variability in maximal capacity (USDHHS 1990). One solution to this inconsistency in terminology is to create consistent categories that equate a variety of measures to the same adjective (Table 2-4). Using such a rubric, the observations of Spelman and colleagues (1993) that brisk walking for healthy adults aged 22–58 years demands 40–60 percent of their aerobic power suggests a correspondence with 3–5 METs and a classification of moderate intensity. Those prescribing an exercise pattern for adults can use the rating of perceived exertion (RPE) scale (ACSM 1991). An RPE of 10–11 corresponds to light intensity, 12–13 to moderate intensity, and 14–16 to hard intensity (Table 2-4), and the approximate

physiologic equivalents can be estimated. This type of subjective scale furnishes a convenient way to monitor performance.

### Measuring Physical Fitness

Perhaps the most highly developed measurement area is the assessment of physical fitness, since it rests on physiologic measurements that have good to excellent accuracy and reliability. The major foci of fitness measurements are endurance (or cardiorespiratory fitness), muscular fitness, and body composition.

#### Endurance

Cardiorespiratory fitness, also referred to as cardiorespiratory capacity, aerobic power, or endurance fitness, is largely determined by habitual physical activity. However, other factors influence cardiorespiratory fitness, including age, sex, heredity, and medical status (Bouchard, Shepard, Stevens 1994).

The best criterion of cardiorespiratory fitness is maximal oxygen uptake or aerobic power ($\dot{V}O_2$ max). Measured in healthy persons during large muscle, dynamic activity (e.g., walking, running, or cycling), $\dot{V}O_2$ max is primarily limited by the oxygen transport capacity of the cardiovascular system (Mitchell and Blomqvist 1971). $\dot{V}O_2$ max is most accurately determined by measuring expired air composition and respiratory volume during maximal exertion. This procedure requires relatively expensive equipment, highly trained technicians, and time and cooperation from the participant, all of which usually limit its use in large epidemiologic studies (Montoye et al. 1970; King et al. 1991).

Because the individual variation in mechanical and metabolic efficiency is for activities that do not require much skill—such as walking or running on a motor-driven treadmill, cycling on a stationary bicycle ergometer, or climbing steps—oxygen uptake can be quite accurately estimated from the rate of work (Siconolfi et al. 1982). Thus, $\dot{V}O_2$ max can be estimated from the peak exercise workload during a maximal exercise test without measuring respiratory gases. Such procedures require an accurately calibrated exercise device, careful adherence to a specific protocol, and good cooperation by the participant. They have been used in numerous exercise training studies for evaluating the effects of exercise on cardiovascular risk factors and performance, in secondary prevention trials for patients after hospitalization for myocardial infarction, and in some large-scale observational studies (Blair et al. 1989; Sidney et al. 1992).

Any maximal test to assess cardiorespiratory fitness imposes a burden on both the participant and the examiner. To reduce this burden, several submaximal exercise testing protocols have been developed. With these protocols, the heart rate response to a specified workload is used to predict the $\dot{V}O_2$ max. The underlying assumption (besides the linear relationship between heart rate and oxygen uptake) is that the participant's maximal heart rate can be estimated accurately. Both assumptions are adequately met when a standardized protocol is used to test a large sample of healthy adults. In some cases, no extrapolation to maximal values is performed, and an individual's cardiorespiratory fitness is expressed as the heart rate at a set workload (e.g., heart rate at 5 kilometers/hour or at 100 watts) or at the workload required to reach a specific submaximal heart rate (workload at a heart rate of 120 beats/minute).

In another approach to assessing cardiorespiratory fitness, participants usually walk, jog, or run a specified time or distance, and their performance is converted to an estimate of $\dot{V}O_2$ max (Cooper 1968). These procedures have been frequently used to test the cardiorespiratory fitness of children, of young adults, or of groups that have occupation-related physical fitness requirements, such as military and emergency service personnel. In many cases, these tests require maximal or near-maximal effort by the participant and thus have not been used for older persons or those at increased risk for CVD. The advantage is that large numbers of participants can be tested rapidly at low cost. However, to obtain an accurate evaluation, participants must be willing to exert themselves and know how to set a proper pace.

### Muscular Fitness

Common measures of muscular fitness are muscular strength, muscular endurance, flexibility, and balance, agility, and coordination. Muscular strength can be measured during performance of either static or dynamic muscle contraction (NCHS, Wilmore 1989). Because muscular strength is specific to the muscle group, the testing of one group does not provide accurate information about the strength of other muscle groups (Clarke 1973). Thus, for a comprehensive assessment, strength testing must involve at least several major muscle groups, including the upper body, trunk, and lower body. Standard tests have included the bench press, leg extension, and biceps curl using free weights. The heaviest weight a person can lift only one time through the full range of motion for a particular muscle group is considered the person's maximum strength for that specific muscle group.

Muscular endurance is specific to each muscle group. Most tests for use in the general population do not distinguish between muscular endurance and muscular strength. Tests of muscular endurance and strength, which include sit-ups, push-ups, bent-arm hangs, and pull-ups, must be properly administered and may not discriminate well in some populations (e.g., pull-ups are not a good test for many populations because a high percentage of those tested will have 0 scores). Few laboratory tests of muscular endurance have been developed, and such tests usually involve having the participant perform a series of contractions at a set percentage of maximal strength and at a constant rate until the person can no longer continue at that rate. The total work performed or the test duration is used as a measure of muscular endurance.

Flexibility is difficult to measure accurately and reliably. Because it is specific to the joint being tested, no one measure provides a satisfactory index of an individual's overall flexibility (Harris 1969). Field testing of flexibility frequently has been limited to the sit-and-reach test, which is considered to be a measure of lower back and hamstring flexibility. The criterion method for measuring flexibility in the laboratory is goniometry, which is used to measure the angle of the joint at both extremes in the range of motion (NCHS, Wilmore 1989).

Balance, agility, and coordination are especially important among older persons, who are more prone to fall and, as a result, suffer fractures due to reduced bone mineral density. Field methods for measuring balance, agility, and coordination have included various balance stands (e.g., one-foot stand with eyes open and with eyes closed; standing on a narrow block) and balance walks on a narrow line or rail (Tse and Bailey 1992). In the laboratory, computer-based technology is now being used to evaluate balance measured on an electronic force platform or to analyze a videotape recording of the participant walking (Lehmann et al. 1990). Agility or coordination are measured most frequently by using a field test, such as an agility walk or run (Cureton 1947). In the laboratory, coordination or reaction/movement time are determined by using electronic signaling and timing devices (Spirduso 1975). More development is needed to establish norms using standardized tests for measuring balance, agility, and coordination, especially of older persons.

*Body Composition*

In most population-based studies that have provided information on the relationship between physical activity and morbidity or mortality, body composition has been estimated by measuring body height and weight and calculating body mass index (weight/height²). The preferred method for determining amount of body fat and lean body mass in exercise training studies has been hydrostatic or underwater weighing (NCHS, Wilmore 1989); however, this method lacks accuracy in some populations, including older persons and children (Lohman 1986). Anthropometric measurements (i.e., girths, diameters, and skinfolds) used to calculate the percentage of body fat have varying degrees of accuracy and reliability (Wilmore and Behnke 1970).

Data now suggest that the distribution of body fat, especially accumulation in the abdominal area, and total body fat are significant risk factors for CVD and diabetes (Bierman and Brunzell 1992; Blumberg and Alexander 1992). Researchers have determined the magnitude of this abdominal or central obesity by calculating the waist-to-hip circumference ratio or by using new electronic methods that can image regional fat tissue. New technologies that measure body composition include total body electrical conductivity (Segal et al. 1985), bioelectrical impedance (Lukaski et al. 1986), magnetic resonance imaging (Lohman 1984), and dual-energy x-ray absorptiometry (DEXA) (Mazess et al. 1990). These new procedures have substantial potential to provide new information on how changes in physical activity affect body composition and fat distribution.

### Validity of Measurements

Health behaviors are difficult to measure, and this is certainly true for the behavior of physical activity. Of particular concern is how well self-reported physical activity accurately represents a person's habitual activity status. Factors that interfere with obtaining accurate assessments include incomplete recall, exaggeration of amount of activity, and nonrepresentative sampling of time intervals during which activity is assessed.

One of the principal difficulties in establishing the validity of a physical activity measure is the lack of a suitable "gold-standard" criterion measure for comparison. In the absence of a true criterion measure, cardiorespiratory fitness has often been used as a validation standard for physical activity surveys. Although habitual physical activity is a major determinant of cardiorespiratory fitness, other factors, such as genetic inheritance, also play a role. Therefore, a perfect correlation between physical activity reporting and cardiorespiratory fitness would not be expected. Nonetheless, correlations of reported physical activity with measured cardiorespiratory fitness have been examined. Table 2-5 shows results from studies

Table 2-5. Correlation of two survey instruments with physiologic measures of caloric exchange

| Study | Sample | Physiologic test | Correlation coefficient |
|---|---|---|---|
| \multicolumn{4}{c}{*Minnesota Leisure-Time Physical Activity Questionnaire*} | | | |
| Taylor et al. (1978) | 175 men | Treadmill endurance | 0.45 |
| Skinner et al. (1966) | 54 men | Submaximal treadmill text | 0.13 NS |
| Leon et al. (1981) | 175 men | Treadmill | 0.41 |
| | | Submaximal heart rate | 0.59 |
| DeBacker et al. (1981) | 1,513 men | Submaximal treadmill test | 0.10 |
| Jacobs et al. (1993) | 64 men | $\dot{V}O_2$ max | 0.43 |
| | & women | Submaximal heart rate | 0.45 |
| Richardson et al. (1995) | 78 men | $\dot{V}O_2$ max | 0.47 |
| | & women | | |
| Albanes et al. (1990) | 21 men | Resting caloric intake | 0.17 NS |
| Montoye et al. (1996) | 28 men | Doubly labeled water | 0.26 NS |
| \multicolumn{4}{c}{*College Alumni Study Survey*} | | | |
| Siconolfi et al. (1985) | 36 men | $\dot{V}O_2$ max | 0.29 |
| | 32 women | $\dot{V}O_2$ max | 0.46 |
| Jacobs et al. (1993) | 64 men | | |
| | & women | $\dot{V}O_2$ max | 0.52 |
| | | Submaximal heart rate | 0.52 |
| Albanes et al. (1990) | 21 men | Resting caloric intake | 0.32 NS |
| Montoye et al. (1996) | 28 men | Doubly labeled water | 0.39 |
| | | Energy intake, 7 days | 0.44 |

NS = nonsignificant correlation coefficient; all others were statistically significant.

in which questionnaire data from the Minnesota Leisure-Time Physical Activity Questionnaire (Taylor et al. 1978) and the College Alumni Study survey (Paffenbarger et al. 1993) are compared with physiological measures, in most cases cardiorespiratory fitness. Although most correlation coefficients (e.g., Pearson's r) are statistically significant, they exhibit considerable variability (range 0.10 to 0.59), and the overall central tendency (median, 0.41) suggests only moderate external validity. However, in a study of predictors of cardiorespiratory fitness among adults (Blair et al. 1989), in all age and sex subgroups, self-reported physical activity was the principal contributor to the predictive models that also included weight, resting heart rate, and current smoking. Thus, self-reported physical activity may not be perfectly correlated with cardiorespiratory fitness, but it may be the predominant predictive factor.

Because misclassification of physical activity, as could occur by using an invalid measure, would tend to bias studies towards finding no association, the consistently found associations between physical activity and lower risk of several diseases (as is discussed in Chapter 4) suggest that the measure has at least some validity. Moreover, they suggest that a more precise measure of physical activity would likely yield even stronger associations with health. Thus, although measurement of physical activity by currently available methods may be far from ideal, it has provided a means to investigate and demonstrate important health benefits of physical activity.

## Chapter Summary

The assertion that frequent participation in physical activity contributes to better health has been a recurring theme in medicine and education throughout much of Western history. Early empirical observations and case studies suggesting that a sedentary life was not healthy have been supported by rigorous scientific investigation that has evolved over the past century. In recent decades, a number of experimental and clinical specialties have contributed substantially to an emerging field that may accurately be described as exercise science. This field includes disciplines ranging from exercise physiology and biomechanics to physical activity epidemiology, exercise psychology, clinical sports medicine, and preventive medicine. Research findings from these specialties provide the basis for this first Surgeon General's report on physical activity and health. Numerous expert panels, committees, and conferences have been convened over the years to evaluate the evidence relating physical activity and health. These gatherings have laid a solid foundation for the current consensus that for optimal health, people of all ages should be physically active on most days. Specific exercise recommendations have emphasized only vigorous activity for cardiorespiratory fitness until recently, when the benefits of moderate-intensity physical activity have been recognized and promoted as well.

## Conclusions

1. Physical activity for better health and well-being has been an important theme throughout much of western history.

2. Public health recommendations have evolved from emphasizing vigorous activity for cardiorespiratory fitness to including the option of moderate levels of activity for numerous health benefits.

3. Recommendations from experts agree that for better health, physical activity should be performed regularly. The most recent recommendations advise people of all ages to include a minimum of 30 minutes of physical activity of moderate intensity (such as brisk walking) on most, if not all, days of the week. It is also acknowledged that for most people, greater health benefits can be obtained by engaging in physical activity of more vigorous intensity or of longer duration.

4. Experts advise previously sedentary people embarking on a physical activity program to start with short durations of moderate-intensity activity and gradually increase the duration or intensity until the goal is reached.

5. Experts advise consulting with a physician before beginning a new physical activity program for people with chronic diseases, such as CVD and diabetes mellitus, or for those who are at high risk for these diseases. Experts also advise men over age 40 and women over age 50 to consult a physician before they begin a vigorous activity program.

6. Recent recommendations from experts also suggest that cardiorespiratory endurance activity should be supplemented with strength-developing exercises at least twice per week for adults, in order to improve musculoskeletal health, maintain independence in performing the activities of daily life, and reduce the risk of falling.

# Appendix A: *Healthy People 2000* Objectives

The nation's public health goals for the 1990s and beyond, as presented in *Healthy People 2000* (USDHHS 1990), aim to increase the span of healthy life for all Americans, to reduce health disparities among Americans, and to achieve access to preventive services for all Americans. Reproduced here are the *Healthy People 2000* objectives for physical activity and fitness as revised in 1995 (USDHHS 1995).

Duplicate objectives that appear in two or more priority areas are marked with an asterisk alongside the objective number.

### Physical Activity and Fitness
*Health Status Objectives*

1.1*    Reduce coronary heart disease deaths to no more than 100 per 100,000 people.

*Special Population Target*

| Coronary Deaths (per 100,000) | 2000 Target |
|---|---|
| 1.1a    Blacks | 115 |

1.2*    Reduce overweight to a prevalence of no more than 20 percent among people aged 20 and older and no more than 15 percent among adolescents aged 12–19.

*Special Population Target*

| Overweight Prevalence | 2000 Target |
|---|---|
| 1.2a    Low-income women aged 20 and older | 25% |
| 1.2b    Black women aged 20 and older | 30% |
| 1.2c    Hispanic women aged 20 and older | 25% |
| 1.2d    American Indians/Alaska Natives | 30% |
| 1.2e    People with disabilities | 25% |
| 1.2f    Women with high blood pressure | 41% |
| 1.2g    Men with high blood pressure | 35% |
| 1.2h    Mexican-American men | 25% |

Note: For people aged 20 and older, overweight is defined as body mass index (BMI) equal to or greater than 27.8 for men and 27.3 for women. For adolescents, overweight is defined as BMI equal to or greater than 23.0 for males aged 12–14, 24.3 for males aged 15–17, 25.8 for males aged 18–19, 23.4 for females aged 12–14, 24.8 for females aged 15–17, and 25.7 for females aged 18–19. The values for adults are the gender-specific 85th percentile values of the 1976–80 National Health and Nutrition Examination Survey (NHANES II), reference population 20–29 years of age. For adolescents, overweight was defined using BMI cutoffs based on modified age- and gender-specific 85th percentile values of the NHANES II. BMI is calculated by dividing weight in kilograms by the square of height in meters. The cut points used to define overweight approximate the 120 percent of desirable body weight definition used in the 1990 objectives.

*Risk Reduction Objectives*

1.3*    Increase to at least 30 percent the proportion of people aged 6 and older who engage regularly, preferably daily, in light to moderate physical activity for at least 30 minutes per day.

*Special Population Targets*

| Moderate Physical Activity | 2000 Target |
|---|---|
| 1.3a    Hispanics aged 18 and older | 25 % |
| 5 or more times per week | |

Note: Light to moderate physical activity requires sustained, rhythmic muscular movements, is at least equivalent to sustained walking, and is performed at less than 60 percent of maximum heart rate for age. Maximum heart rate equals roughly 220 beats per minute minus age. Examples may include walking, swimming, cycling, dancing, gardening and yardwork, various domestic and occupational activities, and games and other childhood pursuits.

## Historical Background, Terminology, Evolution of Recommendations, and Measurement

1.4 Increase to at least 20 percent the proportion of people aged 18 and older and to at least 75 percent the proportion of children and adolescents aged 6–17 who engage in vigorous physical activity that promotes the development and maintenance of cardiorespiratory fitness 3 or more days per week for 20 or more minutes per occasion.

*Special Population Targets*

| *Vigorous Physical Activity* | *2000 Target* |
|---|---|
| 1.4a Lower-income people aged 18 and older (annual family income <$20,000) | 12% |
| 1.4b Blacks aged 18 years and older | 17% |
| 1.4c Hispanics aged 18 years and older | 17% |

*Note: Vigorous physical activities are rhythmic, repetitive physical activities that use large muscle groups at 60 percent or more of maximum heart rate for age. An exercise rate of 60 percent of maximum heart rate for age is about 50 percent of maximal cardiorespiratory capacity and is sufficient for cardiorespiratory conditioning. Maximum heart rate equals roughly 220 beats per minute minus age.*

1.5 Reduce to no more than 15 percent the proportion of people aged 6 and older who engage in no leisure-time physical activity.

*Special Population Targets*

| *No Leisure-Time Physical Activity* | *2000 Target* |
|---|---|
| 1.5a People aged 65 and older | 22% |
| 1.5b People with disabilities | 20% |
| 1.5c Lower-income people (annual family income <$20,000) | 17% |
| 1.5d Blacks aged 18 and older | 20% |
| 1.5e Hispanics aged 18 and older | 25% |
| 1.5f American Indians/Alaska Natives aged 18 and older | 21% |

*Note: For this objective, people with disabilities are people who report any limitation in activity due to chronic conditions.*

1.6 Increase to at least 40 percent the proportion of people aged 6 and older who regularly perform physical activities that enhance and maintain muscular strength, muscular endurance, and flexibility.

1.7* Increase to at least 50 percent the proportion of overweight people aged 12 and older who have adopted sound dietary practices combined with regular physical activity to attain an appropriate body weight.

*Special Population Targets*

| *Adoption of Weight-Loss Practices* | *2000 Target* |
|---|---|
| 1.7a Overweight Hispanic males aged 18 and older | 24% |
| 1.7b Overweight Hispanic females aged 18 and older | 22% |

*Services and Protection Objectives*

1.8 Increase to at least 50 percent the proportion of children and adolescents in 1st–12th grade who participate in daily school physical education.

1.9 Increase to at least 50 percent the proportion of school physical education class time that students spend being physically active, preferably engaged in lifetime physical activities.

## Physical Activity and Health

*Note: Lifetime activities are activities that may be readily carried into adulthood because they generally need only one or two people. Examples include swimming, bicycling, jogging, and racquet sports. Also counted as lifetime activities are vigorous social activities such as dancing. Competitive group sports and activities typically played only by young children such as group games are excluded.*

1.10    Increase the proportion of worksites offering employer-sponsored physical activity and fitness programs as follows:

| Worksite Size | 2000 Target |
|---|---|
| 50–99 employees | 20% |
| 100–249 employees | 35% |
| 250–749 employees | 50% |
| ≥750 employees | 80% |

1.11    Increase community availability and accessibility of physical activity and fitness facilities as follows:

| Facility | 2000 Target |
|---|---|
| Hiking, biking, and fitness trail miles | 1 per 10,000 people |
| Public swimming pools | 1 per 25,000 people |
| Acres of park and recreation open space | 4 per 1,000 people |
|  | (250 people per managed acre) |

1.12    Increase to at least 50 percent the proportion of primary care providers who routinely assess and counsel their patients regarding the frequency, duration, type, and intensity of each patient's physical activity practices.

*Health Status Objective*

1.13*   Reduce to no more than 90 per 1,000 people the proportion of all people aged 65 and older who have difficulty in performing two or more personal care activities thereby preserving independence.

*Special Population Targets*

| Difficulty Performing Self Care (per 1,000) | 2000 Target |
|---|---|
| 1.13a   People aged 85 and older | 325 |
| 1.13b   Blacks aged 65 and older | 98 |

*Note: Personal care activities are bathing, dressing, using the toilet, getting in and out of bed or chair, and eating.*

## Appendix B: NIH Consensus Conference Statement

In Press (3/18/96)

National Institutes of Health
Consensus Development Conference Statement

Physical Activity and Cardiovascular Health
December 18–20, 1995

NIH Consensus Statements are prepared by a nonadvocate, non-Federal panel of experts, based on (1) presentations by investigators working in areas relevant to the consensus questions during a 2-day public session; (2) questions and statements from conference attendees during open discussion periods that are part of the public session; and (3) closed deliberations by the panel during the remainder of the second day and morning of the third. This statement is an independent report of the panel and is not a policy statement of the NIH or the Federal Government.

### Abstract

*Objective.* To provide physicians and the general public with a responsible assessment of the relationship between physical activity and cardiovascular health.

*Participants.* A non-Federal, nonadvocate, 13-member panel representing the fields of cardiology, psychology, exercise physiology, nutrition, pediatrics, public health, and epidemiology. In addition, 27 experts in cardiology, psychology, epidemiology, exercise physiology, geriatrics, nutrition, pediatrics, public health, and sports medicine presented data to the panel and a conference audience of 600.

*Evidence.* The literature was searched through Medline and an extensive bibliography of references was provided to the panel and the conference audience. Experts prepared abstracts with relevant citations from the literature. Scientific evidence was given precedence over clinical anecdotal experience.

*Consensus Process.* The panel, answering predefined questions, developed their conclusions based on the scientific evidence presented in open forum and the scientific literature. The panel composed a draft statement that was read in its entirety and circulated to the experts and the audience for comment. Thereafter, the panel resolved conflicting recommendations and released a revised statement at the end of the conference. The panel finalized the revisions within a few weeks after the conference.

*Conclusions.* All Americans should engage in regular physical activity at a level appropriate to their capacity, needs, and interest. Children and adults alike should set a goal of accumulating at least 30 minutes of moderate-intensity physical activity on most, and preferably, all days of the week. Most Americans have little or no physical activity in their daily lives, and accumulating evidence indicates that physical inactivity is a major risk factor for cardiovascular disease. However, moderate levels of physical activity confer significant health benefits. Even those who currently meet these daily standards may derive additional health and fitness benefits by becoming more physically active or including more vigorous activity. For those with known cardiovascular disease, cardiac rehabilitation programs that combine physical activity with reduction in other risk factors should be more widely used.

### Introduction

Over the past 25 years, the United States has experienced a steady decline in the age-adjusted death toll from cardiovascular disease (CVD), primarily in mortality caused by coronary heart disease and stroke. Despite this decline, coronary heart disease remains the leading cause of death and stroke the third leading cause of death. Lifestyle improvements by the American public and better control of the risk factors for heart disease and stroke have been major factors in this decline.

Coronary heart disease and stroke have many causes. Modifiable risk factors include smoking, high blood pressure, blood lipid levels, obesity, diabetes, and physical inactivity. In contrast to the positive national trends observed with cigarette smoking, high blood pressure, and high blood cholesterol, obesity and physical inactivity in the United States have not improved. Indeed automation and other technologies have contributed greatly to lessening physical activity at work and home.

The purpose of this conference was to examine the accumulating evidence on the role of physical activity in the prevention and treatment of CVD and its risk factors.

Physical activity in this statement is defined as "bodily movement produced by skeletal muscles that requires energy expenditure" and produces healthy benefits. Exercise, a type of physical activity, is defined as "a planned, structured, and repetitive bodily movement done to improve or maintain one or more components of physical fitness." Physical inactivity denotes a level of activity less than that needed to maintain good health.

Physical inactivity characterizes most Americans. Exertion has been systematically engineered out of most occupations and lifestyles. In 1991, 54 percent of adults reported little or no regular leisure physical activity. Data from the 1990 Youth Risk Behavior Survey show that most teenagers in grades 9-12 are not performing regular vigorous activity. About 50 percent of high school students reported they are not enrolled in physical education classes.

Physical activity protects against the development of CVD and also favorably modifies other CVD risk factors, including high blood pressure, blood lipid levels, insulin resistance, and obesity. The type, frequency, and intensity of physical activity that are needed to accomplish these goals remain poorly defined and controversial.

Physical activity is also important in the treatment of patients with CVD or those who are at increased risk for developing CVD, including patients who have hypertension, stable angina, or peripheral vascular disease, or who have had a prior myocardial infarction or heart failure. Physical activity is an important component of cardiac rehabilitation, and people with CVD can benefit from participation. However, some questions remain regarding benefits, risks, and costs associated with becoming physically active.

Many factors influence adopting and maintaining a physically active lifestyle, such as socioeconomic status, cultural influences, age, and health status. Understanding is needed on how such variables influence the adoption of this behavior at the individual level. Intervention strategies for encouraging individuals from different backgrounds to adopt and adhere to a physically active lifestyle need to be developed and tested. Different environments such as schools, worksites, health care settings, and the home can play a role in promoting physical activity. These community-level factors also need to be better understood.

To address these and related issues, the NIH's National Heart, Lung, and Blood Institute and Office of Medical Applications of Research convened a Consensus Development Conference on Physical Activity and Cardiovascular Health. The conference was cosponsored by the NIH's National Institute of Child Health and Human Development, National Institute on Aging, National Institute of Arthritis and Musculoskeletal and Skin Diseases, National Institute of Diabetes and Digestive and Kidney Diseases, National Institute of Nursing Research, Office of Research on Women's Health, and Office of Disease Prevention, as well as the Centers for Disease Control and Prevention and the President's Council on Physical Fitness and Sports.

The conference brought together specialists in medicine, exercise physiology, health behavior, epidemiology, nutrition, physical therapy, and nursing as well as representatives from the public. After a day and a half of presentations and audience discussion, an independent, non-Federal consensus panel weighed the scientific evidence and developed a draft statement that addressed the following five questions.

- What is the health burden of a sedentary lifetye on the population?
- What type, what intensity, and what quantity of physical activity are important to prevent cardiovascular disease?
- What are the benefits and risks of different types of physical activity for people with cardiovascular disease?
- What are the successful approaches to adopting and maintaining a physically active lifestyle?
- What are the important questions for future research?

## 1. What Is the Health Burden of a Sedentary Lifestyle on the Population?

Physical inactivity among the U.S. population is now widespread. National surveillance programs have documented that about one in four adults (more women than men) currently have sedentary lifestyles with no leisure time physical activity. An additional one-third of adults are insufficiently active to achieve health benefits. The prevalence of inactivity varies by gender, age, ethnicity, health status, and geographic region but is common to all demographic groups. Change in physical exertion associated with occupation has declined markedly in this century.

Girls become less active than do boys as they grow older. Children become far less active as they move through adolescence. Obesity is increasing among children, at least in part related to physical inactivity. Data indicate that obese children and adolescents have a high risk of becoming obese adults, and obesity in adulthood is related to coronary artery disease, hypertension, and diabetes. Thus, the prevention of childhood obesity has the potential of preventing CVD in adults. At age 12, 70 percent of children report participation in vigorous physical activity; by age 21 this activity falls to 42 percent for men and 30 percent for women. Furthermore, as adults age, their physical activity levels continue to decline.

Although knowledge about physical inactivity as a risk factor for CVD has come mainly from investigations of middle-aged, white men, more limited evidence from studies in women minority groups and the elderly suggests that the findings are similar in these groups. On the basis of current knowledge, we must note that physical inactivity occurs disproportionately among Americans who are not well educated and who are socially or economically disadvantaged.

Physical activity is directly related to physical fitness. Although the means of measuring physical activity have varied between studies (i.e., there is no standardization of measures), evidence indicates that physical inactivity and lack of physical fitness are directly associated with increased mortality from CVD. The increase in mortality is not entirely explained by the association with elevated blood pressure, smoking, and blood lipid levels.

There is an inverse relationship between measures of physical activity and indices of obesity in most U.S. population studies. Only a few studies have examined the relationship between physical activity and body fat distribution, and these suggest an inverse relationship between levels of physical activity and visceral fat. There is evidence that increased physical activity facilitates weight loss and

that the addition of physical activity to dietary energy restriction can increase and help to maintain loss of body weight and body fat mass.

Middle-aged and older men and women who engage in regular physical activity have significantly higher high-density lipoprotein (HDL) cholesterol levels than do those who are sedentary. When exercise training has extended to at least 12 weeks, beneficial HDL cholesterol level changes have been reported.

Most studies of endurance exercise training of individuals with normal blood pressure and those with hypertension have shown decreases in systolic and diastolic blood pressure. Insulin sensitivity is also improved with endurance exercise.

A number of factors that affect thrombotic function—including hematocrit, fibrinogen, platelet function, and fibrinolysis—are related to the risk of CVD. Regular endurance exercise lowers the risk related to these factors.

The burden of CVD rests most heavily on the least active. In addition to its powerful impact on the cardiovascular system, physical inactivity is also associated with other adverse health effects, including osteoporosis, diabetes, and some cancers.

## 2. What Type, What Intensity, and What Quantity of Physical Activity Are Important to Prevent Cardiovascular Disease?

Activity that reduces CVD risk factors and confers many other health benefits does not require a structured or vigorous exercise program. The majority of benefits of physical activity can be gained by performing moderate-intensity activities. The amount or type of physical activity needed for health benefits or optimal health is a concern due to limited time and competing activities for most Americans. The amount and types of physical activity that are needed to prevent disease and promote health must, therefore, be clearly communicated, and effective strategies must be developed to promote physical activity to the public.

The quantitative relationship between level of activity or fitness and magnitude of cardiovascular benefit may extend across the full range of activity. A moderate level of physical activity confers health benefits. However, physical activity must be performed regularly to maintain these effects.

## Physical Activity and Health

Moderate=intensity activity performed by previously sedentary individuals results in significant improvement in many health-related outcomes. These moderate intensity activities are more likely to be continued than are high-intensity activities.

We recommend that all people in the United States increase their regular physical activity to a level appropriate to their capacities, needs, and interest. We recommend that all children and adults should set a long-term goal to accumulate at least 30 minutes or more of moderate-intensity physical activity on most, or preferably all, days of the week. Intermittent or shorter bouts of activity (at least 10 minutes), including occupational, nonoccupational, or tasks of daily living, also have similar cardiovascular and health benefits if performed at a level of moderate intensity (such as brisk walking, cycling, swimming, home repair, and yardwork) with an accumulated duration of at least 30 minutes per day. People who currently meet the recommended minimal standards may derive additional health and fitness benefits from becoming more physically active or including more vigorous activity.

Some evidence suggests lowered mortality with more vigorous activity, but further research is needed to more specifically define safe and effective levels. The most active individuals have lower cardiovascular morbidity and mortality rates than do those who are least active; however, much of the benefit appears to be accounted for by comparing the least active individuals to those who are moderately active. Further increases in the intensity or amount of activity produce further benefits in some, but not all, parameters of risk. High-intensity activity is also associated with an increased risk of injury, discontinuation of activity, or acute cardiac events during the activity. Current low rates of regular activity in Americans may be partially due to the mis-perception of many that vigorous, continuous exercise is necessary to reap health benefits. Many people, for example, fail to appreciate walking as "exercise" or to recognize the substantial benefits of short bouts (at least 10 minutes) of moderate-level activity.

The frequency, intensity, and duration of activity are interrelated. The number of episodes of activity recommended for health depends on the intensity and/or duration of the activity: higher intensity or longer duration activity could be performed approximately three times weekly and achieve cardiovascular benefits, but low-intensity or shorter duration activities should be performed more often to achieve cardiovascular benefits.

The appropriate type of activity is best determined by the individual's preferences and what will be sustained. Exercise, or a structured program of activity, is a subset of activity that may encourage interest and allow for more vigorous activity. People who perform more formal exercise (i.e., structured or planned exercise programs) can accumulate this daily total through a variety of recreational or sports activities. People who are currently sedentary or minimally active should gradually build up to the recommended goal of 30 minutes of moderate activity daily by adding a few minutes each day until reaching their personal goal to reduce the risk associated with suddenly increasing the amount or intensity of exercise. (The defined levels of effort depend on individual characteristics such as baseline fitness and health status.)

Developing muscular strength and joint flexibility is also important for an overall activity program to improve one's ability to perform tasks and to reduce the potential for injury. Upper extremity and resistance (or strength) training can improve muscular function, and evidence suggests that there may be cardiovascular benefits, especially in older patients or those with underlying CVD, but further research and guidelines are needed. Older people or those who have been deconditioned from recent inactivity or illness may particularly benefit from resistance training due to improved ability in accomplishing tasks of daily living. Resistance training may contribute to better balance, coordination, and agility that may help prevent falls in the elderly.

Physical activity carries risks as well as benefits. The most common adverse effects of activity relate to musculoskeletal injury and are usually mild and self-limited. The risk of injury increases with increased intensity, frequency, and duration of activity and also depends on the type of activity. Exercise-related injuries can be reduced by moderating these parameters. A more serious but rare complication of activity is myocardial infarction or sudden cardiac death. Although persons who engage in vigorous physical activity have a slight increase in risk of sudden cardiac death during activity, the health benefits outweigh this risk because of the large overall risk reduction.

In children and young adults, exertion-related deaths are uncommon and are generally related to congenital heart defects (e.g., hypertrophic cardiomyopathy, Marfan's syndrome, severe aortic valve stenosis, prolonged QT syndromes, cardiac conduction abnormalities) or to acquired myocarditis. It is recommended that patients with those conditions remain active but not participate in vigorous or competitive athletics.

Because the risks of physical activity are very low compared with the health benefits, most adults do not need medical consultation or pretesting before starting a moderate-intensity physical activity program. However, those with known CVD and men over age 40 and women over age 50 with multiple cardiovascular risk factors who contemplate a program of vigorous activity should have a medical evaluation prior to initiating such a program.

## 3. What Are the Benefits and Risks of Different Types of Physical Activity for People with Cardiovascular Disease?

More than 10 million Americans are afflicted with clinically significant CVD, including myocardial infarction, angina pectoris, peripheral vascular disease, and congestive heart failure. In addition, more than 300,000 patients per year are currently subjected to coronary artery bypass surgery and a similar number to percutaneous transluminal coronary angioplasty. Increased physical activity appears to benefit each of these groups. Benefits include reduction in cardiovascular mortality, reduction of symptoms, improvement in exercise tolerance and functional capacity, and improvement in psychological well-being and quality of life.

Several studies have shown that exercise training programs significantly reduce overall mortality, as well as death caused by myocardial infarction. The reported reductions in mortality have been highest—approximately 25 percent—in cardiac rehabilitation programs that have included control of other cardiovascular risk factors. Rehabilitation programs using both moderate and vigorous physical activity have been associated with reductions in fatal cardiac events, although the minimal or optimal level and duration of exercise required to achieve beneficial effects remains uncertain. Data are inadequate to determine whether stroke incidence is affected by physical activity or exercise training.

The risk of death during medically supervised cardiac exercise training programs is very low. However, those who exercise infrequently and have poor functional capacity at baseline may be at somewhat higher risk during exercise training. All patients with CVD should have a medical evaluation prior to participation in a vigorous exercise program.

Appropriately prescribed and conducted exercise training programs improve exercise tolerance and physical fitness in patients with coronary heart disease. Moderate as well as vigorous exercise training regimens are of value. Patients with low basal levels of exercise capacity experience the most functional benefits, even at relatively modest levels of physical activity. Patients with angina pectoris typically experience improvement in angina in association with a reduction in effort-induced myocardial ischemia, presumably as a result of decreased myocardial oxygen demand and increased work capacity.

Patients with congestive heart failure also appear to show improvement in symptoms, exercise capacity, and functional well-being in response to exercise training, even though left ventricular systolic function appears to be unaffected. The exercise program should be tailored to the needs of these patients and supervised closely in view of the marked predisposition of these patients to ischemic events and arrhythmias.

Cardiac rehabilitation exercise training often improves skeletal muscle strength and oxidative capacity and, when combined with appropriate nutritional changes, may result in weight loss. In addition, such training generally results in improvement in measures of psychological status, social adjustment, and functional capacity. However, cardiac rehabilitation exercise training has less influence on rates of return to work than many nonexercise variables, including employer attitudes, prior employment status, and economic incentives. Multifactorial intervention programs, including nutritional changes and medication plus exercise, are needed to improve health status and reduce cardiovascular disease risk.

45

Cardiac rehabilitation programs have traditionally been institutional-based and group-centered (e.g., hospitals, clinics, community centers). Referral and enrollment rates have been relatively low, generally ranging from 10 to 25 percent of patients with CHD. Referral rates are lower for women than for men and lower for non-whites than for whites. Home-based programs have the potential to provide rehabilitative services to a wider population. Home-based programs incorporating limited hospital visits with regular mail or telephone followup by a nurse case manager have demonstrated significant increases in functional capacity, smoking cessation, and improvement in blood lipid levels. A range of options exists in cardiac rehabilitation including site, number of visits, monitoring, and other services.

There are clear medical and economic reasons for carrying out cardiac rehabilitation programs. Optimal outcomes are achieved when exercise training is combined with educational messages and feedback about changing lifestyle. Patients who participate in cardiac rehabilitation programs show a lower incidence of rehospitalization and lower charges per hospitalization. Cardiac rehabilitation is a cost-efficient therapeutic modality that should be used more frequently.

## 4. What Are the Successful Approaches to Adopting and Maintaining a Physically Active Lifestyle?

The cardiovascular benefits from and physiological reactions to physical activity appear to be similar among diverse population subgroups defined by age, sex, income, region of residence, ethnic background, and health status. However, the behavioral and attitudinal factors that influence the motivation for and ability to sustain physical activity are strongly determined by social experiences, cultural background, and physical disability and health status. For example, perceptions of appropriate physical activity differ by gender, age, weight, marital status, family roles and responsibilities, disability, and social class. Thus, the following general guidelines will need to be further refined when one is planning with or prescribing for specific individuals and population groups, but generally physical activity is more likely to be initiated and maintained if the individual

- Perceives a net benefit.
- Chooses an enjoyable activity.
- Feels competent doing the activity.
- Feels safe doing the activity.
- Can easily access the activity on a regular basis.
- Can fit the activity into the daily schedule.
- Feels that the activity does not generate financial or social costs that he or she is unwilling to bear.
- Experiences a minimum of negative consequences such as injury, loss of time, negative peer pressure, and problems with self-identity.
- Is able to successfully address issues of competing time demands.
- Recognizes the need to balance the use of labor-saving devices (e.g., power lawn mowers, golf carts, automobiles) and sedentary activities (e.g., watching television, use of computers) with activities that involve a higher level of physical exertion.

Other people in the individual's social environment can influence the adoption and maintenance of physical activity. Health care providers have a key role in promoting smoking cessation and other risk-reduction behaviors. Preliminary evidence suggests that this also applies to physical activity. It is highly probable that people will be more likely to increase their physical activity if their health care provider counsels them to do so. Providers can do this effectively by learning to recognize stages of behavior change, to communicate the need for increased activity, to assist the patient in initiating activity, and by following up appropriately.

Family and friends can also be important sources of support for behavior change. For example, spouses or friends can serve as "buddies," joining in the physical activity; or a spouse could offer to take on a household task, giving his or her mate time to engage in physical activity. Parents can support their children's activity by providing transportation, praise, and encouragement, and by participating in activities with their children.

Worksites have the potential to encourage increased physical activity by offering opportunities, reminders, and rewards for doing so. For example, an appropriate indoor area can be set aside to enable walking during lunch hours. Signs placed near elevators can encourage the use of the stairs instead. Discounts on parking fees can be offered to employees who elect to park in remote lots and walk.

Schools are a major community resource for increasing physical activity, particularly given the urgent need to develop strategies that affect children and adolescents. As noted previously, there is now clear evidence that U.S. children and adolescents have become more obese. There is also evidence that obese children and adolescents exercise less than their leaner peers. All schools should provide opportunities for physical activities that

- Are appropriate and enjoyable for children of all skill levels and are not limited to competitive sports or physical education classes.
- Appeal to girls as well as to boys, and to children from diverse backgrounds.
- Can serve as a foundation for activities throughout life.
- Are offered on a daily basis.

Successful approaches may involve mass education strategies or changes in institutional policies or community variables. In some environments (e.g., schools, worksites, community centers), policy-level interventions may be necessary to enable people to achieve and maintain an adequate level of activity. Policy changes that increase opportunities for physical activity can facilitate activity maintenance for motivated individuals and increase readiness to change among the less motivated. As in other areas of health promotion, mass communication strategies should be used to promote physical activity. These strategies should include a variety of mainstream channels and techniques to reach diverse audiences that acquire information through different media (e.g., TV, newspaper, radio, Internet).

### 5. What Are the Important Considerations for Future Research?

While much has been learned about the role of physical activity in cardiovascular health, there are many unanswered questions.

- Maintain surveillance of physical activity levels in the U.S. population by age, sex, geographic, and socioeconomic measures.

- Develop better methods for analysis and quantification of activity. These methods should be applicable to both work and leisure time measurements and provide direct quantitative estimates of activity.
- Conduct physiologic, biochemical, and genetic research necessary to define the mechanisms by which activity affects CVD including changes in metabolism as well as cardiac and vascular effects. This will provide new insights into cardiovascular biology that may have broader implications than for other clinical outcomes.
- Examine the effects of physical activity and cardiac rehabilitation programs on morbidity and mortality in elderly individuals.
- Conduct research on the social and psychological factors that influence adoption of a more active lifestyle and the maintenance of that behavior change throughout life.
- Carry out controlled randomized clinical trials among children and adolescents to test the effects of increased physical activity on CVD risk factor levels including obesity. The effects of intensity, frequency, and duration of increased physical activity should be examined in such studies.

## Conclusions

Accumulating scientific evidence indicates that physical inactivity is a major risk factor for CVD. Moderate levels of regular physical activity confer significant health benefits. Unfortunately, most Americans have little or no physical activity in their daily lives.

All Americans should engage in regular physical activity at a level appropriate to their capacities, needs, and interests. All children and adults should set and reach a goal of accumulating at least 30 minutes of moderate-intensity physical activity on most, and preferably all, days of the week. Those who currently meet these standards may derive additional health and fitness benefits by becoming more physically active or including more vigorous activity.

Cardiac rehabilitation programs that combine physical activity with reduction in other risk factors should be more widely applied to those with known CVD. Well-designed rehabilitation programs have benefits that are lost because of these programs' limited use.

Individuals with CVD and men over 40 or women over 50 years of age with multiple cardiovascular risk factors should have a medical evaluation prior to embarking on a vigorous exercise program.

Recognizing the importance of individual and societal factors in initiating and sustaining regular physical activity, the panel recommends the following:

- Development of programs for health care providers to communicate to patients the importance of regular physical activity.

- Community support of regular physical activity with environmental and policy changes at schools, worksites, community centers, and other sites.

- Initiation of a coordinated national campaign involving a consortium of collaborating health organizations to encourage regular physical activity.

- The implementation of the recommendations in this statement has considerable potential to improve the health and well-being of American citizens.

# About the NIH Consensus Development Program

NIH Consensus Development Conferences are convened to evaluate available scientific information and resolve safety and efficacy issues related to a biomedical technology. The resultant NIH Consensus Statements are intended to advance understanding of the technology or issue in question and to be useful to health professionals and the public.

# References

Acheson KJ, Campbell IT, Edholm OG, Miller DS, Stock MJ. The measurement of daily energy expenditure: an evaluation of some techniques. *American Journal of Clinical Nutrition* 1980;33:1155–1164.

Ainsworth BE, Montoye HJ, Leon AS. Methods of assessing physical activity during leisure and work. In: Bouchard C, Shephard RJ, Stephens T, editors. *Physical activity, fitness, and health: international proceedings and consensus statement.* Champaign, IL: Human Kinetics, 1994:146–159.

Albanes D, Conway JM, Taylor PR, Moe PW, Judd J. Validation and comparison of eight physical activity questionnaires. *Epidemiology* 1990;1:65–71.

Allen W, Pepys WH. On respiration. *Philosophical Transactions of the Royal Society of London* 1809(Pt 2):404–429.

American Academy of Pediatrics, Committee on Sports Medicine and Fitness. Assessing physical activity and fitness in the office setting. *Pediatrics* 1994;93:686–689.

American Academy of Pediatrics, Committee on Sports Medicine and Fitness. Fitness, activity, and sports participation in the preschool child. *Pediatrics* 1992;90:1002–1004.

American Association of Cardiovascular and Pulmonary Rehabilitation. *Guidelines for cardiac rehabilitation programs.* Champaign, IL: Human Kinetics, 1991.

American Association of Cardiovascular and Pulmonary Rehabilitation. *Guidelines for pulmonary rehabilitation programs.* Champaign, IL: Human Kinetics, 1993.

American Association of Cardiovascular and Pulmonary Rehabilitation. *Guidelines for cardiac rehabilitation programs.* 2nd ed. Champaign, IL: Human Kinetics, 1995.

American College of Sports Medicine. ACSM position stand on osteoporosis and exercise. *Medicine and Science in Sports and Exercise* 1995a;27:i–vii.

American College of Sports Medicine. *ACSM's guidelines for exercise testing and prescription.* 5th ed. Baltimore: Williams and Wilkins, 1995b.

American College of Sports Medicine. *Guidelines for exercise testing and prescription.* 3rd ed. Philadelphia: Lea and Febiger, 1986.

American College of Sports Medicine. *Guidelines for exercise testing and prescription.* 4th ed. Philadelphia: Lea and Febiger, 1991.

American College of Sports Medicine. *Guidelines for graded exercise testing and exercise prescription.* Philadelphia: Lea and Febiger, 1975.

American College of Sports Medicine. *Guidelines for graded exercise testing and exercise prescription.* 2nd ed. Philadelphia: Lea and Febiger, 1980.

American College of Sports Medicine. Physical activity, physical fitness, and hypertension. *Medicine and Science in Sports and Exercise* 1993;25:i–x.

American College of Sports Medicine. Position stand: exercise for patients with coronary artery disease. *Medicine and Science in Sports and Exercise* 1994;26:i–v.

American College of Sports Medicine. Position stand: the recommended quantity and quality of exercise for developing and maintaining cardiorespiratory and muscular fitness in healthy adults. *Medicine and Science in Sports and Exercise* 1990;22:265–274.

American College of Sports Medicine. The recommended quantity and quality of exercise for developing and maintaining fitness in healthy adults. *Medicine and Science in Sports* 1978;10:vii–x.

American Heart Association. Cardiac rehabilitation programs: a statement for healthcare professionals from the American Heart Association. *Circulation* 1994;90:1602–1610.

American Heart Association. Exercise standards: a statement for healthcare professionals from the American Heart Association. *Circulation* 1995;91:580–615.

American Heart Association. *Exercise testing and training of apparently healthy individuals: a handbook for physicians.* Dallas: American Heart Association, 1972.

American Heart Association. *Exercise testing and training of individuals with heart disease or at high risk for its development: a handbook for physicians.* Dallas: American Heart Association, 1975.

American Heart Association. Statement on exercise: benefits and recommendations for physical activity programs for all Americans: a statement for health professionals by the Committee on Exercise and Cardiac Rehabilitation of the Council on Clinical Cardiology, American Heart Association. *Circulation* 1992;86:340–344.

American Heart Association, Blair SN, Powell KE, Bazzarre TL, Early JL, Epstein LH, et al. AHA prevention conference. III. Behavior change and compliance: key to improving cardiovascular health. Physical inactivity: workshop V. *Circulation* 1993;88:1402–1405.

American Medical Association, Elster AB, Kuznets NJ. *AMA guidelines for adolescent preventive services (GAPS): recommendations and rationale.* Chicago, IL: Williams and Wilkins, 1994.

## Physical Activity and Health

Balogun JA, Amusa LO, Onyewadume IU. Factors affecting Caltrac® and Calcount® accelerometer output. *Physical Therapy* 1988;68:1500–1504.

Baranowski T. Methodologic issues in self-report of health behavior. *Journal of School Health* 1985;55:179–182.

Beecher CE. *Physiology and calisthenics for schools and families.* New York: Harper and Brothers, 1856.

Benedict FG, Cathcart EP. *Muscular work: a metabolic study with special reference to the efficiency of the human body as a machine.* Washington, DC: Carnegie Institution of Washington, 1913.

Berryman JW. Exercise and the medical tradition from Hippocrates through antebellum America: a review essay. In: Berryman JW, Park RJ, editors. *Sport and exercise science: essays in the history of sports medicine.* Urbana, IL: University of Illinois Press, 1992:1–56.

Berryman JW. *Out of many, one: a history of the American College of Sports Medicine.* Champaign, IL: Human Kinetics, 1995.

Bierman EL, Brunzell JD. Obesity and atherosclerosis. In: Björntorp P, Brodoff BN, editors. *Obesity.* Philadelphia: J.B. Lippincott Company, 1992:512–516.

Blair SN. 1993 C.H. McCloy research lecture: physical activity, physical fitness, and health. *Research Quarterly for Exercise and Sport* 1993;64:365–376.

Blair SN, Dowda M, Pate RR, Kronenfeld J, Howe HG Jr, Parker G, et al. Reliability of long-term recall of participation in physical activity by middle-aged men and women. *American Journal of Epidemiology* 1991;133:266–275.

Blair SN, Falls HB, Pate RR. A new physical fitness test. *Physician and Sportsmedicine* 1983;11:87–95.

Blair SN, Kannel WB, Kohl HW, Goodyear N, Wilson PWF. Surrogate measures of physical activity and physical fitness: evidence for sedentary traits of resting tachycardia, obesity, and low vital capacity. *American Journal of Epidemiology* 1989;129:1145–1156.

Blair SN, Kohl HW, Gordon NF. How much physical activity is good for health? *Annual Reviews of Public Health* 1992;13:99–126.

Blair SN, Kohl HW III, Paffenbarger RS Jr, Clark DG, Cooper KH, Gibbons LW. Physical fitness and all-cause mortality: a prospective study of healthy men and women. *Journal of the American Medical Association* 1989;262:2395–2401.

Blumberg VS, Alexander J. Obesity and the heart. In: Björntorp P, Brodoff BN, editors. *Obesity.* Philadelphia: J.B. Lippincott Company, 1992:517–531.

Borg GA. Psychophysical bases of perceived exertion. *Medicine and Science in Sports and Exercise* 1982;14:377–381.

Bouchard C, Shephard RJ, Stephens T, editors. *Physical activity, fitness, and health: international proceedings and consensus statement.* Champaign, IL: Human Kinetics, 1994.

Bouchard C, Shephard RJ, Stephens T, Sutton JR, McPherson BD. Exercise, fitness, and health: the consensus statement. In: Bouchard C, Shephard RJ, Stephens T, Sutton JR, McPherson BD, editors. *Exercise, fitness, and health.* Champaign, IL: Human Kinetics, 1990:4–28.

Brown RG, Davidson LAG, McKeown T, Whitfield AGW. Coronary-artery disease—influences affecting its incidence in males in the seventh decade. *Lancet* 1957;2:1073–1077.

Buchan W. *Domestic medicine: or, a treatise on the prevention and cure of diseases, by regimen and simple medicines* [1769]. Reprint, Boston: Joseph Bumstead, 1813.

Burns CR. The nonnaturals: a paradox in the western concept of health. *Journal of Medicine and Philosophy* 1976;1:202–211.

Byford WH. On the physiology of exercise. *American Journal of Medical Sciences* 1855;30:32–42.

Bylebyl JJ. The school of Padua: humanistic medicine in the sixteenth century. In: Webster C, editor. *Health, medicine, and mortality in the sixteenth century.* Cambridge, MA: Cambridge University Press, 1979:335–370.

Caldwell C. *Thoughts on physical education: being a discourse delivered to a convention of teachers in Lexington, Kentucky, on the 6th and 7th of November 1833.* Boston: Marsh, Capen, and Lyon, 1834.

Caspersen CJ. Physical activity epidemiology: concepts, methods, and applications to exercise science. *Exercise and Sport Sciences Reviews* 1989;17:423–473.

Caspersen CJ, Pollard RA. Validity of global self-reports of physical activity in epidemiology. *CVD Epidemiology Newsletter* 1988;43:15.

Caspersen CJ, Powell KE, Christensen GM. Physical activity, exercise, and physical fitness: definitions and distinctions for health-related research. *Public Health Reports* 1985;100:126–131.

Cassedy JH. Why self-help? Americans alone with their diseases, 1800–1850. In: Risse GB, Numbers RL, Leavitt JW, editors. *Medicine without doctors: home health care in American history.* New York: Science History Publications, 1977:31–48.

Chapman CB, Mitchell JH. The physiology of exercise. *Scientific America* 1965;212:88–96.

Cheyne G. *An essay of health and long life* [1724]. Reprint, London: George Strahan, 1734.

Christensen EH. Intervallarbeit und intervalltraining. *Arbeitsphysiologie* 1960;18:345–356.

Clarke HH, editor. Toward a better understanding of muscular strength. *Physical Fitness Research Digest* 1973;3:1–20.

Cogan T. *The haven of health* [1584]. Reprint, London: Bonham Norton, 1596.

Cooper KH. A means of assessing maximal oxygen intake: correlation between field and treadmill testing. *Journal of the American Medical Association* 1968;203:135–138.

Corbin CB, Lindsey R. *Concepts in physical education with laboratories.* 8th ed. Dubuque, IA: Times Mirror Higher Education Group, 1994.

Cornaro L. *The art of living long* [1558]. Reprint, Milwaukee: William F. Butler, 1905.

Crampton CW. A test of condition: preliminary report. *Medical News* 1905;87:529–535.

Crampton CW. *Start today: your guide to physical fitness.* New York: A.S. Barnes, 1941.

Cureton TK. *Physical fitness workbook: a manual of conditioning exercises and standards, tests, and rating scales for evaluating physical fitness.* 3rd ed. St. Louis: C.V. Mosby Company, 1947.

Cyriax RJ. A short history of mechano-therapeutics in Europe until the time of Ling. *Janus* 1914;19:178–240.

DeBacker G, Kornitzer M, Sobolski J, Dramaix M, Degre S, de Marneffe M. Physical activity and physical fitness levels of Belgian males aged 40–55 years. *Cardiology* 1981;67:110–128.

Dill DB. The Harvard Fatigue Laboratory: its development, contributions, and demise. In: Chapman CB, editor. *Physiology of muscular exercise.* New York: American Heart Association, 1967.

DiPietro L, Caspersen CJ, Ostfeld AM, Nadel ER. A survey for assessing physical activity among older adults. *Medicine and Science in Sports and Exercise* 1993;25:628–642.

Dishman RK, editor. *Exercise adherence: its impact on public health.* Champaign, IL: Human Kinetics, 1988.

Dublin L. Longevity of college athletes. *Statistical Bulletin of the Metropolitan Insurance Company* 1932;13:5–7.

Eaton SB, Shostak M, Konner M. *The paleolithic prescription: a program of diet and exercise and a design for living.* New York: Harper and Row, 1988.

Edwards JE, Stager JM, Updyke W, Elizondo R. Validity of the doubly labeled water method of measuring energy expenditure with rest and exercise in non-human primates. *Medicine and Science in Sports and Exercise* 1990;22:550–557.

Fitz GW. *Principles of physiology and hygiene.* New York: H. Holt and Company, 1908.

Fishbein M. *A history of the American Medical Association, 1847 to 1947.* Philadelphia: W.B. Saunders, 1947.

Fishbein M. Health of young men under selective service. *Journal of the American Medical Association* 1941;116:54–55.

Fletcher GF, Blair SN, Blumenthal J, Caspersen C, Chaitman B, Epstein S, et al. Statement on exercise: benefits and recommendations for physical activity programs for all Americans: a statement for health professionals by the Committee on Exercise and Cardiac Rehabilitation of the Council on Clinical Cardiology, American Heart Association. *Circulation* 1992;86:340–344.

Foster WL. A test of physical efficiency. *American Physical Education Review* 1914;19:632–636.

Freedson PS. Field monitoring of physical activity in children. *Pediatric Exercise Science* 1989;1:8–18.

Gemmill C, Booth W, Detrick J, Schiebel H. Muscular training. II. The effects of training on the recovery period following severe muscular exercise. *American Journal of Physiology* 1931;96:265–277.

Gilliam TB, Freedson PS, Geenen DL, Shahraray B. Physical activity patterns determined by heart rate monitoring in 6–7 year-old children. *Medicine and Science in Sports and Exercise* 1981;13:65–67.

Green RM. *A translation of Galen's hygiene (De sanitate tuenda).* Springfield, IL: Charles C. Thomas, 1951.

Gruman GJ. The rise and fall of prolongevity hygiene, 1558–1873. *Bulletin of the History of Medicine* 1961; 35:221–229.

Gunn JC. *Gunn's domestic medicine, or poor man's friend* [1830]. Reprint, with an introduction by Charles E. Rosenberg. Knoxville, TN: University of Tennessee Press, 1986.

Hackensmith CW. *History of physical education.* New York: Harper and Row, 1966.

Harris ML. A factor analytic study of flexibility. *Research Quarterly* 1969;40:62–70.

Harris SS, Caspersen CJ, DeFriese GH, Estes EH Jr. Physical activity counseling for healthy adults as a primary preventive intervention in the clinical setting: report for the U.S. Preventive Services Task Force. *Journal of the American Medical Association* 1989;261:3588–3598.

Hartwell EM. On the physiology of exercise. *Boston Medical and Surgical Journal* 1887;116:13:297–302.

Haskell WL. Physical activity and health: the need to define the required stimulus. *American Journal of Cardiology* 1984;55:4D–9D.

Haskell WL, Yee MC, Evans A, Irby PJ. Simultaneous measurement of heart rate and body motion to quantitate physical activity. *Medicine and Science in Sports and Exercise* 1993;25:109–115.

Hill AV. *Living machinery: eight lectures delivered at the Lowell Institute, Boston, March 1927*. New York: Harcourt, Brace, and Company, 1927.

Hill AV. *Muscular activity*. Baltimore: Williams and Wilkins, 1926.

Hill AV. The physiological basis of athletic records. *Lancet* 1925a;2:481–486.

Hill AV. The physiological basis of athletic records. *Scientific Monthly* 1925b;21:409–428.

Hippocrates. *Regimen I*. Translated by W.H.S. Jones. Cambridge, MA: Harvard University Press, 1953.

Hitchcock E. *Elementary anatomy and physiology*. Rev. ed. New York: Ivison, Phinney, 1861.

Horvath SM, Horvath EC. *The Harvard Fatigue Laboratory: its history and contributions*. Englewood Cliffs, NJ: Prentice-Hall, 1973.

Huang Ti. *Nei Ching Su Wen: the Yellow Emperor's classic of internal medicine*. Translated by Ilza Veith. Baltimore: Williams and Wilkins, 1949.

Huard P, Wong M. *Chinese medicine*. Translated by Bernard Fielding. London: Weidenfeld and Nicolson, 1968.

Jacobs DR, Ainsworth BE, Hartman TJ, Leon AS. A simultaneous evaluation of 10 commonly used physical activity questionnaires. *Medicine and Science in Sports and Exercise* 1993;25:81–91.

Jaeger W. *Paideia: the ideals of Greek culture*. Translated by Gilbert Highet. Vol. 1. *Archaic Greece—the mind of Athens*. 2nd ed. New York: Oxford University Press, 1965.

Kannel WB, Wilson P, Blair SN. Epidemiological assessment of the role of physical activity and fitness in development of cardiovascular disease. *American Heart Journal* 1985;109:876–885.

Karvonen MJ, Kentala E, Mustala O. The effects of training on heart rate. *Acta Medica Exp Fenn* 1957;35:308–315.

Kashiwazaki H, Inaoka T, Suzuki T, Kondo Y. Correlations of pedometer readings with energy expenditure in workers during free-living daily activities. *European Journal of Applied Physiology* 1986;54:585–590.

Katzenstein G. Ueber die Einwirkung der Muskelthätigkeit auf den Stoffverbrauch des Menschen. Pflüger EFW. *Archiv für die gesammte Physiologie des Menschen und der Thiere*. Bonn: M. Hager, 1891:49:330–404.

King AC, Haskell WL, Taylor CB, Kraemer HC, DeBusk RF. Group- vs home-based exercise training in healthy older men and women: a community-based clinical trial. *Journal of the American Medical Association* 1991;266:1535–1542.

Klein PD, James WPT, Wong WW, Irving CS, Murgatroyd PR, Cabrera M, et al. Calorimetric validation of the doubly labelled water method for determination of energy expenditure in man. *Human Nutrition, Clinical Nutrition* 1984;38C:95–106.

Klesges LM, Klesges RC. The assessment of children's physical activity: a comparison of methods. *Medicine and Science in Sports and Exercise* 1987;19:511–517.

Knehr CA, Dill DB, Neufeld W. Training and its effects on man at rest and at work. *American Journal of Physiology* 1942;136:148–156.

Kraus H, Hirschland RP. Muscular fitness and health. *Journal for Health, Physical Education, and Recreation* 1953;24:17–19.

Kriska AM, Sandler RB, Cauley JA, LaPorte RE, Hom DL, Pambianco G. The assessment of historical physical activity and its relation to adult bone parameters. *American Journal of Epidemiology* 1988;127:1053–1063.

Lagrange F. *Physiology of bodily exercise* [188]. Reprint, New York: D. Appleton, 1890.

Lakka TA, Nyyssonen K, Salonen JT. Higher levels of conditioning leisure-time physical activity are associated with reduced levels of stored iron in Finnish men. *American Journal of Epidemiology* 1994;140:148–160.

Langenfeld H. Auf dem wege zur sportwissenschaft: mediziner und leibesübungen im 19. jahrhundert. *Stadion* 1988;14:125–148.

LaPorte RE, Black-Sandler R, Cauley JA, Link M, Bayles C, Marks B. The assessment of physical activity in older women: analysis of the interrelationship and reliability of activity monitoring, activity surveys, and caloric intake. *Journal of Gerontology* 1983;38:394–397.

LaPorte RE, Montoye HJ, Caspersen CJ. Assessment of physical activity in epidemiologic research: problems and prospects. *Public Health Reports* 1985;100:131–146.

Larson LA, Yocom RD. *Measurement and evaluation in physical, health, and recreation education.* St. Louis: C.V. Mosby, 1951.

Lavoisier AL. Expériences sur la respiration des animaux, et sur les changemens qui arrivent à l'air en passant par leur poumon. *Histoire de l'Académie Royale des Sciences.* Paris: Académie des Sciences, 1777:185–194.

Lavoisier AL, de LaPlace PS. Mémoire sur la chaleur. *Histoire de l'Académie Royale des Sciences.* Paris: Académie des Sciences, 1780:355–408.

Lehmann JF, Boswell S, Price R, Burleigh A, de Lateur BJ, Jaffe KM, et al. Quantitative evaluation of sway as an indicator of functional balance in post-traumatic brain injury. *Archives of Physical Medicine and Rehabilitation* 1990;71:955–962.

Leon AS, Jacobs DR Jr, DeBacker G, Taylor HL. Relationship of physical characteristics and life habits to treadmill exercise capacity. *American Journal of Epidemiology* 1981;113:653–660.

Leonard FE, Affleck GB. *A guide to the history of physical education.* 3rd ed. Philadelphia: Lea and Febiger, 1947.

Lewis D. *The new gymnastics for men, women, and children.* New York: Clarke Brothers, 1883.

Licht S. History [of therapeutic exercise]. In: Basmajian JV, editor. *Therapeutic exercise.* 4th ed. Baltimore: Williams and Wilkins, 1984:1–44.

Lohman TG. Applicability of body composition techniques and constants for children and youths. *Exercise and Sport Sciences Reviews* 1986;14:325–357.

Lohman TG. Research progress in validation of laboratory methods of assessing body composition. *Medicine and Science in Sports and Exercise* 1984;16:596–603.

Lukaski HC, Bolonchuk WW, Hall CB, Siders WA. Validation of tetrapolar bioelectric impedance method to assess human body composition. *Journal of Applied Physiology* 1986;60:1327–1332.

Mazess RB, Barden HS, Bisek JP, Hanson J. Dual-energy x-ray absorptiometry for total-body and regional bone-mineral and soft-tissue composition. *American Journal of Clinical Nutrition* 1990;51:1106–1112.

McCloy CH. Physical fitness and citizenship. *Journal of Health and Physical Education* 1938;9:298.

McCurdy JH. The effect of maximum muscular effort on blood pressure. *American Journal of Physiology* 1901; 5:95–103.

McKenzie RT. *Exercise in education and medicine.* Philadelphia: W.B. Saunders, 1909.

McKenzie RT. The influence of exercise on the heart. *American Journal of the Medical Sciences* 1913;145: 69–74.

Mendez C. *Book of bodily exercise* [1553]. translated by F. Guerra. New Haven, CT: Elizabeth Licht, 1960.

Mercurialis H. *De arte gymnastica* [1569]. 2nd ed. Paris: Du Puys, 1577.

Mitchell JH, Blomqvist G. Maximal oxygen uptake. *New England Journal of Medicine* 1971;284:1018–1022.

Montoye HJ. The Raymond Pearl memorial lecture, 1991: health, exercise, and athletics: a millennium of observations—a century of research. *American Journal of Human Biology* 1992;4:69–82.

Montoye HJ, Cunningham DA, Welch HG, Epstein FH. Laboratory methods of assessing metabolic capacity in a large epidemiologic study. *American Journal of Epidemiology* 1970;91:38–47.

Montoye HJ, Kemper HCG, Saris WHM, Washburn RA. *Measuring physical activity and energy expenditure.* Champaign, IL: Human Kinetics, 1996.

Montoye HJ, Taylor HL. Measurement of physical activity in population studies: a review. *Human Biology* 1984;56:195–216.

Montoye HJ, Van Huss WD, Brewer WD, Jones EM, Ohlson MA, MaLoney E, et al. The effects of exercise on blood cholesterol of middle-aged men. *American Journal of Clinical Nutrition* 1959;7:139–145.

Morantz RM. Making women modern: middle-class women and health reform in 19th-century America. In: Leavitt JW, editor. *Women and health in America: historical readings.* Madison, WI: University of Wisconsin Press, 1984:346–358.

Morris JN, Heady JA, Raffle PAB, Roberts CG, Parks JW. Coronary heart disease and physical activity of work. *Lancet* 1953;2:1053–1057, 1111–1120.

Nabokov P. *Indian running: Native American history and tradition.* Santa Barbara, CA: Capra Press, 1981.

# Physical Activity and Health

National Center for Health Statistics, Bloom B. *Current estimates from the National Health Interview Survey, United States, 1981*. Vital and Health Statistics: Series 10, No. 141. Hyattsville, MD: U.S. Department of Health and Human Services, Public Health Service, National Center for Health Statistics, 1982. DHHS Publication No. (PHS)82-1569.

National Center for Health Statistics, Wilmore JH. Design issues and alternatives in assessing physical fitness among apparently healthy adults in a health examination survey of the general population. In: *Assessing physical fitness and physical activity in population-based surveys*. Hyattsville, MD: U.S. Department of Health and Human Services, Public Health Service, National Center for Health Statistics, 1989:107–153. DHHS Publication No. (PHS)89-1253.

National Council of Young Men's Christian Associations of the United States. *Y's way to physical fitness: the complete guide to fitness testing and instruction*. Champaign, IL: Human Kinetics, 1989.

National Institutes of Health. Consensus development conference statement on physical activity and cardiovascular health, December 20, 1995, Bethesda, MD (draft statement).

Noland M, Danner F, DeWalt K, McFadden M, Kotchen JM. The measurement of physical activity in young children. *Research Quarterly for Exercise and Sport* 1990;61:146–153.

Numbers RL. Do-it-yourself the sectarian way. In: Risse GB, Numbers RL, Leavitt JW, editors. *Medicine without doctors: home health care in American history*. New York: Science History Publications, 1977:49–72.

Olivova V. Scientific and professional gymnastics. In: Olivova V, editor. *Sports and games in the ancient world*. New York: St. Martin's Press, 1985:135–145.

Paffenbarger RS Jr, Hyde RT, Wing AL, Lee IM, Jung DL, Kampert JB. The association of changes in physical activity level and other lifestyle characteristics with mortality among men. *New England Journal of Medicine* 1993;328:538–545.

Park RJ. Athletes and their training in Britain and America, 1800–1914. In: Berryman JW, Park RJ, editors. *Sport and exercise science: essays in the history of sports medicine*. Urbana, IL: University of Illinois Press, 1992:57–107.

Park RJ. *Measurement of physical fitness: a historical perspective*. Office of Disease Prevention and Health Promotion Monograph Series. Washington, DC: U.S. Department of Health and Human Services, Public Health Service, 1989:1–35.

Park RJ. The emergence of the academic discipline of physical education in the United States. In: Brooks GA, editor. *Perspectives on the academic discipline of physical education*. Champaign, IL: Human Kinetics, 1981:20–45.

Pate RR. A new definition of youth fitness. *Physician and Sportsmedicine* 1983;11:77–83.

Pate RR, Pratt M, Blair SN, Haskell WL, Macera CA, Bouchard C, et al. Physical activity and public health: a recommendation from the Centers for Disease Control and Prevention and the American College of Sports Medicine. *Journal of the American Medical Association* 1995;273:402–407.

Pollock ML. The quantification of endurance training programs. *Exercise and Sport Sciences Reviews* 1973;1:155–188.

Pomeroy WC, White PD. Coronary heart disease in former football players. *Journal of the American Medical Association* 1958;167:711–714.

Powell KE, Thompson PD, Caspersen CJ, Kendrick JS. Physical activity and the incidence of coronary heart disease. *Annual Review of Public Health* 1987;8:253–287.

Precope J. *Hippocrates on diet and hygiene*. London: Williams, Lea, and Company, 1952.

President's Council on Physical Fitness. *Adult physical fitness: a program for men and women*. Washington, DC: U.S. Government Printing Office, 1965.

Progress of physical education. *American Journal of Education* 1826;1:19–23.

Ramazzini B. *Diseases of workers*.[1713]. Translated by W.C. Wright. New York: Hafner, 1964.

Reindell H, Roskamm H, Gerschler W. *Das intervalltraining: physiologische Grundlagen, praktische Anwendungen und Schädigungsmöglichkeiten*. München: Bath, 1962.

Reiser SJ. Responsibility for personal health: a historical perspective. *Journal of Medicine and Philosophy* 1985;10:7–17.

Richardson MT, Leon AS, Jacobs DR, Ainsworth BE, Serfass R. Ability of the Caltrac® accelerometer to assess daily physical activity levels. *Journal of Cardiopulmonary Rehabilitation* 1995;15:107–113.

Ricketson S. *Means of preserving health and preventing diseases*. New York: Collins, Perkins, and Company, 1806.

Robinson S, Harmon PM. The lactic acid mechanism and certain properties of the blood in relation to training. *American Journal of Physiology* 1941;132:757–769.

Rogers F, Juneau M, Taylor CB, Haskell WL, Kraemer HC, Ahn DK, et al. Assessment by a microprocessor of adherence to home-based moderate-intensity exercise training in healthy, sedentary middle-aged men and women. *American Journal of Cardiology* 1987;60:71–75.

Rogers FB. Shadrach Ricketson (1768–1839): Quaker hygienist. *Journal of the History of Medicine* 1965;20:140–150.

Rogers JE. How has the depression in education affected physical education? *Journal of Health and Physical Education* 1934;5:12–3, 57–58.

Rook A. An investigation into the longevity of Cambridge sportsmen. *British Medical Journal* 1954;4:773–777.

Sallis JF, Buono MJ, Roby JJ, Carlson D, Nelson JA. The Caltrac® accelerometer as a physical activity monitor for school-age children. *Medicine and Science in Sports and Exercise* 1990;22:698–703.

Sallis JF, Condon SA, Goggin KJ, Roby JJ, Kolody B, Alcaraz JE. The development of self-administered physical activity surveys for 4th grade students. *Research Quarterly for Exercise and Sport* 1993;64:25–31.

Sallis JF, Patrick K. Physical activity guidelines for adolescents: consensus statement. *Pediatric Exercise Science* 1994;6:302–314.

Scharling EA. Versuche über die Quantität der, von einem Menschen in 24 Stunden ausgeathmeten, Kohlensäure. *Annalen der Chemie und Pharmacie* 1843;45:214–242.

Schneider EC, Ring GC. The influence of a moderate amount of physical training on the respiratory exchange and breathing during physical exercise. *American Journal of Physiology* 1929;91:103–114.

Segal KR, Gutin B, Presta E, Wang J, Van Itallie TB. Estimation of human body composition by electrical impedance methods: a comparative study. *Journal of Applied Physiology* 1985;58:1565–1571.

Shampo MA, Kyle RA. Nei Ching—oldest known medical book. *Mayo Clinic Proceedings* 1989;64:134.

Shea EJ. In memoriam: Thomas K. Cureton, Jr. *Journal of Physical Education, Recreation, and Dance* 1993;64:15.

Siconolfi SF, Cullinane EM, Carleton RA, Thompson PD. Assessin V̇O$_2$max in epidemiologic studies: modification of the Åstrand-Ryhming test. *Medicine and Science in Sports and Exercise* 1982;14:335–338.

Siconolfi SF, Lasater TM, Snow RC, Carleton RA. Self-reported physical activity compared with maximal oxygen uptake. *American Journal of Epidemiology* 1985;122:101–105.

Sidney S, Haskell WL, Crow R, Sternfeld B, Oberman A, Armstrong MA, et al. Symptom-limited graded treadmill exercise testing in young adults in the CARDIA study. *Medicine and Science in Sports and Exercise* 1992;24:177–183.

Sinasalo UV, Juurtola T. Comparative study of the physiological effects of two ski-training methods. *Research Quarterly* 1957;28:288–294.

Skinner JS, Benson H, McDonough JR, Hames CG. Social status, physical activity, and coronary proneness. *Journal of Chronic Diseases* 1966;19:773–783.

Sloan AW, Keen EN. Physical fitness of oarsmen and rugby players before and after training. *Journal of Applied Physiology* 1959;14:635–636.

Smith E. The influence of the labour of the tread-wheel over respiration and pulsation, and its relation to the waste of the system, and the dietary of the prisoners. *Medical Times and Gazette* 1857;14:601–603.

Smith G. Prescribing the rules of health: self-help and advice in the late eighteenth century. In: Porter R, editor. *Patients and practitioners: lay perceptions of medicine in pre-industrial society.* Cambridge: Cambridge University Press, 1985:249–282.

Snook GA. The history of sports medicine. Part 1. *American Journal of Sports Medicine* 1984;12:252–254.

Speck K. Ueber den Einfluss der Muskelthätigkeit auf dem Athemprocess. *Deutsche Archiv fur Klinische Medicin* 1889;45:461–528.

Spelman CC, Pate RR, Macera CA, Ward DS. Self-selected exercise intensity of habitual walkers. *Medicine and Science in Sports and Exercise* 1993;25:1174–1179.

Spirduso WW. Reaction and movement time as a function of age and physical activity level. *Journal of Gerontology* 1975;30:435–440.

Steinhaus AH. Health and physical fitness from the standpoint of the physiologist. *Journal of Health, Physical Education, and Recreation* 1936;7:224–227, 286–289.

Steinhaus AH, Bauer WW, Hellerbrandt FA, Kranz L, Miller A. The role of exercise in physical fitness. *Journal of Health, Physical Education, and Recreation* 1943;14:299–300, 345.

Storey TA. The influence of fatigue upon the speed of voluntary contraction of human muscle. *American Journal of Physiology* 1903;8:355–375.

## Physical Activity and Health

Taylor CB, Kraemer HC, Bragg DA, Miles LE, Rule B, Savin WM, et al. A new system for long-term recording and processing of heart rate and physical activity in outpatients. *Computers and Biomedical Research* 1982;15:7–17.

Taylor HL, Anderson JT, Keys A. Physical activity, serum cholesterol and other lipids in man. *Proceedings of the Society for Experimental Biology and Medicine* 1957;95:383–388.

Taylor HL, Jacobs DR, Schucker B, Knudsen J, Leon AS, Debacker G. A questionnaire for the assessment of leisure-time physical activities. *Journal of Chronic Diseases* 1978;31:741–755.

Tse SK, Bailey DM. T'ai chi and postural control in the well elderly. *American Journal of Occupational Therapy* 1992;46:295–300.

U.S. Department of Agriculture, U.S. Department of Health and Human Services. *Nutrition and your health: dietary guidelines for Americans.* 4th ed. Washington, DC: U.S. Department of Agriculture, 1995. Home and Garden Bulletin No. 232.

U.S. Department of Health and Human Services. *Healthy people 2000: midcourse review and 1995 revisions.* Washington, DC: U.S. Department of Health and Human Services, Public Health Service, 1995.

U.S. Department of Health and Human Services. *Healthy people 2000: national health promotion and disease prevention objectives, full report, with commentary.* Washington, DC: U.S. Department of Health and Human Services, Public Health Service, 1990. DHHS Publication No. (PHS)91–50212.

U.S. Department of Health and Human Services. *The Surgeon General's report on nutrition and health.* Washington, DC: U.S. Department of Health and Human Services, Public Health Service, 1988. DHHS Publication No. (PHS)88–50210.

U.S. Preventive Services Task Force. *Guide to clinical preventive services.* Baltimore: Williams and Wilkins, 1989.

U.S. Preventive Services Task Force. *Guide to clinical preventive services.* 2nd ed. Baltimore: Williams and Wilkins, 1996.

Van Dalen DB, Bennett BL. *A world history of physical education: cultural, philosophical, comparative.* Englewood Cliffs, NJ: Prentice-Hall, 1971.

Verbrugge MH. Healthy animals and civic life: Sylvester Graham's physiology of subsistence. *Reviews in American History* 1981;9:359–364.

Voorrips LE, Ravelli AC, Dongelmans PCA, Deurenberg P, Van Staveren WA. A physical activity questionnaire for the elderly. *Medicine and Science in Sports and Exercise* 1991;23:974–979.

Warner JH. *The therapeutic perspective: medical practice, knowledge, and identity in America, 1820–1885.* Cambridge, MA: Harvard University Press, 1986.

Washburn RA, Adams LL, Haile GT. Physical activity assessment for epidemiologic research: the utility of two simplified approaches. *Preventive Medicine* 1987;16:636–646.

Washburn RA, Janney CA, Fenster JR. The validity of objective physical activity monitoring in older individuals. *Research Quarterly for Exercise and Sport* 1990;61:114–117.

Washburn RA, Smith KW, Jette AM, Janney CA. The Physical Activity Scale for the Elderly (PASE): development and evaluation. *Journal of Clinical Epidemiology* 1993;46:153–162.

Wesley J. *Primitive physic: or, an easy and natural method of curing most diseases* [1747]. Reprint, Philadelphia: Parry Hall, 1793.

Westerterp KR, Brouns F, Saris WHM, ten Hoor F. Comparison of doubly labeled water with respirometry at low- and high-activity levels. *Journal of Applied Physiology* 1988;65:53–56.

Whorton JC. *Crusaders for fitness: the history of American health reformers.* Princeton, NJ: Princeton University Press, 1982.

Willich AFM. *Lectures on diet and regimen.* New York: T. and J. Swords, 1801.

Wilmore JH, Behnke AR. An anthropometric estimation of body density and lean body weight in young women. *American Journal of Clinical Nutrition* 1970;23:267–274.

Wilmore JH, Costill DL. *Physiology of sport and exercise.* Champaign, IL: Human Kinetics, 1994.

Wilson PWF, Paffenbarger RS, Morris JN, Havlik RJ. Assessment methods for physical activity and physical fitness in population studies: a report of an NHLBI Workshop. *American Heart Journal* 1986;111:1177–1192.

Wong TC, Webster JG, Montoye HJ, Washburn R. Portable accelerometer device for measuring human energy expenditure. *IEEE Transactions on Biomedical Engineering* 1981;28:467–471.

Yakovlev NN, Kaledin SV, Krasnova AF, Leshkevich LG, Popova NK, Rogozkin VA, et al. Physiological and chemical adaptation to muscular activity in relation to length of rest periods between exertions during training. *Sechenov-Physiological Journal of the USSR* 1961;47:56–59.

Zukel WJ, Lewis RH, Enterline PE, Painter RC, Ralston LS, Fawcett RM, et al. A short-term community study of the epidemiology of coronary heart disease: a preliminary report on the North Dakota study. *American Journal of Public Health* 1959;49:1630–1639.

# CHAPTER 3
# PHYSIOLOGIC RESPONSES AND LONG-TERM ADAPTATIONS TO EXERCISE

## Contents

# Contents, *continued*

# PHYSIOLOGIC RESPONSES AND LONG-TERM ADAPTATIONS TO EXERCISE

## Introduction

When challenged with any physical task, the human body responds through a series of integrated changes in function that involve most, if not all, of its physiologic systems. Movement requires activation and control of the musculoskeletal system; the cardiovascular and respiratory systems provide the ability to sustain this movement over extended periods. When the body engages in exercise training several times a week or more frequently, each of these physiologic systems undergoes specific adaptations that increase the body's efficiency and capacity. The magnitude of these changes depends largely on the intensity and duration of the training sessions, the force or load used in training, and the body's initial level of fitness. Removal of the training stimulus, however, will result in loss of the efficiency and capacity that was gained through these training-induced adaptations; this loss is a process called detraining.

This chapter provides an overview of how the body responds to an episode of exercise and adapts to exercise training and detraining. The discussion focuses on aerobic or cardiorespiratory endurance exercise (e.g., walking, jogging, running, cycling, swimming, dancing, and in-line skating) and resistance exercise (e.g., strength-developing exercises). It does not address training for speed, agility, and flexibility. In discussing the multiple effects of exercise, this overview will orient the reader to the physiologic basis for the relationship of physical activity and health. Physiologic information pertinent to specific diseases is presented in the next chapter. For additional information, the reader is referred to the selected textbooks shown in the sidebar.

### Selected Textbooks on Exercise Physiology

Åstrand PO, Rodahl K. *Textbook of work physiology.* 3rd edition. New York: McGraw-Hill Book Company, 1986.

Brooks GA, Fahey TD, White TP. *Exercise physiology: human bioenergetics and its applications.* 2nd edition. Mountain View, CA: Mayfield Publishing Company, 1996.

Fox E, Bowers R, Foss M. *The physiological basis for exercise and sport.* 5th edition. Madison, WI: Brown and Benchmark, 1993.

McArdle WD, Katch FI, Katch VL. *Essentials of exercise physiology.* Philadelphia, PA: Lea and Febiger, 1994.

Powers SK, Howley ET. *Exercise physiology: theory and application to fitness and performance.* Dubuque, IA: William C. Brown, 1990.

Wilmore JH, Costill DL. *Physiology of sport and exercise.* Champaign, IL: Human Kinetics, 1994.

## Physiologic Responses to Episodes of Exercise

The body's physiologic responses to episodes of aerobic and resistance exercise occur in the musculoskeletal, cardiovascular, respiratory, endocrine, and immune systems. These responses have been studied in controlled laboratory settings, where exercise stress can be precisely regulated and physiologic responses carefully observed.

### Cardiovascular and Respiratory Systems

The primary functions of the cardiovascular and respiratory systems are to provide the body with oxygen ($O_2$) and nutrients, to rid the body of carbon dioxide ($CO_2$) and metabolic waste products, to maintain body temperature and acid-base balance, and to transport hormones from the endocrine glands to their target organs (Wilmore and Costill 1994). To be effective and efficient, the cardiovascular system should be able to respond to increased skeletal muscle activity. Low rates of work, such as walking at 4 kilometers per hour (2.5 miles per hour), place relatively small demands on the cardiovascular and respiratory systems. However, as the rate of muscular work increases, these two systems will eventually reach their maximum capacities and will no longer be able to meet the body's demands.

### Cardiovascular Responses to Exercise

The cardiovascular system, composed of the heart, blood vessels, and blood, responds predictably to the increased demands of exercise. With few exceptions, the cardiovascular response to exercise is directly proportional to the skeletal muscle oxygen demands for any given rate of work, and oxygen uptake ($\dot{V}O_2$) increases linearly with increasing rates of work.

### Cardiac Output

Cardiac output ($\dot{Q}$) is the total volume of blood pumped by the left ventricle of the heart per minute. It is the product of heart rate (HR, number of beats per minute) and stroke volume (SV, volume of blood pumped per beat). The arterial-mixed venous oxygen ($A\text{-}\bar{v}O_2$) difference is the difference between the oxygen content of the arterial and mixed venous blood. A person's maximum oxygen uptake ($\dot{V}O_2$ max) is a function of cardiac output ($\dot{Q}$) multiplied by the $A\text{-}\bar{v}O_2$ difference. Cardiac output thus plays an important role in meeting the oxygen demands for work. As the rate of work increases, the cardiac output increases in a nearly linear manner to meet the increasing oxygen demand, but only up to the point where it reaches its maximal capacity ($\dot{Q}$ max).

To visualize how cardiac output, heart rate, and stroke volume change with increasing rates of work, consider a person exercising on a cycle ergometer, starting at 50 watts and increasing 50 watts every 2 minutes up to a maximal rate of work (Figure 3-1 A, B, and C). In this scenario, cardiac output and heart rate increase over the entire range of work, whereas stroke volume only increases up to approximately 40

**Figure 3-1. Changes in cardiac output (A), heart rate (B), and stroke volume (C) with increasing rates of work on the cycle ergometer**

**(A)**

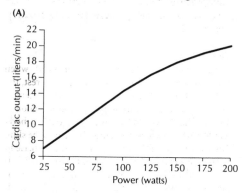

**(B)**

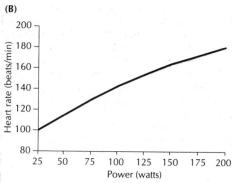

**(C)**

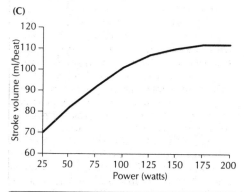

to 60 percent of the person's maximal oxygen uptake ($\dot{V}O_2$ max), after which it reaches a plateau. Recent studies have suggested that stroke volume in highly trained persons can continue to increase up to near maximal rates of work (Scruggs et al. 1991; Gledhill, Cox, Jamnik 1994).

## Blood Flow

The pattern of blood flow changes dramatically when a person goes from resting to exercising. At rest, the skin and skeletal muscles receive about 20 percent of the cardiac output. During exercise, more blood is sent to the active skeletal muscles, and, as body temperature increases, more blood is sent to the skin. This process is accomplished both by the increase in cardiac output and by the redistribution of blood flow away from areas of low demand, such as the splanchnic organs. This process allows about 80 percent of the cardiac output to go to active skeletal muscles and skin at maximal rates of work (Rowell 1986). With exercise of longer duration, particularly in a hot and humid environment, progressively more of the cardiac output will be redistributed to the skin to counter the increasing body temperature, thus limiting both the amount going to skeletal muscle and the exercise endurance (Rowell 1986).

## Blood Pressure

Mean arterial blood pressure increases in response to dynamic exercise, largely owing to an increase in systolic blood pressure, because diastolic blood pressure remains at near-resting levels. Systolic blood pressure increases linearly with increasing rates of work, reaching peak values of between 200 and 240 millimeters of mercury in normotensive persons. Because mean arterial pressure is equal to cardiac output times total peripheral resistance, the observed increase in mean arterial pressure results from an increase in cardiac output that outweighs a concomitant decrease in total peripheral resistance. This increase in mean arterial pressure is a normal and desirable response, the result of a resetting of the arterial baroreflex to a higher pressure. Without such a resetting, the body would experience severe arterial hypotension during intense activity (Rowell 1993). Hypertensive patients typically reach much higher systolic blood pressures for a given rate of work, and they can also experience increases in diastolic blood pressure. Thus, mean arterial pressure

is generally much higher in these patients, likely owing to a lesser reduction in total peripheral resistance.

For the first 2 to 3 hours following exercise, blood pressure drops below preexercise resting levels, a phenomenon referred to as postexercise hypotension (Isea et al. 1994). The specific mechanisms underlying this response have not been established. The acute changes in blood pressure after an episode of exercise may be an important aspect of the role of physical activity in helping control blood pressure in hypertensive patients.

## Oxygen Extraction

The A-$\bar{v}O_2$ difference increases with increasing rates of work (Figure 3-2) and results from increased oxygen extraction from arterial blood as it passes through exercising muscle. At rest, the A-$\bar{v}O_2$ difference is approximately 4 to 5 ml of $O_2$ for every 100 ml of blood (ml/100 ml); as the rate of work approaches maximal levels, the A-$\bar{v}O_2$ difference reaches 15 to 16 ml/100 ml of blood.

## Coronary Circulation

The coronary arteries supply the myocardium with blood and nutrients. The right and left coronary arteries curve around the external surface of the heart, then branch and penetrate the myocardial muscle bed, dividing and subdividing like branches of a tree to form a dense vascular and capillary network to supply each myocardial muscle fiber. Generally one capillary supplies each myocardial fiber in adult humans and animals; however, evidence suggests that the capillary density of the ventricular myocardium can be increased by endurance exercise training.

At rest and during exercise, myocardial oxygen demand and coronary blood flow are closely linked. This coupling is necessary because the myocardium depends almost completely on aerobic metabolism and therefore requires a constant oxygen supply. Even at rest, the myocardium's oxygen use is high relative to the blood flow. About 70 to 80 percent of the oxygen is extracted from each unit of blood crossing the myocardial capillaries; by comparison, only about 25 percent is extracted from each unit crossing skeletal muscle at rest. In the healthy heart, a linear relationship exists between myocardial oxygen demands, consumption, and coronary blood flow, and adjustments are made on a beat-to-beat

**Figure 3-2. Changes in arterial and mixed venous oxygen content with increasing rates of work on the cycle ergometer**

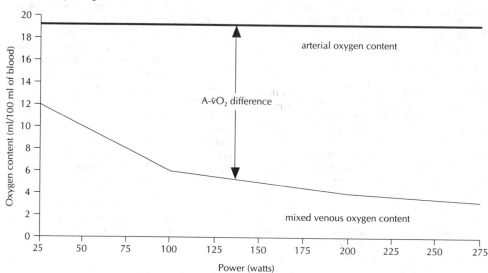

basis. The three major determinants of myocardial oxygen consumption are heart rate, myocardial contractility, and wall stress (Marcus 1983; Jorgensen et al. 1977). Acute increases in arterial pressure increase left ventricular pressure and wall stress. As a result, the rate of myocardial metabolism increases, necessitating an increased coronary blood flow. A very high correlation exists between both myocardial oxygen consumption and coronary blood flow and the product of heart rate and systolic blood pressure (SBP) (Jorgensen et al. 1977). This so-called double product (HR • SBP) is generally used to estimate myocardial oxygen and coronary blood flow requirements. During vigorous exercise, all three major determinants of myocardial oxygen requirements increase above their resting levels.

The increase in coronary blood flow during exercise results from an increase in perfusion pressure of the coronary artery and from coronary vasodilation. Most important, an increase in sympathetic nervous system stimulation leads to an increase in circulating catecholamines. This response triggers metabolic processes that increase both perfusion pressure of the

coronary artery and coronary vasodilation to meet the increased need for blood flow required by the increase in myocardial oxygen use.

### Respiratory Responses to Exercise
The respiratory system also responds when challenged with the stress of exercise. Pulmonary ventilation increases almost immediately, largely through stimulation of the respiratory centers in the brain stem from the motor cortex and through feedback from the proprioceptors in the muscles and joints of the active limbs. During prolonged exercise, or at higher rates of work, increases in $CO_2$ production, hydrogen ions (H[+]), and body and blood temperatures stimulate further increases in pulmonary ventilation. At low work intensities, the increase in ventilation is mostly the result of increases in tidal volume. At higher intensities, the respiratory rate also increases. In normal-sized, untrained adults, pulmonary ventilation rates can vary from about 10 liters per minute at rest to more than 100 liters per minute at maximal rates of work; in large, highly trained male athletes, pulmonary

ventilation rates can reach more than 200 liters per minute at maximal rates of work.

### Resistance Exercise

The cardiovascular and respiratory responses to episodes of resistance exercise are mostly similar to those associated with endurance exercise. One notable exception is the exaggerated blood pressure response that occurs during resistance exercise. Part of this response can be explained by the fact that resistance exercise usually involves muscle mass that develops considerable force. Such high, isolated force leads to compression of the smaller arteries and results in substantial increases in total peripheral resistance (Coyle 1991). Although high-intensity resistance training poses a potential risk to hypertensive patients and to those with cardiovascular disease, research data suggest that the risk is relatively low (Gordon et al. 1995) and that hypertensive persons may benefit from resistance training (Tipton 1991; American College of Sports Medicine 1993).

## Skeletal Muscle

The primary purpose of the musculoskeletal system is to define and move the body. To provide efficient and effective force, muscle adapts to demands. In response to demand, it changes its ability to extract oxygen, choose energy sources, and rid itself of waste products. The body contains three types of muscle tissue: skeletal (voluntary) muscle, cardiac muscle or myocardium, and smooth (autonomic) muscle. This section focuses solely on skeletal muscle.

Skeletal muscle is composed of two basic types of muscle fibers distinguished by their speed of contraction—slow-twitch and fast-twitch—a characteristic that is largely dictated by different forms of the enzyme myosin adenosinetriphosphatase (ATPase). Slow-twitch fibers, which have relatively slow contractile speed, have high oxidative capacity and fatigue resistance, low glycolytic capacity, relatively high blood flow capacity, high capillary density, and high mitochondrial content (Terjung 1995). Fast-twitch muscle fibers have fast contractile speed and are classified into two subtypes, fast-twitch type "a" ($FT_a$) and fast-twitch type "b" ($FT_b$). $FT_a$ fibers have moderately high oxidative capacity, are relatively fatigue resistant, and have high glycolytic capacity, relatively high blood flow capacity, high capillary density, and high mitochondrial content (Terjung 1995). $FT_b$ fibers have low oxidative capacity, low fatigue resistance, high glycolytic capacity, and fast contractile speed. Further, they have relatively low blood flow capacity, capillary density, and mitochondrial content (Terjung 1995).

There is a direct relationship between predominant fiber type and performance in certain sports. For example, in most marathon runners, slow-twitch fibers account for up to or more than 90 percent of the total fibers in the leg muscles. On the other hand, the leg muscles in sprinters are often more than 80 percent composed of fast-twitch fibers. Although the issue is not totally resolved, muscle fiber type appears to be genetically determined; researchers have shown that several years of either high-intensity sprint training or high-intensity endurance training do not significantly alter the percentage of the two major types of fibers (Jolesz and Sreter 1981).

## Skeletal Muscle Energy Metabolism

Metabolic processes are responsible for generating adenosine triphosphate (ATP), the body's energy source for all muscle action. ATP is generated by three basic energy systems: the ATP-phosphocreatine (ATP-PCr) system, the glycolytic system, and the oxidative system. Each system contributes to energy production in nearly every type of exercise. The relative contribution of each will depend on factors such as the intensity of work rate at the onset of exercise and the availability of oxygen in the muscle.

### Energy Systems

The ATP-PCr system provides energy from the ATP stored in all of the body's cells. PCr, also found in all cells, is a high-energy phosphate molecule that stores energy. As ATP concentrations in the cell are reduced by the breakdown of ATP to adenosine diphosphate (ADP) to release energy for muscle contraction, PCr is broken down to release both energy and a phosphate to allow reconstitution of ATP from ADP. This process describes the primary energy system for short, high-intensity exercise, such as a 40- to 200-meter sprint; during such exercise, the system can produce energy at very high rates, and ATP and PCr stores, which are depleted in 10–20 seconds, will last just long enough to complete the exercise.

At high rates of work, the active muscle cell's oxygen demand exceeds its supply. The cell must then rely on the glycolytic energy system to produce ATP in the absence of oxygen (i.e., anaerobically). This system can only use glucose, available in the blood plasma and stored in both muscle and the liver as glycogen. The glycolytic energy system is the primary energy system for all-out bouts of exercise lasting from 30 seconds to 2 minutes, such as an 800-meter run. The major limitation of this energy system is that it produces lactate, which lowers the pH of both the muscle and blood. Once the pH drops below a value of 6.4 to 6.6, enzymes critical for producing energy are no longer able to function, and ATP production stops (Wilmore and Costill 1994).

The oxidative energy system uses oxygen to produce ATP within the mitochondria, which are special cell organelles within muscle. This process cannot generate ATP at a high enough rate to sustain an all-out sprint, but it is highly effective at lower rates of work (e.g., long distance running). ATP can also be produced from fat and protein metabolism through the oxidative energy system. Typically, carbohydrate and fat provide most of the ATP; under most conditions, protein contributes only 5 to 10 percent at rest and during exercise.

## Metabolic Rate

The rate at which the body uses energy is known as the metabolic rate. When measured while a person is at rest, the resulting value represents the lowest (i.e., basal) rate of energy expenditure necessary to maintain basic body functions. Resting metabolic rate is measured under highly controlled resting conditions following a 12-hour fast and a good night's sleep (Turley, McBride, Wilmore 1993). To quantify the rate of energy expenditure during exercise, the metabolic rate at rest is defined as 1 metabolic equivalent (MET); a 4 MET activity thus represents an activity that requires four times the resting metabolic rate. The use of METs to quantify physical activity intensity is the basis of the absolute intensity scale. (See Chapter 2 for further information.)

## Maximal Oxygen Uptake

During exercise, $\dot{V}O_2$ increases in direct proportion to the rate of work. The point at which a person's $\dot{V}O_2$ is no longer able to increase is defined as the maximal oxygen uptake ($\dot{V}O_2$max) (Figure 3-3). A person's $\dot{V}O_2$max is in part genetically determined; it can be increased through training until the point that the genetically possible maximum is reached. $\dot{V}O_2$max is considered the best estimate of a person's cardiorespiratory fitness or aerobic power (Jorgensen et al. 1977).

## Lactate Threshold

Lactate is the primary by-product of the anaerobic glycolytic energy system. At lower exercise intensities, when the cardiorespiratory system can meet the oxygen demands of active muscles, blood lactate levels remain close to those observed at rest, because some lactate is used aerobically by muscle and is removed as fast as it enters the blood from the muscle. As the intensity of exercise is increased, however, the rate of lactate entry into the blood from muscle eventually exceeds its rate of removal from the blood, and blood lactate concentrations increase above resting levels. From this point on, lactate levels continue to increase as the rate of work increases, until the point of exhaustion. The point at which the concentration of lactate in the blood begins to increase above resting levels is referred to as the lactate threshold (Figure 3-3).

Lactate threshold is an important marker for endurance performance, because distance runners set their race pace at or slightly above the lactate threshold (Farrell et al. 1979). Further, the lactate thresholds of highly trained endurance athletes occur at a much higher percentage of their $\dot{V}O_2$max, and thus at higher relative workloads, than do the thresholds of untrained persons. This key difference is what allows endurance athletes to perform at a faster pace.

## Hormonal Responses to Exercise

The endocrine system, like the nervous system, integrates physiologic responses and plays an important role in maintaining homeostatic conditions at rest and during exercise. This system controls the release of hormones from specialized glands throughout the body, and these hormones exert their actions on targeted organs and cells. In response to an episode of exercise, many hormones, such as catecholamines, are secreted at an increased rate, though insulin is secreted at a decreased rate (Table 3-1). The actions of some of these hormones, as well as

Figure 3-3. Changes in oxygen uptake and blood lactate concentrations with increasing rates of work on the cycle ergometer*

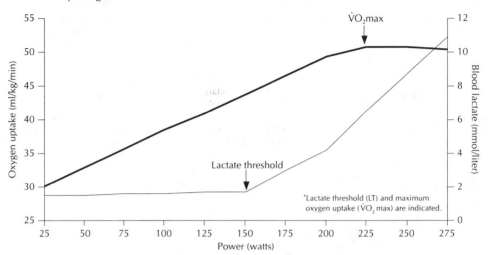

*Lactate threshold (LT) and maximum oxygen uptake ($\dot{V}O_2$ max) are indicated.

their specific responses to exercise, are discussed in more detail in Chapter 4.

## Immune Responses to Exercise

The immune system is a complex adaptive system that provides surveillance against foreign proteins, viruses, and bacteria by using the unique functions of cells produced by the bone marrow and the thymus gland. By interacting with neural and endocrine factors, the immune system influences the body's overall response to exercise (Reichlin 1992). A growing body of literature indicates that the incidence of some infections may be influenced by the exercise history of the individual (Nieman 1994; Hoffman-Goetz and Pedersen 1994).

Moderate exercise has been shown to bolster the function of certain components of the human immune system—such as natural killer cells, circulating T- and B-lymphocytes, and cells of the monocyte-macrophage system—thereby possibly decreasing the incidence of some infections (Keast, Cameron, Morton 1988; Pedersen and Ullum 1994; Woods and Davis 1994) and perhaps of certain types of cancer (Shephard and Shek 1995).

Exercise of high intensity and long duration or exercise that involves excessive training may have adverse effects on immune function. In general, a high-intensity, single episode of exercise results in a marked decline in the functioning of all major cells of the immune system (Newsholme and Parry-Billings 1994; Shephard and Shek 1995). In addition, over-training may reduce the response of T-lymphocytes to mutagenic stimulation, decrease antibody synthesis and plasma level of immunoglobins and complement, and impair macrophage phagocytosis. The reduced plasma glutamine levels that occur with high-intensity exercise or excessive training are postulated to contribute to these adverse effects on the immune system (Newsholme and Parry-Billings 1994).

## Long-Term Adaptations to Exercise Training

### Adaptations of Skeletal Muscle and Bone

Skeletal muscle adapts to endurance training chiefly through a small increase in the cross-sectional area of slow-twitch fibers, because low- to moderate-

**Table 3-1. A summary of hormonal changes during an episode of exercise**

| Hormone | Exercise response | Special relationships | Probable importance |
|---|---|---|---|
| Catecholamines | Increases | Greater increase with intense exercise; norepinephrine > epinephrine; increases less after training | Increased blood glucose; increased skeletal muscle and liver glycogenolysis; increased lipolysis |
| Growth hormone (GH) | Increases | Increases more in untrained persons; declines faster in trained persons | Unknown |
| Adrenocorticotropic hormone (ACTH)-cortisol | Increases | Greater increase with intense exercise; increases less after training with submaximal exercise | Increased gluconeogenesis in liver; increased mobilization of fatty acids |
| Thyroid-stimulating hormone (TSH)-thyroxine | Increases | Increased thyroxine turnover with training but no toxic effects are evident | Unknown |
| Luteinizing hormone (LH) | No change | None | None |
| Testosterone | Increases | None | Unknown |
| Estradiol-progesterone | Increases | Increases during luteal phase of the menstrual cycle | Unknown |
| Insulin | Decreases | Decreases less after training | Decreased stimulus to use blood glucose |
| Glucagon | Increases | Increases less after training | Increased blood glucose via glycogenolysis and gluconeogenesis |
| Renin-angiotensin-aldosterone | Increases | Same increase after training in rats | Sodium retention to maintain plasma volume |
| Antidiuretic hormone (ADH) | Expected increase | None | Water retention to maintain plasma volume |
| Parathormone (PTH)-calcitonin | Unknown | None | Needed to establish proper bone development |
| Erythropoietin | Unknown | None | Would be important to increase erythropoiesis |
| Prostaglandins | May increase | May increase in response to sustained isometric contractions; may need ischemic stress | May be local vasodilators |

Adapted from Wilmore JH, Costill DL. *Physiology of sport and exercise.* Champaign, IL: Human Kinetics, 1994, p. 136.

intensity aerobic activity primarily recruits these fibers (Abernethy, Thayer, Taylor 1990). Prolonged endurance training (i.e., months to years) can lead to a transition of $FT_h$ fibers to $FT_a$ fibers, which have a higher oxidative capacity (Abernethy, Thayer, Taylor 1990). No substantive evidence indicates that fast-twitch fibers will convert to slow-twitch fibers under normal training conditions (Jolesz and Sreter 1981). Endurance training also increases the number of capillaries in trained skeletal muscle, thereby allowing a greater capacity for blood flow in the active muscle (Terjung 1995).

Resistance-trained skeletal muscle exerts considerably more force because of both increased muscle size (hypertrophy) and increased muscle fiber recruitment. Fiber hypertrophy is the result of increases in both the size and number of myofibrils in both fast-twitch and slow-twitch muscle fibers (Kannus et al. 1992). Hyperplasia, or increased fiber number, has been reported in animal studies, where the number of individual muscle fibers can be counted (Gonyea et al. 1986), and has been indirectly demonstrated during autopsies on humans by using direct fiber counts to compare dominant and nondominant paired muscles (Sjöström et al. 1991).

During both aerobic and resistance exercise, active muscles can undergo changes that lead to muscle soreness. Some soreness is felt immediately after exercise, and some can even occur during exercise. This muscle soreness is generally not physically limiting and dissipates rapidly. A more limiting soreness, however, may occur 24 to 48 hours following exercise. This delayed-onset muscle soreness is primarily associated with eccentric-type muscle action, during which the muscle exerts force while lengthening, as can happen when a person runs down a steep hill or lowers a weight from a fully flexed to a fully extended position (e.g., the two-arm curl). Delayed-onset muscle soreness is the result of structural damage to the muscle; in its most severe form, this damage may include rupture of the cell membrane and disruption of the contractile elements of individual muscle fibers (Armstrong, Warren, Warren 1991). Such damage appears to result in an inflammatory response (MacIntyre, Reid, McKenzie 1995).

Total inactivity results in muscle atrophy and loss of bone mineral and mass. Persons who are sedentary generally have less bone mass than those who exercise, but the increases in bone mineral and mass that result from either endurance or resistance training are relatively small (Chesnut 1993). The role of resistance training in increasing or maintaining bone mass is not well characterized. Endurance training has little demonstrated positive effect on bone mineral and mass. Nonetheless, even small increases in bone mass gained from endurance or resistance training can help prevent or delay the process of osteoporosis (Drinkwater 1994). (See Chapter 4 for further information on the effects of exercise on bone.)

The musculoskeletal system cannot function without connective tissue linking bones to bones (ligaments) and muscles to bones (tendons). Extensive animal studies indicate that ligaments and tendons become stronger with prolonged and high-intensity exercise. This effect is the result of an increase in the strength of insertion sites between ligaments, tendons, and bones, as well as an increase in the cross-sectional areas of ligaments and tendons. These structures also become weaker and smaller with several weeks of immobilization (Tipton and Vailas 1990), which can have important implications for musculoskeletal performance and risk of injury.

## Metabolic Adaptations

Significant metabolic adaptations occur in skeletal muscle in response to endurance training. First, both the size and number of mitochondria increase substantially, as does the activity of oxidative enzymes. Myoglobin content in the muscle can also be augmented, increasing the amount of oxygen stored in individual muscle fibers (Hickson 1981), but this effect is variable (Svedenhag, Henriksson, Sylvén 1983). Such adaptations, combined with the increase in capillaries and muscle blood flow in the trained muscles (noted in a previous section), greatly enhance the oxidative capacity of the endurance-trained muscle.

Endurance training also increases the capacity of skeletal muscle to store glycogen (Kiens et al. 1993). The ability of trained muscles to use fat as an energy source is also improved, and this greater reliance on fat spares glycogen stores (Kiens et al. 1993). The increased capacity to use fat following endurance training results from an enhanced ability to mobilize free-fatty acids from fat depots and an improved capacity to oxidize fat consequent to the increase in the muscle enzymes responsible for fat oxidation (Wilmore and Costill 1994).

These changes in muscle and in cardiorespiratory function are responsible for increases in both $\dot{V}O_2$max and lactate threshold. The endurance-trained person can thus perform at considerably higher rates of work than the untrained person. Increases in $\dot{V}O_2$max generally range from 15 to 20 percent following a 6-month training period (Wilmore and Costill 1994). However, individual variations in this response are considerable. In one study of 60- to 71-year-old men and women who endurance trained for 9 to 12 months, the improvement in $\dot{V}O_2$max varied from 0 to 43 percent; the mean increase was 24 percent

(Kohrt et al. 1991). This variation in response may be due in part to genetic factors and to initial levels of fitness. To illustrate the changes that can be expected with endurance training, a hypothetical sedentary man's pretraining values have been compared with his values after a 6-month period of endurance training and with the values of a typical elite endurance runner (Table 3-2).

Responses to endurance training are similar for men and women. At all ages, women and men show similar gains in strength from resistance training (Rogers and Evans 1993; Holloway and Baechle 1990)

**Table 3-2.** A hypothetical example of alterations in selected physiological variables consequent to a 6-month endurance training program in a previously sedentary man compared with those of a typical elite endurance runner

| Variable | Sedentary man | | Runner |
|---|---|---|---|
| | Pretraining | Posttraining | |
| **Cardiovascular** | | | |
| HR at rest (beats • min$^{-1}$) | 71 | 59 | 36 |
| HR max (beats • min$^{-1}$) | 185 | 183 | 174 |
| SV rest (ml) | 65 | 80 | 125 |
| SV max (ml) | 120 | 140 | 200 |
| $\dot{Q}$ rest (L • min$^{-1}$) | 4.6 | 4.7 | 4.5 |
| $\dot{Q}$ max (L • min$^{-1}$) | 22.2 | 25.6 | 32.5 |
| Heart volume (ml) | 750 | 820 | 1,200 |
| Blood volume (L) | 4.7 | 5.1 | 6.0 |
| Systolic BP rest (mmHg) | 135 | 130 | 120 |
| Systolic BP max (mmHg) | 210 | 205 | 210 |
| Diastolic BP rest (mmHg) | 78 | 76 | 65 |
| Diastolic BP max (mmHg) | 82 | 80 | 65 |
| **Respiratory** | | | |
| $\dot{V}_E$ rest (L • min$^{-1}$) | 7 | 6 | 6 |
| $\dot{V}_E$ rest (L • min$^{-1}$) | 110 | 135 | 195 |
| TV rest (L) | 0.5 | 0.5 | 0.5 |
| TV max (L) | 2.75 | 3.0 | 3.9 |
| RR rest (breaths • min$^{-1}$) | 14 | 12 | 12 |
| RR max (breaths • min$^{-1}$) | 40 | 45 | 50 |
| **Metabolic** | | | |
| A-$\bar{v}O_2$ diff rest (ml • 100 ml$^{-1}$) | 6.0 | 6.0 | 6.0 |
| A-$\bar{v}O_2$ diff max (ml • 100 ml$^{-1}$) | 14.5 | 15.0 | 16.0 |
| $\dot{V}O_2$ rest (ml • kg$^{-1}$ • min$^{-1}$) | 3.5 | 3.5 | 3.5 |
| $\dot{V}O_2$ max (ml • kg$^{-1}$ • min$^{-1}$) | 40.5 | 49.8 | 76.5 |
| Blood lactate rest (mmol • L$^{-1}$) | 1.0 | 1.0 | 1.0 |
| Blood lactate max (mmol • L$^{-1}$) | 7.5 | 8.5 | 9.0 |

Adapted from Wilmore JH, Costill DL. *Physiology of sport and exercise.* Champaign, IL: Human Kinetics, 1994, p. 230.

HR = heart rate; max = maximal; SV = stroke volume; $\dot{Q}$ = cardiac output; BP = blood pressure; $\dot{V}_E$ = ventilatory volume; TV = tidal volume; RR = respiration rate; A-$\bar{v}O_2$ diff = arterial-mixed venous oxygen difference; $\dot{V}O_2$ = oxygen consumption.

and similar gains in $\dot{V}O_2$max from aerobic endurance training (Kohrt et al. 1991; Mitchell et al. 1992).

## Cardiovascular and Respiratory Adaptations

Endurance training leads to significant cardiovascular and respiratory changes at rest and during steady-state exercise at both submaximal and maximal rates of work. The magnitude of these adaptations largely depends on the person's initial fitness level; on mode, intensity, duration, and frequency of exercise; and on the length of training (e.g., weeks, months, years).

### Long-Term Cardiovascular Adaptations

Cardiac output at rest and during submaximal exercise is essentially unchanged following an endurance training program. At or near maximal rates of work, however, cardiac output is increased substantially, up to 30 percent or more (Saltin and Rowell 1980). There are important differences in the responses of stroke volume and heart rate to training. After training, stroke volume is increased at rest, during submaximal exercise, and during maximal exercise; conversely, posttraining heart rate is decreased at rest and during submaximal exercise and is usually unchanged at maximal rates of work. The increase in stroke volume appears to be the dominant change and explains most of the changes observed in cardiac output.

Several factors contribute to the increase in stroke volume from endurance training. Endurance training increases plasma volume by approximately the same percentage that it increases stroke volume (Green, Jones, Painter 1990). An increased plasma volume increases the volume of blood available to return to the right heart and, subsequently, to the left ventricle. There is also an increase in the end-diastolic volume (the volume of blood in the heart at the end of the diastolic filling period) because of increased amount of blood and increased return of blood to the ventricle during exercise (Seals et al. 1994). This acute increase in the left ventricle's end-diastolic volume stretches its walls, resulting in a more elastic recoil.

Endurance training also results in long-term changes in the structure of the heart that augment stroke volume. Short-term adaptive responses include ventricular dilatation; this increase in the volume of the ventricles allows end-diastolic volume to increase without excessive stress on the ventricular walls. Long-term adaptive responses include hypertrophy of the cardiac muscle fibers (i.e., increases in the size of each fiber). This hypertrophy increases the muscle mass of the ventricles, permitting greater force to be exerted with each beat of the heart. Increases in the thickness of the posterior and septal walls of the left ventricle can lead to a more forceful contraction of the left ventricle, thus emptying more of the blood from the left ventricle (George, Wolfe, Burggraf 1991).

Endurance training increases the number of capillaries in trained skeletal muscle, thereby allowing a greater capacity for blood flow in the active muscle (Terjung 1995). This enhanced capacity for blood flow is associated with a reduction in total peripheral resistance; thus, the left ventricle can exert a more forceful contraction against a lower resistance to flow out of the ventricle (Blomqvist and Saltin 1983).

Arterial blood pressure at rest, blood pressure during submaximal exercise, and peak blood pressure all show a slight decline as a result of endurance training in normotensive individuals (Fagard and Tipton 1994). However, decreases are greater in persons with high blood pressure. After endurance training, resting blood pressure (systolic/diastolic) will decrease on average -3/-3 mmHg in persons with normal blood pressure; in borderline hypertensive persons, the decrease will be -6/-7 mmHg; and in hypertensive persons, the decrease will be -10/-8 mmHg (Fagard and Tipton 1994). (See Chapter 4 for further information.)

### Respiratory Adaptations

The major changes in the respiratory system from endurance training are an increase in the maximal rate of pulmonary ventilation, which is the result of increases in both tidal volume and respiration rate, and an increase in pulmonary diffusion at maximal rates of work, primarily due to increases in pulmonary blood flow, particularly to the upper regions of the lung.

## Maintenance, Detraining, and Prolonged Inactivity

Most adaptations that result from both endurance and resistance training will be reversed if a person stops or reduces training. The greatest deterioration in physiologic function occurs during prolonged bed rest and immobilization by casts. A basic maintenance training program is necessary to prevent these losses in function.

## Maintaining Fitness and Muscular Strength

Muscle strength and cardiorespiratory capacity are dependent on separate aspects of exercise. After a person has obtained gains in $\dot{V}O_2$max by performing cardiorespiratory exercise six times per week, two to four times per week is the optimal frequency of training to maintain those gains (Hickson and Rosenkoetter 1981). Further, a substantial part of the gain can be retained when the duration of each session is reduced by as much as two-thirds, but only if the intensity during these abbreviated sessions is maintained at $\geq$70 percent of $\dot{V}O_2$max (Hickson et al. 1985). If training intensity is reduced by as little as one-third, however, a substantial reduction in $\dot{V}O_2$max can be expected over the next 15 weeks (Hickson et al. 1985).

In previously untrained persons, gains in muscular strength can be sustained by as little as a single session per week of resistance training, but only if the intensity is not reduced (Graves et al. 1988).

## Detraining

With complete cessation of exercise training, a significant reduction in $\dot{V}O_2$max and a decrease in plasma volume occur within 2 weeks; all prior functional gains are dissipated within 2 to 8 months, even if routine low- to moderate-intensity physical activity has taken the place of training (Shephard 1994). Muscular strength and power are reduced at a much slower rate than $\dot{V}O_2$max, particularly during the first few months after an athlete discontinues resistance training (Fleck and Kraemer 1987). In fact, no decrement in either strength or power may occur for the first 4 to 6 weeks after training ends (Neufer et al. 1987). After 12 months, almost half of the strength gained might still be retained if the athlete remains moderately active (Wilmore and Costill 1994).

## Prolonged Inactivity

The effects of prolonged inactivity have been studied by placing healthy young male athletes and sedentary volunteers in bed for up to 3 weeks after a control period during which baseline measurements were made. The resulting detrimental changes in physiologic function and performance are similar to those resulting from reduced gravitational forces during space flight and are more dramatic than those resulting from detraining studies in which routine daily activities in the upright position (e.g., walking, stair climbing, lifting, and carrying) are not restricted.

Results of bed rest studies show numerous physiologic changes, such as profound decrements in cardiorespiratory function proportional to the duration of bed rest (Shephard 1994; Saltin et al. 1968). Metabolic disturbances evident within a few days of bed rest include reversible glucose intolerance and hyperinsulinemia in response to a standard glucose load, reflecting cell insulin resistance (Lipman et al. 1972); reduced total energy expenditure; negative nitrogen balance, reflecting loss of muscle protein; and negative calcium balance, reflecting loss of bone mass (Bloomfield and Coyle 1993). There is also a substantial decrease in plasma volume, which affects aerobic power.

From one study, a decline in $\dot{V}O_2$max of 15 percent was evident within 10 days of bed rest and progressed to 27 percent in 3 weeks; the rate of loss was approximately 0.8 percent per day of bed rest (Bloomfield and Coyle 1993). The decrement in $\dot{V}O_2$max from bed rest and reduced activity results from a decrease in maximal cardiac output, consequent to a reduced stroke volume. This, in turn, reflects the decrease in end-diastolic volume resulting from a reduction in total blood and plasma volume, and probably also from a decrease in myocardial contractility (Bloomfield and Coyle 1993). Maximal heart rate and A-$\bar{v}O_2$ difference remain unchanged (Bloomfield and Coyle 1993). Resting heart rate remains essentially unchanged or is slightly increased, whereas resting stroke volume and cardiac output remain unchanged or are slightly decreased. However, the heart rate for submaximal exertion is generally increased to compensate for the sizable reduction in stroke volume.

Physical inactivity associated with bed rest or prolonged weightlessness also results in a progressive decrement in skeletal muscle mass (disuse atrophy) and strength, as well as an associated reduction in bone mineral density that is approximately proportional to the duration of immobilization or weightlessness (Bloomfield and Coyle 1993). The loss of muscle mass is not as great as that which occurs with immobilization of a limb by a plaster cast, but it exceeds that associated with cessation of resistance exercise training. The muscle groups most affected by prolonged immobilization are the antigravity postural muscles of the lower extremities (Bloomfield and Coyle 1993). The loss of normal mechanical strain patterns from contraction of these muscles results in a corresponding loss of density in the bones of the lower extremity, particularly the heel and the spine (Bloomfield and Coyle 1993). Muscles atrophy faster than bones lose their density. For example, 1 month of bed rest by healthy young men resulted in a 10 to 20 percent decrease in muscle fiber cross-sectional area and a 21 percent reduction in peak isokinetic torque of knee extensors (Bloomfield and Coyle 1993), whereas a similar period of bed rest resulted in a reduction in bone mineral density of only 0.3 to 3 percent for the lumbar spine and 1.5 percent for the heel.

Quantitative histologic examination of muscle biopsies of the vastus lateralis of the leg following immobilization shows reduced cross-sectional area for both slow-twitch and fast-twitch fibers, actual necrotic changes in affected fibers, loss of capillary density, and a decline in aerobic enzyme activity, creatinine phosphate, and glycogen stores (Bloomfield and Coyle 1993). On resuming normal activity, reversibility of these decrements in cardiorespiratory, metabolic, and muscle function is fairly rapid (within days to weeks) (Bloomfield and Coyle 1993). By contrast, the reversal of the decrement of bone mineral density requires weeks to months.

## Special Considerations

The physiologic responses to exercise and physiologic adaptations to training and detraining, reviewed in the preceding sections, can be influenced by a number of factors, including physical disability, environmental conditions, age, and sex.

### Disability

Although there is a paucity of information about physiologic responses to exercise among persons with disabilities, existing information supports the notion that the capacity of these persons to adapt to increased levels of physical activity is similar to that of persons without disabilities. Many of the acute effects of physical activity on the cardiovascular, respiratory, endocrine, and musculoskeletal systems have been demonstrated to be similar among persons with disabilities, depending on the specific nature of the disability. For example, physiologic responses to exercise have been studied among persons with paraplegia (Davis 1993), quadriplegia (Figoni 1993), mental retardation (Fernhall 1993), multiple sclerosis (Ponichtera-Mulcare 1993), and postpolio syndrome (Birk 1993).

### Environmental Conditions

The basic physiologic responses to an episode of exercise vary considerably with changes in environmental conditions. As environmental temperature and humidity increase, the body is challenged to maintain its core temperature. Generally, as the body's core temperature increases during exercise, blood vessels in the skin begin to dilate, diverting more blood to the body's surface, where body heat can be passed on to the environment (unless environmental temperature exceeds body temperature). Evaporation of water from the skin's surface significantly aids in heat loss; however, as humidity increases, evaporation becomes limited.

These methods for cooling can compromise cardiovascular function during exercise. Increasing blood flow to the skin creates competition with the active muscles for a large percentage of the cardiac output. When a person is exercising for prolonged periods in the heat, stroke volume will generally decline over time consequent to dehydration and increased blood flow in the skin (Rowell 1993; Montain and Coyle 1992). Heart rate increases substantially to try to maintain cardiac output to compensate for the reduced stroke volume.

High air temperature is not the only factor that stresses the body's ability to cool itself in the heat. High humidity, low air velocity, and the radiant heat from the sun and reflective surfaces also contribute to the total effect. For example, exercising under conditions of 32°C (90°F) air temperature, 20 percent relative humidity, 3.0 kilometers per hour (4.8 miles per hour) air velocity, and cloud cover is much more comfortable and less stressful to the body than the same exercise under conditions of 24°C (75°F) air temperature, 90 percent relative humidity, no air movement, and direct exposure to the sun.

Children respond differently to heat than adults do. Children have a higher body surface area to body mass ratio (surface area/mass), which facilitates heat loss when environmental temperatures are below skin temperature. When environmental temperature exceeds skin temperature, children are at an even greater disadvantage because these mechanisms then become avenues of heat gain. Children also have a lower rate of sweat production; even though they have more heat-activated sweat glands, each gland produces considerably less sweat than that of an adult (Bar-Or 1983).

The inability to maintain core temperature can lead to heat-related injuries. Heat cramps, characterized by severe cramping of the active skeletal muscles, is the least severe of three primary heat disorders. Heat exhaustion results when the demand for blood exceeds what is available, leading to competition for the body's limited blood supply. Heat exhaustion is accompanied by symptoms including extreme fatigue, breathlessness, dizziness, vomiting, fainting, cold and clammy or hot and dry skin, hypotension, and a weak, rapid pulse (Wilmore and Costill 1994). Heatstroke, the most extreme of the three heat disorders, is characterized by a core temperature of 40°C (104°F) or higher, cessation of sweating, hot and dry skin, rapid pulse and respiration, hypertension, and confusion or unconsciousness. If left untreated, heatstroke can lead to coma, then death. People experiencing symptoms of heat-related injury should be taken to a shady area, cooled with by whatever means available, and if conscious given nonalcoholic beverages to drink. Medical assistance should be sought. To reduce the risk of developing heat disorders, a person should drink enough fluid to try to match that which is lost through sweating, avoid extreme heat, and reduce the intensity of activity in hot weather. Because children are less resistant to the adverse effects of heat during exercise, special attention should be given to protect them when they exercise in the heat and to provide them with extra fluids to drink.

Stresses associated with exercising in the extreme cold are generally less severe. For most situations, the problems associated with cold stress can be eliminated by adequate clothing. Still, cold stress can induce a number of changes in the physiologic response to exercise (Doubt 1991; Jacobs, Martineau, Vallerand 1994; Shephard 1993). These include the increased generation of body heat by vigorous activity and shivering, increased production of catecholamines, vasoconstriction in both the cutaneous and nonactive skeletal muscle beds to provide insulation for the body's core, increased lactate production, and a higher oxygen uptake for the same work (Doubt 1991). For the same absolute temperature, exposure to cold water is substantially more stressful than exposure to cold air because the heat transfer in water is about 25 times greater than in air (Toner and McArdle 1988). Because the ratio of surface area to mass is higher in children than in adults, children lose heat at a faster rate when exposed to the same cold stress. The elderly tend to have a reduced response of generating body heat and are thus more susceptible to cold stress.

Altitude also affects the body's physiologic responses to exercise. As altitude increases, barometric pressure decreases, and the partial pressure of inhaled oxygen is decreased proportionally. A decreased partial pressure of oxygen reduces the driving force to unload oxygen from the air to the blood and from the blood to the muscle, thereby compromising oxygen delivery (Fulco and Cymerman 1988). $\dot{V}O_2$max is significantly reduced at altitudes greater than 1,500 meters. This effect impairs the performance of endurance activities. The body makes both short-term and long-term adaptations to altitude exposure that enable it to at least partially adapt to this imposed stress. Because oxygen delivery is the primary concern, the initial adaptation that occurs within the first 24 hours of exposure to altitude is an increased cardiac output both at rest and during submaximal exercise. Ventilatory volumes are also increased. An ensuing reduction in plasma volume increases the concentration of red blood cells (hemoconcentration), thus providing more oxygen molecules per unit of blood (Grover, Weil, Reeves 1986). Over several weeks, the red blood cell mass is increased through stimulation of the bone marrow by the hormone erythropoietin.

Exercising vigorously outdoors when air quality is poor can also produce adverse physiologic responses. In addition to decreased tolerance for exercise, direct respiratory effects include increased airway reactivity and potential exposure to harmful vapors and airborne dusts, toxins, and pollens (Wilmore and Costill 1994).

74

## Effects of Age

When absolute values are scaled to account for differences in body size, most differences in physiologic function between children and adults disappear. The exceptions are notable. For the same absolute rate of work on a cycle ergometer, children will have approximately the same metabolic cost, or $\dot{V}O_2$ demands, but they meet those demands differently. Because children have smaller hearts, their stroke volume is lower than that for adults for the same rate of work. Heart rate is increased to compensate for the lower stroke volume; but because this increase is generally inadequate, cardiac output is slightly lower (Bar-Or 1983). The A-$\bar{v}O_2$ difference is therefore increased to compensate for the lower cardiac output to achieve the same $\dot{V}O_2$. The $\dot{V}O_2$max, expressed in liters per minute, increases during the ages of 6–18 years for boys and 6–14 years for girls (Figure 3-4) before it reaches a plateau (Krahenbuhl, Skinner, Kohrt 1985). When expressed relative to body weight (milliliters per kilogram per minute), $\dot{V}O_2$max remains fairly stable for boys from 6–18 years of age but decreases

steadily for girls during those years (Figure 3-4) (Krahenbuhl, Skinner, Kohrt 1985). Most likely, different patterns of physical activity contribute to this variation because the difference in aerobic capacity between elite female endurance athletes and elite male endurance athletes is substantially less than the difference between boys and girls in general (e.g., 10 percent vs. 25 percent) (Wilmore and Costill 1994).

The deterioration of physiologic function with aging is almost identical to the change in function that generally accompanies inactivity. Maximal heart rate and maximal stroke volume are decreased in older adults; maximal cardiac output is thus decreased, which results in a $\dot{V}O_2$max lower than that of a young adult (Raven and Mitchell 1980). The decline in $\dot{V}O_2$max approximates 0.40 to 0.50 milliliters per kilogram per minute per year in men, according to data from cross-sectional studies; this rate of decline is less in women (Buskirk and Hodgson 1987). Through training, both older men and women can increase their $\dot{V}O_2$max values by approximately the same percentage as those seen

**Figure 3-4. Changes in $\dot{V}O_2$ max with increasing age from 6 to 18 years of age in boys and girls***

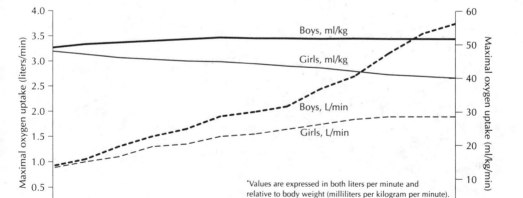

*Values are expressed in both liters per minute and relative to body weight (milliliters per kilogram per minute).

Data were taken from Krahenbuhl GS, Skinner JS, Kohrt WM 1985 and Bar-Or O 1983.

in younger adults (Kohrt et al. 1991). The interrelationships of age, $\dot{V}O_2$max, and training status are evident when the loss in $\dot{V}O_2$max with age is compared for active and sedentary individuals (Figure 3-5).

When the cardiorespiratory responses of an older adult are compared with those of a young or middle-aged adult at the same absolute submaximal rate of work, stroke volume for an older person is generally lower and heart rate is higher from the attempt to maintain cardiac output. Because this attempt is generally insufficient, the A-$\bar{v}O_2$ difference must increase to provide the same submaximal oxygen uptake (Raven and Mitchell 1980; Thompson and Dorsey 1986). Some researchers have shown, however, that cardiac output can be maintained at both submaximal and maximal rates of work through a higher stroke volume in older adults (Rodeheffer et al. 1984).

The deterioration in physiological function normally associated with aging is, in fact, caused by a combination of reduced physical activity and the aging process itself. By maintaining an active lifestyle, or by increasing levels of physical activity if previously sedentary, older persons can maintain relatively high levels of cardiovascular and metabolic function, including $\dot{V}O_2$max (Kohrt et al. 1991), and of skeletal muscle function (Rogers and Evans 1993). For example, Fiatarone and colleagues (1994) found an increase of 113 percent in the strength of elderly men and women (mean age of 87.1 years) following a 10-week training program of progressive resistance exercise. Cross-sectional thigh muscle area was increased, as was stair-climbing power, gait velocity, and level of spontaneous activity. Increasing endurance and strength in the elderly contributes to their ability to live independently.

## Differences by Sex

For the most part, women and men who participate in exercise training have similar responses in cardiovascular, respiratory, and metabolic function (providing that size and activity level are normalized). Relative increases in $\dot{V}O_2$max are equivalent

---

**Figure 3-5.** Changes in $\dot{V}O_2$ max with aging, comparing an active population and sedentary population (the figure also illustrates the expected increase in $\dot{V}O_2$ max when a previously sedentary person begins an exercise program)

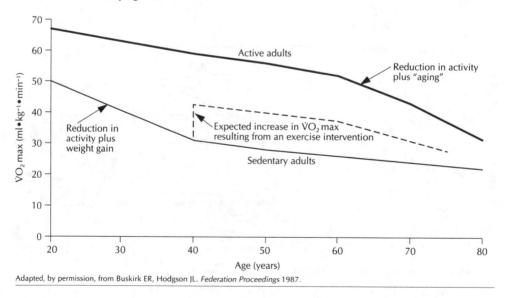

Adapted, by permission, from Buskirk ER, Hodgson JL. *Federation Proceedings* 1987.

for women and men (Kohrt et al. 1991; Mitchell et al. 1992). Some evidence suggests that older women accomplish this increase in $\dot{V}O_2$max mainly through an increase in the A-$\bar{v}O_2$ difference, whereas younger women and men have substantial increases in stroke volume, which increases maximal cardiac output (Spina et al. 1993). With resistance training, women experience equivalent increases in strength (Rogers and Evans 1993; Holloway and Baechle 1990), although they gain less fat-free mass due to less muscle hypertrophy.

Several sex differences have been noted in the acute response to exercise. At the same absolute rate of exercise, women have a higher heart rate response than men, primarily because of a lower stroke volume. This lower stroke volume is a function of smaller heart size and smaller blood volume. In addition, women have less potential to increase the A-$\bar{v}O_2$ difference because of lower hemoglobin content. Those differences, in addition to greater fat mass, result in a lower $\dot{V}O_2$max in women, even when normalized for size and level of training (Lewis, Kamon, Hodgson 1986).

## Conclusions

1. Physical activity has numerous beneficial physiologic effects. Most widely appreciated are its effects on the cardiovascular and musculoskeletal systems, but benefits on the functioning of metabolic, endocrine, and immune systems are also considerable.

2. Many of the beneficial effects of exercise training—from both endurance and resistance activities—diminish within 2 weeks if physical activity is substantially reduced, and effects disappear within 2 to 8 months if physical activity is not resumed.

3. People of all ages, both male and female, undergo beneficial physiologic adaptations to physical activity.

### Research Needs

1. Explore individual variations in response to exercise.

2. Better characterize mechanisms through which the musculoskeletal system responds differentially to endurance and resistance exercise.

3. Better characterize the mechanisms by which physical activity reduces the risk of cardiovascular disease, hypertension, and non–insulin-dependent diabetes mellitus.

4. Determine the minimal and optimal amount of exercise for disease prevention.

5. Better characterize beneficial activity profiles for people with disabilities.

## References

Abernethy PJ, Thayer R, Taylor AW. Acute and chronic responses of skeletal muscle to endurance and sprint exercise: a review. *Sports Medicine* 1990;10:365–389.

American College of Sports Medicine. Position stand: physical activity, physical fitness, and hypertension. *Medicine and Science in Sports and Exercise* 1993;25:i–x.

Armstrong RB, Warren GL, Warren JA. Mechanisms of exercise-induced muscle fibre injury. *Sports Medicine* 1991;12:184–207.

Bar-Or O. *Pediatric sports medicine for the practitioner: from physiologic principles to clinical applications.* New York: Springer-Verlag, 1983.

Birk TJ. Poliomyelitis and the post-polio syndrome: exercise capacities and adaptations—current research, future directions, and widespread applicability. *Medicine and Science in Sports and Exercise* 1993;25:466–472.

Blomqvist CG, Saltin B. Cardiovascular adaptations to physical training. *Annual Review of Physiology* 1983;45:169–189.

Bloomfield SA, Coyle EF. Bed rest, detraining, and retention of training-induced adaptation. In: Durstine JL, King AC, Painter PL, Roitman JL, Zwiren LD, editors. *ACSM's resource manual for guidelines for exercise testing and prescription.* 2nd ed. Philadelphia: Lea and Febiger, 1993:115–128.

Buskirk ER, Hodgson JL. Age and aerobic power: the rate of change in men and women. *Federation Proceedings* 1987;46:1824–1829.

Chesnut CH III. Bone mass and exercise. *American Journal of Medicine* 1993;95(5A Suppl):34S–36S.

## Physical Activity and Health

Coyle EF. Cardiovascular function during exercise: neural control factors. *Sports Science Exchange* 1991;4:1–6.

Davis GM. Exercise capacity of individuals with paraplegia. *Medicine and Science in Sports and Exercise* 1993;25:423–432.

Doubt TJ. Physiology of exercise in the cold. *Sports Medicine* 1991;11:367–381.

Drinkwater BL. Physical activity, fitness, and osteoporosis. In: Bouchard C, Shephard RJ, Stephens T, editors. *Physical activity, fitness, and health: international proceedings and consensus statement.* Champaign, IL: Human Kinetics, 1994:724–736.

Fagard RH, Tipton CM. Physical activity, fitness, and hypertension. In: Bouchard C, Shephard RJ, Stephens T, editors. *Physical activity, fitness, and health: international proceedings and consensus statement.* Champaign, IL: Human Kinetics, 1994:633–655.

Farrell PA, Wilmore JH, Coyle EF, Billing JE, Costill DL. Plasma lactate accumulation and distance running performance. *Medicine and Science in Sports* 1979;11:338–344.

Fernhall B. Physical fitness and exercise training of individuals with mental retardation. *Medicine and Science in Sports and Exercise* 1993;25:442–450.

Fiatarone MA, O'Neill EF, Ryan ND, Clements KM, Solares GR, Nelson ME, et al. Exercise training and nutritional supplementation for physical frailty in very elderly people. *New England Journal of Medicine* 1994;330:1769–1775.

Figoni SF. Exercise responses and quadriplegia. *Medicine and Science in Sports and Exercise* 1993;25:433–441.

Fleck SJ, Kraemer WJ. *Designing resistance training programs.* Champaign, IL: Human Kinetics, 1987:264.

Fulco CS, Cymerman A. Human performance and acute hypoxia. In: Pandolf KB, Sawka MN, Gonzalez RR, editors. *Human performance physiology and environmental medicine at terrestrial extremes.* Indianapolis: Benchmark Press, 1988:467–495.

George KP, Wolfe LA, Burggraf GW. The "athletic heart syndrome": a critical review. *Sports Medicine* 1991;11:300–331.

Gledhill N, Cox D, Jamnik R. Endurance athletes' stroke volume does not plateau: major advantage is diastolic function. *Medicine and Science in Sports and Exercise* 1994;26:1116–1121.

Gonyea WJ, Sale DG, Gonyea FB, Mikesky A. Exercise-induced increases in muscle fiber number. *European Journal of Applied Physiology* 1986;55:137–141.

Gordon NF, Kohl HW III, Pollock ML, Vaandrager H, Gibbons LW, Blair SN. Cardiovascular safety of maximal strength testing in healthy adults. *American Journal of Cardiology* 1995;76:851–853.

Graves JE, Pollock ML, Leggett SH, Braith RW, Carpenter DM, Bishop LE. Effect of reduced training frequency on muscular strength. *International Journal of Sports Medicine* 1988;9:316–319.

Green HJ, Jones LL, Painter DC. Effects of short-term training on cardiac function during prolonged exercise. *Medicine and Science in Sports and Exercise* 1990;22:488–493.

Grover RF, Weil JV, Reeves JT. Cardiovascular adaptation to exercise at high altitude. *Exercise and Sport Sciences Reviews* 1986;14:269–302.

Hickson RC. Skeletal muscle cytochrome *c* and myoglobin, endurance, and frequency of training. *Journal of Applied Physiology* 1981;51:746–749.

Hickson RC, Foster C, Pollock ML, Galassi TM, Rich S. Reduced training intensities and loss of aerobic power, endurance, and cardiac growth. *Journal of Applied Physiology* 1985;58:492–499.

Hickson RC, Rosenkoetter MA. Reduced training frequencies and maintenance of increased aerobic power. *Medicine and Science in Sports and Exercise* 1981;13:13–16.

Hoffman-Goetz L, Pedersen BK. Exercise and the immune system: a model of the stress response? *Immunology Today* 1994;15:382–387.

Holloway JB, Baechle TR. Strength training for female athletes: a review of selected aspects. *Sports Medicine* 1990;9:216–228.

Isea JE, Piepoli M, Adamopoulos S, Pannarale G, Sleight P, Coats AJS. Time course of haemodynamic changes after maximal exercise. *European Journal of Clinical Investigation* 1994;24:824–829.

Jacobs I, Martineau L, Vallerand AL. Thermoregulatory thermogenesis in humans during cold stress. *Exercise and Sport Sciences Reviews* 1994;22:221–250.

Jolesz F, Sreter FA. Development, innervation, and activity-pattern induced changes in skeletal muscle. *Annual Review of Physiology* 1981;43:531–552.

Jorgensen CR, Gobel FL, Taylor HL, Wang Y. Myocardial blood flow and oxygen consumption during exercise. *Annals of the New York Academy of Sciences* 1977;301:213–223.

Kannus P, Jozsa L, Renström P, Järvinen M, Kvist M, Lehto M, et al. The effects of training, immobilization, and remobilization on musculoskeletal tissue. *Scandinavian Journal of Medicine and Science in Sports* 1992;2:100–118.

Keast D, Cameron K, Morton AR. Exercise and the immune response. *Sports Medicine* 1988;5:248–267.

Kiens B, Éssen-Gustavsson B, Christensen NJ, Saltin B. Skeletal muscle substrate utilization during submaximal exercise in man: effect of endurance training. *Journal of Physiology* 1993;469:459–478.

Kohrt WM, Malley MT, Coggan AR, Spina RJ, Ogawa T, Ehsani AA, et al. Effects of gender, age, and fitness level on response of $VO_2$ max to training in 60–71 yr olds. *Journal of Applied Physiology* 1991;71:2004–2011.

Krahenbuhl GS, Skinner JS, Kohrt WM. Developmental aspects of maximal aerobic power in children. *Exercise and Sport Sciences Reviews* 1985;13:503–538.

Lewis DA, Kamon E, Hodgson JL. Physiological differences between genders: implications for sports conditioning. *Sports Medicine* 1986;3:357–369.

Lipman RL, Raskin P, Love T, Triebwasser J, Lecocq FR, Schnure JJ. Glucose intolerance during decreased physical activity in man. *Diabetes* 1972;21:101–107.

MacIntyre DL, Reid WD, McKenzie DC. Delayed muscle soreness: the inflammatory response to muscle injury and its clinical implications. *Sports Medicine* 1995;20:24–40.

Marcus ML. *The coronary circulation in health and disease.* New York: McGraw Hill, 1983.

Mitchell JH, Tate C, Raven P, Cobb F, Kraus W, Moreadith R, et al. Acute response and chronic adaptation to exercise in women. *Medicine and Science in Sports and Exercise* 1992;24(6 Suppl):S258–S265.

Montain SJ, Coyle EF. Influence of graded dehydration on hyperthermia and cardiovascular drift during exercise. *Journal of Applied Physiology* 1992;73:1340–1350.

Neufer PD, Costill DL, Fielding RA, Flynn MG, Kirwan JP. Effect of reduced training on muscular strength and endurance in competitive swimmers. *Medicine and Science in Sports and Exercise* 1987;19:486–490.

Newsholme EA, Parry-Billings M. Effects of exercise on the immune system. In: Bouchard C, Shephard RJ, Stephens T, editors. *Physical activity, fitness, and health: international proceedings and consensus statement.* Champaign, IL: Human Kinetics, 1994:451–455.

Nieman DC. Exercise, infection, and immunity. *International Journal of Sports Medicine* 1994;15(3 Suppl):S131–S141.

Pedersen BK, Ullum H. NK cell response to physical activity: possible mechanisms of action. *Medicine and Science in Sports and Exercise* 1994;26:140–146.

Ponichtera-Mulcare JA. Exercise and multiple sclerosis. *Medicine and Science in Sports and Exercise* 1993;25:451–465.

Raven PB, Mitchell J. The effect of aging on the cardiovascular response to dynamic and static exercise. In: Weisfeldt ML, editor. *The aging heart.* New York: Raven Press, 1980:269–296.

Reichlin S. Neuroendocrinology. In: Wilson JD, Foster DW, editors. *Williams' textbook of endocrinology.* 8th ed. Philadelphia: W.B. Saunders, 1992:201.

Rodeheffer RJ, Gerstenblith G, Becker LC, Fleg JL, Weisfeldt ML, Lakatta EG. Exercise cardiac output is maintained with advancing age in healthy human subjects: cardiac dilatation and increased stroke volume compensate for a diminished heart rate. *Circulation* 1984;69:203–213.

Rogers MA, Evans WJ. Changes in skeletal muscle with aging: effects of exercise training. *Exercise and Sport Sciences Reviews* 1993;21:65–102.

Rowell LB. *Human cardiovascular control.* New York: Oxford University Press, 1993.

Rowell LB. *Human circulation regulation during physical stress.* New York: Oxford University Press, 1986.

Saltin B, Blomqvist G, Mitchell JH, Johnson RL, Wildenthal K, Chapman CB. Response to exercise after bed rest and after training: a longitudinal study of adaptive changes in oxygen transport and body composition. *Circulation* 1968;38(Suppl 7):1–78.

Saltin B, Rowell LB. Functional adaptations to physical activity and inactivity. *Federation Proceedings* 1980;39:1506–1513.

Scruggs KD, Martin NB, Broeder CE, Hofman Z, Thomas EL, Wambsgans KC, et al. Stroke volume during submaximal exercise in endurance-trained normotensive subjects and in untrained hypertensive subjects with beta blockade (propranolol and pindolol). *American Journal of Cardiology* 1991;67:416–421.

Seals DR, Hagberg JM, Spina RJ, Rogers MA, Schechtman KB, Ehsani AA. Enhanced left ventricular performance in endurance trained older men. *Circulation* 1994;89:198–205.

## Physical Activity and Health

Shephard RJ. *Aerobic fitness and health*. Champaign, IL: Human Kinetics, 1994.

Shephard RJ. Metabolic adaptations to exercise in the cold: an update. *Sports Medicine* 1993;16:266–289.

Shephard RJ, Shek PN. Cancer, immune function, and physical activity. *Canadian Journal of Applied Physiology* 1995;20:1–25.

Sjöström M, Lexell J, Eriksson A, Taylor CC. Evidence of fibre hyperplasia in human skeletal muscles from healthy young men? A left-right comparison of the fibre number in whole anterior tibialis muscles. *European Journal of Applied Physiology* 1991;62:301–304.

Spina RJ, Ogawa T, Miller TR, Kohrt WM, Ehsani AA. Effect of exercise training on left ventricular performance in older women free of cardiopulmonary disease. *American Journal of Cardiology* 1993;71:99–104.

Svedenhag J, Henriksson J, Sylvén C. Dissociation of training effects on skeletal muscle mitochondrial enzymes and myoglobin in man. *Acta Physiologica Scandinavica* 1983;117:213–218.

Terjung RL. Muscle adaptations to aerobic training. *Sports Science Exchange* 1995;8:1–4.

Thompson PD, Dorsey DL. The heart of the masters athlete. In: Sutton JR, Brock RM, editors. *Sports medicine for the mature athlete*. Indianapolis: Benchmark Press, 1986:309–318.

Tipton CM. Exercise, training, and hypertension: an update. *Exercise and Sport Sciences Reviews* 1991;19: 447–505.

Tipton CM, Vailas AC. Bone and connective tissue adaptations to physical activity. In: Bouchard C, Shephard RJ, Stephens T, Sutton JR, McPherson BD, editors. *Exercise, fitness, and health: a consensus of current knowledge*. Champaign, IL: Human Kinetics, 1990:331–344.

Toner MM, McArdle WD. Physiological adjustments of man to the cold. In: Pandolf KB, Sawka MN, Gonzalez RR, editors. *Human performance physiology and environmental medicine at terrestrial extremes*. Indianapolis: Benchmark Press, 1988:361–399.

Turley KR, McBride PJ, Wilmore JH. Resting metabolic rate measured after subjects spent the night at home vs at a clinic. *American Journal of Clinical Nutrition* 1993;58:141–144.

Wilmore JH, Costill DL. *Physiology of sport and exercise*. Champaign, IL: Human Kinetics, 1994.

Woods JA, Davis JM. Exercise, monocyte/macrophage function, and cancer. *Medicine and Science in Sports and Exercise* 1994;26:147–157.

# CHAPTER 4

# THE EFFECTS OF PHYSICAL ACTIVITY ON HEALTH AND DISEASE

## Contents

**Contents,** *continued*

**Contents,** *continued*

# THE EFFECTS OF PHYSICAL ACTIVITY ON HEALTH AND DISEASE

## Introduction

This chapter examines the relationship of physical activity and cardiorespiratory fitness to a variety of health problems. The primary focus is on diseases and conditions for which sufficient data exist to evaluate an association with physical activity, the strength of such relationships, and their potential biologic mechanisms. Because most of the research to date has addressed the health effects of endurance-type physical activity (involving repetitive use of large muscle groups, such as in walking and bicycling), this chapter focuses on that type of activity. Unless otherwise specified, the term physical activity should be understood to refer to endurance-type physical activity. Less well studied are the health effects of resistance-type physical activity (i.e., that which develops muscular strength); when this type of physical activity is discussed, it is specified as such. Much of the research summarized is based on studies having only white men as participants; it remains to be clarified whether the relationships described here are the same for women, racial and ethnic minority groups, and people with disabilities.

Physical activity is difficult to measure directly. Three types of physical activity measures have been used in observational studies over the last 40 years. Most studies have relied on self-reported level of physical activity, as recalled by people prompted by a questionnaire or interview. A more objectively measured characteristic is cardiorespiratory fitness (also referred to as cardiorespiratory endurance) which is measured by aerobic power (see Chapter 2 for more information on measurement issues). Some studies have relied on occupation to classify people according to how likely they were to be physically active at work.

Epidemiologic studies of physical activity and health have compared the activity levels of people who have or develop diseases and those who do not. Cohort studies follow populations forward in time to observe how physical activity habits affect disease occurrence or death. In case-control studies, groups of persons who have disease and separate groups of people who do not have disease are asked to recall their previous physical activity. Cross-sectional studies assess the association between physical activity and disease at the same point in time. Clinical trials, on the other hand, attempt to alter physical activity patterns and then assess whether disease occurrence is modified as a result.

Results from epidemiologic studies can be used to estimate the relative magnitude or strength of an association between physical activity and a health outcome. Two such measures used in this chapter are risk ratio (RR) and odds ratio (OR). For these measures, an estimate of 1.0 indicates no association, when the risk of disease is equivalent in the two groups being compared. RR or OR estimates greater than 1.0 indicate an increase in risk; those less than 1.0 indicate a decreased risk. Confidence intervals (CI) reported with estimates of association indicate the precision of the estimate, as well as its statistical significance. When the CI range includes 1.0, the effect is considered likely to have occurred by chance; therefore the estimate of association is not considered statistically significantly different from the null value of 1.0.

## Overall Mortality

Persons with moderate to high levels of physical activity or cardiorespiratory fitness have a lower mortality rate than those with sedentary habits or low cardiorespiratory fitness. For example, compared with people who are most active, sedentary people experience between a 1.2-fold to a 2-fold increased risk of dying during the follow-up interval (Slattery and Jacobs 1988; Slattery, Jacobs, Nichaman 1989; Leon and Connett 1991; Stender et al. 1993; Sandvik et al. 1993; Chang-Claude and Frentzel-Beyme 1993; Kaplan et al. 1987; Arraiz, Wigle, Mao 1992; Paffenbarger et al. 1993).

Associations are generally stronger for measured cardiorespiratory fitness than for reported physical activity (Blair, Kohl, Paffenbarger 1989). Blair, Kohl, and Barlow (1993) showed that low levels of cardiorespiratory fitness were strongly associated with overall mortality for both women (RR = 5.35; 95% CI, 2.44–11.73) and men (RR = 3.16; 95% CI, 1.92–5.20). The association with physical inactivity was weaker for men (RR = 1.70; 95% CI, 1.06–2.74), and there was no association for women (RR = 0.95; 95% CI, 0.54–1.70).

Though cardiorespiratory fitness may be the better indicator of regular physical activity, the level of reported physical activity has been associated with reduced all-cause mortality. Paffenbarger, Lee, and Leung (1994) evaluated several types of recalled activity (walking, stair climbing, all sports, moderate-level sports, and total energy expended in activity per week) as predictors of all-cause mortality among male Harvard alumni. Among these men, the relative risk of death within the follow-up period was reduced to 0.67 with walking 15 or more kilometers per week (reference group, < 5 kilometers/week), to 0.75 with climbing 55 or more flights of stairs per week (reference group, < 20 flights/week), to 0.63 with involvement in moderate sports (reference group, no involvement), and to 0.47 with 3 or more hours of moderate sports activities per week (reference group, < 1 hour/week). Most importantly, there was a significant trend of decreasing risk of death across increasing categories of distance walked, flights of stairs climbed, and degree of intensity of sports play.

Researchers have also examined age-specific effects of different levels of physical activity on all-cause mortality. Kaplan and colleagues (1987) have shown that physical activity level has an effect on death rates among both older and younger persons. Data from a study of 9,484 Seventh-Day Adventist men aged 30 years or older in 1958 who were

followed through 1985 indicated that both moderate and intense levels of activity reduced overall risk of death even late in life (Lindsted, Tonstad, Kuzma 1991). Both moderate and vigorous levels of activity were equally protective at age 50 years. The protective effect of high levels of activity lasted only until age 70, but the protective effect for moderate activity lasted beyond age 80.

The studies cited thus far in this section assessed physical activity or cardiorespiratory fitness at baseline only and then followed up for mortality. A stronger test for a causal relationship is to examine the effect that changing from lower to higher levels of physical activity or cardiorespiratory fitness has on subsequent mortality. Two large studies provide such evidence. Among middle-aged Harvard male alumni who were sedentary in 1962 or 1966, those who took up moderately intense sports activity during the study's 11 years of follow-up had a 23 percent lower death rate (RR = 0.77; 95% CI, 0.58–0.96) than those who remained sedentary (Paffenbarger et al. 1993). (By comparison, men who quit smoking during the interval had a 41 percent decrease in death rate [RR = 0.59; 95% CI, 0.43–0.80].) Men 45–84 years of age who took up moderately intense sports extended their longevity on average by 0.72 years; added years of life were observed in all age groups, including men 75–84 years of age (Paffenbarger et al. 1993).

Similar reductions in death rates with increases in cardiorespiratory fitness were reported for men in the Aerobics Center Longitudinal Study. Blair and colleagues (1995) reported a reduction in death rates among healthy men (aged 20–82 years) who improved their initially low levels of cardiorespiratory fitness. The men performed two maximal exercise tests an average of 4.8 years apart; follow-up for mortality after the second test occurred an average of 4.7 years later. Among men in the bottom fifth of the cardiorespiratory fitness distribution, those who improved to at least a moderate fitness level had a 44 percent lower death rate than their peers who remained in the bottom fifth (RR = 0.56; 95% CI, 0.41–0.75). After multivariate adjustment, those who became fit had a significant 64 percent reduction in their relative mortality rate. In comparison, men who stopped smoking reduced their adjusted RR by about 50 percent.

## Conclusions

The data reviewed here suggest that regular physical activity and higher cardiorespiratory fitness decrease overall mortality rates in a dose-response fashion. Whereas most studies of physical activity and health address specific diseases and health conditions, the studies in this chapter provide more insight into the biologic mechanisms by which mortality rate reduction occurs.

## Cardiovascular Diseases

Despite a progressive decline since the late 1960s, cardiovascular diseases (CVDs), including coronary heart disease (CHD) and stroke, remain major causes of death, disability, and health care expenditures in the United States (NCHS 1994; Gillum 1994). In 1992, more than 860,000 deaths in the United States were attributed to heart disease and stroke (DHHS 1994). High blood pressure, a major risk factor for CVD, affects about 50 million Americans (National Institutes of Health [NIH] 1993), including an estimated 2.8 million children and adolescents 6–17 years of age (Task Force on Blood Pressure Control in Children 1987). The prevalence of CVD increases with age and is higher among African Americans than whites. The majority of population-based research in the area of physical activity and health has focused on some aspect of CVD.

### Cardiovascular Diseases Combined

Most of the reported studies relating physical activity to CVD have reported CVD mortality as an endpoint; two also reported on nonfatal disease, and one reported on CVD hospitalization (Table 4-1). Seven cohort studies evaluated the association between level of physical activity and the risk of total CVD (Kannel and Sorlie 1979; Paffenbarger et al. 1984; Kannel et al. 1986; Lindsted, Tonstad, Kuzma 1991; Arraiz, Wigle, Mao 1992; Sherman et al. 1994; LaCroix et al. 1996). All relied on a single point-in-time estimate of physical activity, in some cases assessed as long as 26 years before the end of the observational period, and four had follow-up periods of ≥ 14 years. Four of the seven studies found both an inverse association and a dose-response gradient between level of physical activity and risk of CVD outcome (Kannel and Sorlie 1979; Paffenbarger et al. 1984;

Kannel et al. 1986; LaCroix et al. 1996). One study among men found an inverse association among the moderately active group but less of an effect in the vigorously active group (Lindsted, Tonstad, Kuzma 1991). One study of women 50–74 years of age found no relationship of physical activity with CVD mortality (Sherman et al. 1994).

Five large cohort studies have related cardiorespiratory fitness to the risk of CVD mortality (Arraiz, Wigle, Mao 1992; Ekelund et al. 1988; Blair, Kohl, Paffenbarger 1989; Sandvik et al. 1993; Blair et al. 1995), but only one provided a separate analysis for women (Blair, Kohl, Paffenbarger 1989). Each of these studies demonstrated an inverse dose-response relationship between level of cardiorespiratory fitness and CVD mortality. Three of the five studies relied on a maximal or near-maximal exercise test to estimate cardiorespiratory fitness. One study (Blair et al. 1995) demonstrated that men with low cardiorespiratory fitness who became fit had a lower risk of CVD mortality than men who remained unfit.

Taken together, these major cohort studies indicate that low levels of physical activity or cardiorespiratory fitness increase risk of CVD mortality. Findings seem to be more consistent for studies of cardiorespiratory fitness, perhaps because of its greater precision of measurement, than for those of reported physical activity. The demonstrated dose-response relationship indicates that the benefit derived from physical activity occurs at moderate levels of physical activity or cardiorespiratory fitness and increases with increasing levels of physical activity or higher levels of fitness.

### Coronary Heart Disease

Numerous studies have examined the relationship between physical activity and CHD as a specific CVD outcome. Reviews of the epidemiologic literature (Powell et al. 1987; Berlin and Colditz 1990; Blair 1994) have concluded that physical activity is strongly and inversely related to CHD risk. Although physical exertion may transiently increase the risk of an acute coronary event among persons with advanced coronary atherosclerosis, particularly among those who do not exercise regularly (Mittleman et al. 1993; Willich et al. 1993; Siscovick et al. 1984), physically active people have a substantially lower overall risk for major coronary events.

Table 4-1.  Population-based studies of association of physical activity or cardiorespiratory fitness with total cardiovascular diseases

| Study | Population | Definition of physical activity or cardiorespiratory fitness | Definition of cardiovascular disease |
|---|---|---|---|
| **Physical activity** | | | |
| Kannel and Sorlie (1979) | 1,909 Framingham (MA) men and 2,311 women aged 35–64 years at 14-year follow-up | Physical activity index based on hours per day spent at activity-specific intensity | CVD fatal and nonfatal in men (n = 140 deaths, n = 435 total cases) and women (n = 101 deaths) |
| Paffenbarger et al. (1984) | 16,936 US male college alumni who entered college between 1916 and 1950; followed from 1962–1978 | Physical activity index estimated from reports of stairs climbed, city blocks walked, and sports played each week | Death due to CVD (n = 640) |
| Kannel et al. (1986) | 1,166 Framingham (MA) men aged 45–64 years; 24-year follow-up | Physical activity index based on hours per day at activity-specific intensity; occupational physical activity classified by physical demand of work | Death due to CVD (n = 325) |
| Lindsted, Tonstad, Kuzma (1991) | 9,484 Seventh-Day Adventist men aged ≥ 30 years; 26-year follow-up | Self-report to single physical activity question | Death due to CVD (ICD-8 410–458) (n = 410) |
| Arraiz, Wigle, Mao (1992) | Stratified probability sample of Canadians aged 30–69 years, conducted in 1978–1979; 7-year follow-up | Physical activity index summarizing frequency, intensity, and duration of leisure-time activity and household chores | Death due to CVD (n = 256) |
| Sherman et al. (1994) | 1,404 Framingham (MA) women aged 50–74 years; 16-year follow-up | Physical activity index based on hours per day spent at activity-specific intensity | CVD incidence (n = 994) and mortality (n = 303) |
| LaCroix et al. (1996) | 1,645 HMO members age ≥ 65 years; 4.2-year average follow-up | Hours of walking per week | CVD hospitalization (ICD-9 390–448) (n = 359) |
| **Cardiorespiratory fitness** | | | |
| Ekelund et al. (1988) | 3,106 North American men aged 30–69 years; 8.5-year average follow-up | Submaximal aerobic capacity estimated from exercise test | Death due to CVD (ICD-8 390–458) (n = 45) |
| Blair et al. (1989) | 10,244 men and 3,120 women aged ≥ 20 years; 8.1-year average follow-up | Maximal aerobic capacity estimated by exercise test | Death due to CVD (ICD-9 390–448) in men (n = 66) and women (n = 7) |

| Main findings | Dose response* | Adjustment for confounders and other comments |
|---|---|---|
| Inverse association between physical activity index and CVD mortality for both men and women | Yes | Control for several confounding variables; statistical significance only for men after multivariate adjustment |
| Inverse association; relative to highest category (2,000+ kcal/week), relative risk estimates were 1.28 and 1.84, respectively | Yes | Significant dose-response after adjusting for age, smoking, and hypertension prevalence |
| Inverse association; for physical activity index, age-adjusted RR relative to high activity category = 1.62 for low activity, 1.30 for moderate; for occupational activity, age-adjusted RR relative to heavy physical demand category = 1.34 for sedentary, 1.26 for light, 1.09 for medium | Yes | Inverse association constant across all analyses; inverse association maintained after multivariate analyses |
| Inverse association relative to inactive group; moderately active RR = 0.79 (95% CI, 0.58–1.07), highly active RR = 1.02 (95% CI,0.66–1.58) | No | No statistical significance after controlling for sociodemographic variables, BMI, and dietary pattern |
| Null association across categories of physical activity index | No | Point estimates adjusted for age, BMI, sex, and smoking |
| Null association across quartiles of physical activity index | No | No statistical significance after controlling for several clinical and sociodemographic confounding variables |
| Inverse association; compared with walking 4 hrs/week, RR = 0.90 (95% CI 0.69–1.17) for walking 1–4 hrs/week; RR = 0.73 (95% CI 0.55–0.96) for walking > 4 hrs/week | Yes | Multivariate analysis adjusted for age, sex, functional status, BMI, smoking, chronic illnesses, and alcohol |
| Inverse association; adjusted risk estimate of 2.7-fold increased risk of CVD death for a 35 beat/min increase in heart rate for stage II of exercise test | Yes | Extensive control for clinical and sociodemographic confounding influences |
| Inverse association; for men, age-adjusted RR for lowest 20% compared with upper 40% = 7.9; for middle 40% = 2.5; for women, 9.2 and 3.6 | Yes | Significant linear dose-response association; adjusted for age |

**Table 4-1.** *Continued*

| Study | Population | Definition of physical activity or cardiorespiratory fitness | Definition of cardiovascular disease |
|---|---|---|---|
| Arraiz, Wigle, Mao (1992) | Stratified probability sample of Canadians aged 30–69 years, conducted in 1978–1979; 7-year follow-up | Submaximal aerobic capacity estimated from home step test | Death due to CVD (n = 37) |
| Sandvik et al. (1993) | 1,960 Norwegian men aged 40–59 years; average 16-year follow-up | Maximal aerobic capacity estimated by exercise test | Death due to CVD (n = 144) |
| Blair et al. (1995) | 9,777 US men aged 20–82 years with 2 evaluations; 5.1-year average follow-up | Maximal aerobic capacity estimated by exercise test | Death due to CVD (ICD-9 390–449.9) (n = 87) |

Thirty-six studies examining the relationship of physical activity level to risk of CHD have been published since 1953 (Table 4-2). Studies published before 1978 predominantly classified physical activity level by job title or occupational activities. Studies thereafter usually defined activity level by recall of leisure-time activity or by such activity combined with occupational activity. These later studies were also able to control statistically for many potentially confounding variables in addition to age. Most of these studies focused on men in the age ranges associated with increasing risk of CHD (30–75 years); only four included women. Although in several studies, CHD mortality was the sole outcome variable, most included both fatal and nonfatal disease. All but one (Morris et al. 1973) were cohort studies; lengths of follow-up from baseline assessment ranged from 4 to 25 years. All studies related a single baseline estimate of physical activity level to risk of CHD during the follow-up period.

Some study populations have had more than one follow-up assessment for CHD. For example, three follow-up assessments (at 10, 12, and 23 years) have been reported for men in the Honolulu Heart Program (Yano, Reed, McGee 1984; Donahue et al. 1988; Rodriguez et al. 1994). Each represented follow-up further removed from the original determination of physical activity. Thus, the diminishing effect seen over time might indicate changing patterns of physical activity—and thereby a lessening of validity of the original physical activity classification (Table 4-2). Oddly, in the 12-year follow-up, the reduction in CHD risk observed among both active middle-aged men (RR = 0.7) and active older men (RR = 0.4) when compared with their least active counterparts was not diminished by bivariate adjustment for serum cholesterol, body mass index (BMI), or blood pressure (Donahue et al. 1988). In the 23-year follow-up, however, the reduction in CHD risk among active men (RR = 0.8) was greatly diminished by simultaneous adjustment for serum cholesterol, BMI, blood pressure, and diabetes (RR = 0.95), leading the authors to conclude that the beneficial effect of physical activity on CHD risk is likely mediated by the beneficial effect of physical activity on these other factors (Rodriguez et al. 1994). These reports thus illustrate not only the problem of lengthy follow-up without repeated assessments of physical activity but also the problem of lack of uniformity in adjustment for potential confounding factors, as well as the underlying, thorny problem of adjustment for multiple factors that may be in the causal pathway between physical activity and disease. Studies have in fact varied greatly in the extent to which they have controlled for potential confounding and in the factors selected for adjustment.

Although early studies were not designed to demonstrate a dose-response gradient between physical

| Main findings | Dose response[*] | Adjustment for confounders and other comments |
|---|---|---|
| Inverse association; relative to highest fitness level, persons in "moderate" and "low" categories had risks of 0.8 (95% CI, 0.1–7.6) and 5.4 (95% CI, 1.9–15.9), respectively | No | Point estimates adjusted for age, BMI, sex, and smoking |
| Inverse association; relative to men in lowest fitness quartile, multivariate adjusted RR in quartiles 2, 3, and 4 were 0.59, 0.45, and 0.41, respectively | Yes | Extensive control for confounding influences |
| Inverse association; relative to men who remained unfit (lowest 20% of distribution), those who improved had an age-adjusted RR of 0.48 (95% CI, 0.31–0.74) | Yes | For each minute of improvement in exercise test time, adjusted CVD mortality risk was reduced 8.6% |

Abbreviations: BMI = body mass index (wt [kg] /ht [m]$^2$); CVD = cardiovascular disease; CI = confidence interval; HMO = health maintenance organization; ICD = International Classification of Diseases (8 and 9 refer to editions); RR = relative risk.

[*]A dose-response relationship requires more than 2 levels of comparison. In this column, "NA" means that there were only 2 levels of comparison; "No" means that there were more than 2 levels but no dose-response gradient was found; "Yes" means that there were more than 2 levels and a dose-response gradient was found.

activity level and CHD, most found an inverse association: more active persons were found to be at lower risk of CHD than their more sedentary counterparts. Of the 17 recent studies that found an inverse relationship and were able to examine dose-response relationships, 13 (76 percent) demonstrated an inverse dose-response gradient between level of physical activity and risk of CHD, whereas 2 showed a dose-response gradient only for some subgroups.

The relationship between cardiorespiratory fitness and risk of CHD was examined in seven cohort studies (follow-up range, 4–20 years). All but two (Lie, Mundal, Erikssen 1985; Erikssen 1986) used estimates of aerobic power based on submaximal exercise testing. None of these studies included women. Similar to the studies of physical activity and CHD, these all related a single baseline assessment of cardiorespiratory fitness to risk of CHD during the follow-up period. Most controlled statistically for possible confounding variables. All seven studies showed an inverse association between cardiorespiratory fitness and CHD. Of the six studies that had more than two categories of cardiorespiratory fitness, all demonstrated an inverse dose-response gradient.

Two recent meta-analyses of studies of physical activity and CHD have included independent scoring for the quality of the methods used in each study (Powell et al. 1987; Berlin and Colditz 1990). Both concluded that studies with higher-quality scores tended to show higher relative risk estimates than those with lower-quality scores. In the Berlin and Colditz quantitative meta-analysis, the pooled relative risk for CHD—comparing risk for the lowest level of physical activity with risk for the highest level—was 1.8 among the studies judged to be of higher quality. In contrast, the pooled relative risk for the studies with low-quality scores was in the null range.

## CVD Risk Factors in Children

Because CHD is rare in children, the cardiovascular effects of physical activity in children are assessed through the relationship of physical activity with CHD risk factors such as elevated low-density lipoprotein cholesterol (LDL-C), lowered high-density lipoprotein cholesterol (HDL-C), and elevated blood pressure. The presence of CHD risk factors in children is of concern because of evidence that atherosclerosis begins in childhood (Stary 1989), that presence of CHD in adults is related to elevated blood

Table 4-2.  Population-based studies of association of physical activity or cardiorespiratory fitness with coronary heart disease

| Study | Population | Definition of physical activity or cardiorespiratory fitness | Definition of coronary heart disease |
|---|---|---|---|
| **Physical activity** | | | |
| Morris et al. (1953) | 31,000 male employees of London Transport Executive aged 35–64 years | Occupational classification of job duties: sedentary drivers and active conductors | First clinical episode of CHD |
| Morris and Crawford (1958) | 3,731 case necropsy studies (decedents aged 45–70 years) conducted in Scotland, England, and Wales | Physical activity at work defined by coding of last known job title before death (light, active, heavy) | Necropsy evaluation of IMF among persons dying from noncoronary causes |
| Taylor et al. (1962) | 191,609 US white male railroad industry employees aged 40–64 years | Physical activity at work defined by job title for clerks, switchmen, and section men | Death due to arteriosclerotic disease (ICD 420, 422) in 1955–1956 |
| Kahn (1963) | 2,240 Postal Service employees in the Washington, D.C., Post Office between 1906 and 1940; followed through December 1961 | Physical activity at work defined by job title for clerks and carriers | Death due to CHD |
| Morris et al. (1966) | 667 London bus conductors and drivers aged 30–69 years; 5-year follow-up | Occupational classification of job duties as sedentary drivers and active conductors | Incidence of CHD (n = 47) |
| Cassel et al. (1971) | 3,009 male residents of Evans County, Georgia, aged over 40 years in 1960–1962; 7.25-year average follow-up | Occupational classification of job duties as active or sedentary | Incidence of CHD (n = 337) |
| Morris et al. (1973) | British male executive grade civil servants aged 40–60 years; 232 heart attack case-patients and 428 matched controls | 48-hour recall of leisure-time physical activities; activities defined as capable of reaching 7.5 kcal/min were defined as vigorous | First CHD attack (fatal and nonfatal) |
| Brunner et al. (1974) | 5,288 male and 5,229 female residents of 58 Israeli kibbutzim aged 40–69 years; 15-year follow-up | Work types classified as sedentary or nonsedentary | Fatal and nonfatal CHD, males (n = 281) and females (n = 70) |

| Main findings | Dose response[*] | Adjustment for confounders and other comments |
|---|---|---|
| Inverse association; relative to men whose main job responsibility was driving buses, conductors had an age-adjusted risk of first coronary episode of 0.70 | NA | No control for confounding; results were similar in subgroup of men who died of CHD-associated conditions |
| Inverse association; RR for IMF for persons in light occupations was 1.97 relative to heavy group; active group rate was intermediate | Yes | No control for confounding; one of few pathology studies |
| Inverse association; RR for arteriosclerotic disease among clerks was 2.03 relative to that for section men; risk estimate for switchmen was 1.46 | Yes | No control for confounding; specific analyses were consistent with overall results |
| Inverse and null associations; among employees classified by their original occupational category, the age-adjusted risk for CHD death for clerks relative to carriers was 1.26 | NA | No control for confounding; extensive efforts made to consider and evaluate job transfers |
| Inverse association; age-adjusted risk of CHD incidence among drivers was 1.8 relative to that for conductors | NA | Medical evaluation data used to control for confounding variables |
| Inverse association; age-adjusted risk of CHD among sedentary, nonfarm occupations relative to that for active nonfarm occupations was 1.8 | NA | Data also available on black residents; comparisons between sedentary and active occupations not possible |
| Inverse association; RR estimate for first attack among vigorous group = 0.33 compared with nonvigorous group | NA | Only study to analyze 48-hour recall of leisure-time physical activity (5-minute intervals) |
| Inverse association; risk for CHD incidence among those engaged in sedentary work compared with that for nonsedentary peers was 2.52 for men and 3.28 for women | NA | No differences in serum cholesterol and body weight between groups |

**Table 4-2.** *Continued*

| Study | Population | Definition of physical activity or cardiorespiratory fitness | Definition of coronary heart disease |
|-------|-----------|-----------------------------------------------|------------------------|
| Paffenbarger and Hale (1975) | 6,351 San Francisco Bay Area longshoremen aged 35–74 years; followed for 22 years, from 1951 to death or to age 75 | Work-years according to required energy output: heavy (5.2–7.5 kcal/min), moderate (2.4–5.0 kcal/min), and light (1.5–2.0 kcal/min) | CHD death (ICD-7 420) (n = 598) |
| Paffenbarger et al. (1977) | 3,686 San Francisco Bay Area longshoremen aged 35–74 years; followed for 22 years, from 1951 to death or to age 75 | Work-years according to required energy output: high (5.2–7.5 kcal/min), intermediate (2.4–5.0 kcal/min), and light (1.5–2.0 kcal/min) | CHD death (ICD-7 420) (n = 395) |
| Rosenman, Bawol, Oscherwitz (1977) | 2,065 white male San Francisco Bay Area federal employees aged 35–59 years; 4-year follow-up | Occupational physical activity; estimated caloric expenditure for work and nonwork activity | Fatal and nonfatal CHD (n = 65) |
| Chave et al. (1978) | 3,591 British male executive-grade civil servants aged 40–64 years; 8.5-year average follow-up from 1968 to 1970 | 48-hour leisure-time physical activity recall; activities capable of reaching 7.5 kcal/min defined as vigorous | Fatal and nonfatal first CHD attack (n = 268) |
| Paffenbarger, Wing, Hyde (1978) | 16,936 Harvard male alumni aged 35–74 years; followed up for 6–10 years | Physical activity index based on self-report of stairs climbed, blocks walked, and strenuous sports play | Fatal and nonfatal first heart attack (n = 572) |
| Morris et al. (1980) | 17,944 British male executive grade civil servants aged 40–64 years; 8.5-year average follow-up from 1968 to 1970 | 48-hour recall of leisure-time physical activities; activities defined as capable of reaching 7.5 kcal/min were defined as vigorous | Fatal and nonfatal first heart attack (n =1,138) |
| Salonen et al. (1982) | 3,829 women and 4,110 men aged 30–59 years from Eastern Finland; 7-year follow-up | Dichotomous assessment of occupational and leisure-time physical activity (low/high) | Fatal acute ischemic heart disease (ICD-8, 410–412) (n = 89 men and 14 women) and acute myocardial infarction (ICD-8, 410–411) (n = 210 men and 63 women) |
| Pomrehn et al. (1982) | 61,922 deaths from 1964–1978 among Iowa men aged 20 to 64 years | Occupational classification; farmers vs. nonfarmers | Death from ischemic heart disease |

| Main findings | Dose response* | Adjustment for confounders and other comments |
|---|---|---|
| Inverse association; relative to heavy category, age-adjusted RR of CHD death was 1.70 in moderate and 1.80 in light categories | Yes | No control for confounding variables; efforts made to evaluate job changes in the cohort over time |
| Inverse association overall, inverse for younger birth cohorts and null for older cohorts; relative to high category, age-adjusted RRs of CHD death were 1.8 in intermediate and 1.60 in light categories | No/Yes | Dose response noted in age-adjusted rates only for two younger groups; two older groups exhibited no association |
| Null association | No | Relatively short-term follow-up |
| Inverse association; risk of CHD attack among men reporting nonvigorous exercise relative to men reporting vigorous exercise was 2.2 | NA | Preliminary report of further data of Morris et al. 1980 |
| Inverse association; age-adjusted RR of first heart attack for men who expended fewer than 2,000 kcal/week was 1.64 compared with men who expended 2,000 or more kcal/week | Yes | History of athleticism not associated with lower risk unless there was also current energy expenditure |
| Inverse association; age-adjusted risk of CHD attack among men reporting nonvigorous exercise relative to those reporting vigorous exercise was 2.2 | NA | Increased risk similar for fatal and nonfatal attacks |
| Inverse association; RR of acute myocardial infarction for men and women with low levels of physical activity at work = 1.5 (90% CI, 1.2–2.0) for men and 2.4 (90% CI, 1.5–3.7) for women | NA | No associations with leisure-time physical activity; extensive adjustment for confounding |
| Farm men had significantly less mortality than expected from the experience in the general population of Iowa men (SMR = 0.89) | NA | No adjustment for confounding |

**Table 4-2.** *Continued*

| Study | Population | Definition of physical activity or cardiorespiratory fitness | Definition of coronary heart disease |
|---|---|---|---|
| Garcia-Palmieri et al. (1982) | 8,793 Puerto Rican men aged 45–64 years; followed for up to 8.25 years | Usual 24-hour physical activity index based on hours/day at specific intensity | CHD incidence other than angina pectoris (n = 335) |
| Paffenbarger et al. (1984) | 16,936 US male college alumni who entered college between 1916 and 1950; followed from 1962 to 1978 | Physical activity index estimated from reports of stairs climbed, city blocks walked, and sports played each week | Death due to CHD (n = 441) |
| Yano, Reed, McGee (1984) | 7,705 Hawaiian men of Japanese ancestry aged 45–68 years with no history of heart disease; 10-year follow-up | Self-report of 24-hour habitual physical activity in 1965–1968 | Incident cases of fatal and nonfatal CHD (n = 511) |
| Menotti and Seccareccia (1985) | 99,029 Italian male railroad employees aged 40–59 years; 5-year follow-up | Occupational physical activity (heavy, moderate, sedentary) | Fatal myocardial infarction (n = 614) |
| Kannel et al. (1986) | 1,166 Framingham (MA) men aged 45–64 years; 24-year follow-up | Physical activity index based on hours per day at activity-specific intensity; occupational physical activity classified by physical demand of work | Death due to CHD (n = 220) |
| Lapidus and Bengtsson (1986) | 1,462 Swedish women aged 38–60 years; follow-up between 1968 and 1981 | Physical activity at work and during leisure hours, lifetime, and during previous years | Nonfatal myocardial infarction and angina pectoris |
| Leon et al. (1987) | 12,138 North American men at high risk for CHD, aged 35–57 years; 7-year average follow-up | Leisure-time physical activity index; energy expenditure (minutes/week) | Fatal and nonfatal CHD (n = 781; 368 fatal) |
| Pekkanen et al. (1987) | 636 apparently healthy Finnish men aged 45–64 years, followed for 20 years from 1964 baseline | Occupational and transport/recreational physical activity (high or low) | Death due to CHD (n = 106) |
| Sobolski et al. (1987) | 2,109 Belgian men aged 40–55 years in 1976–1978; 5-year follow-up | Occupational and leisure-time physical activity (4 categories each) | Incident cases of fatal and nonfatal myocardial infarction and sudden death (n = 36) |

| Main findings | Dose response[*] | Adjustment for confounders and other comments |
|---|---|---|
| Inverse association; physical activity index was significantly related to lower risk of CHD in urban as well as rural men | Yes | Significant inverse relationship for CHD after multivariate adjustment |
| Inverse association; relative to highest category of index (2,000+ kcal/week), risk estimates in next two lower categories were 1.28 and 1.84, respectively | Yes | Significant dose-response after adjusting for age, smoking, and hypertension prevalence |
| Inverse association; significant only for all CHD; no significant association for various subtypes | NA | Adjusted for age, blood pressure, cholesterol, BMI, serum glucose, vital capacity, etc. |
| Inverse association; relative to sedentary, men in moderate and heavy occupational activity had RRs of 0.97 and 0.64, respectively | Yes | Adjusted for age |
| Inverse association; age-adjusted RR (relative to high category) = 1.38 (low), 1.21 (moderate); for occupational activity, age-adjusted RR (relative to heavy category) = 1.27 (sedentary), 1.22 (light), 0.99 (medium) | Yes | Inverse association constant across all analyses and maintained after controlling for multivariate confounding |
| Inverse association only for leisure-time physical activity; RR = 2.8 (95% CI, 1.2–6.5) comparing low leisure-time physical activity with all other categories | NA | Adjusted for age |
| Inverse association; multivariate adjusted risk estimate (relative to low activity tertile) was 0.90 (95% CI, 0.76–1.06) for more active and 0.83 (95% CI, 0.70–0.99) for most active | Yes | Dose response for fatal and nonfatal cases combined but not for CHD death or sudden death separately |
| Inverse association; adjusted RR for men in low physical activity group was 1.30 (p = 0.17) | NA | Association limited to second half of follow-up period |
| Null association for both leisure-time and occupational physical activity | No | One of two studies to simultaneously evaluate associations of physical activity, fitness, and CHD |

**Table 4-2.** *Continued*

| Study | Population | Definition of physical activity or cardiorespiratory fitness | Definition of coronary heart disease |
|---|---|---|---|
| Donahue et al. (1988) | 7,644 Hawaiian men of Japanese ancestry aged 45–64 years with no history of heart disease; 12-year follow-up | Self-report of 24-hour habitual physical activity in 1965–1968; 3-point scale defined by tertiles of distribution | Incident cases of fatal and nonfatal CHD (n = 444) |
| Salonen et al. (1988) | 15,088 Eastern Finnish men and women aged 30–59 years; 6-year follow-up | Self-reported leisure-time and occupational physical activity (4 levels collapsed into 2 categories each) | Death due to CHD (ICD-8 410–414) (n = 102 90 men, 12 women) |
| Johansson et al. (1988) | 7,495 Göteburg men aged 47–55 years at entry; 11.8-year average follow-up | Physical activity at work and physical activity during leisure time (4-point scale for each) | Incident cases of fatal and nonfatal CHD |
| Slattery, Jacobs, Nichaman (1989) | 3,043 US male railroad employees; followed for 17–20 years | Leisure-time physical activity index (kcal/week) | Death due to CHD (ICD-8 410–414) |
| Morris et al. (1990) | 9,376 British male middle grade executives aged 45–64 years; 9.3-year average follow-up | Leisure-time physical activity reported over previous 4 weeks; energy expenditure values ascribed to reported activities | Fatal and nonfatal CHD (ICD-8 410–414) (n = 474) |
| Lindsted, Tonstad, Kuzma (1991) | 9,484 Seventh-Day Adventist men aged ≥ 30 years; 26-year follow-up | Self-report to single physical activity question | Ischemic heart disease mortality (ICD-8 410–414) (n = 1,351) |
| Shaper and Wannamethee (1991) | 7,735 British men aged 40–59 years; 8.5-year follow-up | Self-report of physical activity at baseline; 6-point scale | Fatal and nonfatal heart attack (n = 488) |
| Seccareccia and Menotti (1992) | 1,712 men from Northern and Central Italy, aged 40–59 years, initially examined in 1960; 25-year follow-up | Occupational physical activity (self-report): sedentary, moderate, and heavy | Death due to CHD |
| Hein, Suadicani, Gyntelberg (1992) | 4,999 Copenhagen men aged 40–59 years; 17-year follow-up from 1970/1971 | Leisure-time physical activity (4-point scale) | Fatal myocardial infarction (ICD-8 410–414) (n = 266) |

98

| Main findings | Dose response* | Adjustment for confounders and other comments |
|---|---|---|
| Inverse association; RR among active men relative to sedentary men was 0.69 (95% CI, 0.53–0.88) for men aged 45–64 and 0.43 (95% CI, 0.19–0.99) for older men aged 65–74 | Yes | Adjusted for age, alcohol use, and smoking; bivariate adjustment for cholesterol, BMI, and blood pressure did not alter findings; follow-up to Yano, Reed, McGee (1984) |
| Inverse association; occupational: adjusted RR among inactive was 1.3 (95% CI, 1.1–1.6) relative to active; adjusted RR of CHD among leisure-time active was 1.2 (95% CI, 1.0–1.5) | NA | Point estimate for low leisure-time physical activity was adjusted toward the null after consideration of other CHD risk factors |
| Null association between physical activity at work and CHD risk; inverse association (not statistically significant) between leisure-time physical activity and CHD | No | Extensive control for confounding variables; ancillary analysis on postinfarction patients also yielded null association |
| Inverse association; adjusted risk estimate (relative to highest physical activity category) was 1.28 for sedentary group (not statistically significant) | Yes | Adjusted for age, smoking, cholesterol, and blood pressure |
| Inverse association; age-adjusted RR for 3 episodes per week of vigorous physical activity relative to sedentary group was 0.36 | Yes | No adjustment for confounding; association only noted for vigorous physical activity |
| Null association; risk estimates of CHD death exhibited a U-shaped relationship with increasing physical activity levels | No | Possible protective association among moderate activity group |
| Inverse association only for 2 activity levels; RR compared with sedentary for increasing physical activity levels: occasional 0.9 (95%CI, 0.5–1.3), light 0.9 (95% CI, 0.6–1.4), moderate 0.5 (95% CI, 0.2–0.8), moderately vigorous 0.5 (95% CI, 0.3–0.9), and vigorous 0.9 (95% CI, 0.5–1.8) | No | No clear linear trend |
| Inverse association; age-adjusted RR for moderate and heavy categories compared with that for sedentary group was 0.69 and 0.58, respectively | Yes | Inverse association remained statistically significant after adjustment for confounding |
| Inverse association; relative to more active men (categories 2–4 of index), least active men had an adjusted RR of CHD of 1.59 (95% CI, 1.14–2.21) | No | One of two studies to simultaneously evaluate activity and fitness in relation to CHD mortality |

**Table 4-2.** *Continued*

| Study | Population | Definition of physical activity or cardiorespiratory fitness | Definition of coronary heart disease |
|---|---|---|---|
| Shaper, Wannamethee, Walker (1994) | 5,694 British men aged 40–59 years; 9.5-year follow-up | Self-report of physical activity at baseline; 6-point scale data analyzed by hypertensive status | Fatal and nonfatal heart attack (n = 311; 165 normotensive, 146 hypertensive) |
| Rodriguez et al. (1994) | 7,074 Hawaiian men of Japanese ancestry aged 45–68 years; 23-year follow-up | Self-report of 24-hour habitual physical activity in 1965–1968 | Incident cases of fatal and nonfatal CHD (n = 340) |
| **Cardiorespiratory fitness** | | | |
| Peters et al. (1983) | 2,779 male Los Angeles County public safety employees aged < 55 years; 4.8-year average follow-up | Submaximal aerobic capacity estimated from cycle ergometer test; age-specific median split used to determine low/high fitness | Incident cases of fatal and nonfatal myocardial infarction (n = 36) |
| Lie, Mundal, Erikssen (1985) | 2,014 Norwegian employed men aged 40–59 years; 7-year follow-up | Near maximal cycle ergometer exercise test; total work in quartiles | Incident cases of fatal and nonfatal CHD |
| Erikssen (1986) | 1,832 Norwegian men aged 40–59 years; 7-year average follow-up | Near maximal cycle ergometer exercise test; total work in quartiles | Incident cases of fatal and nonfatal myocardial infarction and CHD death |
| Sobolski et al. (1987) | 2,109 Belgian men aged 40–55 years in 1976–1978; 5-year follow-up | Submaximal aerobic capacity estimated from cycle ergometry test | Incident cases of fatal and nonfatal myocardial infarction and sudden death (n = 36) |
| Ekelund et al. (1988) | 3,106 North American men aged 30–69 years; 8.5-year average follow-up | Submaximal aerobic capacity estimated from exercise test | Death due to CHD (ICD-8 410–414) |
| Slattery et al. (1988) | 2,431 US male railroad employees; 17- through 20-year follow-up | Submaximal exercise heart rate on standard (3 min) treadmill test evaluation | Death due to CHD (ICD-8 410–414) |
| Hein, Suadicani, Gyntelberg (1992) | 4,999 Copenhagen men aged 40–59 years; 17-year follow-up from 1970/1971 | Submaximal aerobic capacity estimated from cycle ergometer exercise test | Fatal myocardial infarction (ICD-8 410–414) (n = 266) |

| Main findings | Dose response* | Adjustment for confounders and other comments |
|---|---|---|
| Inverse association; statistically significant trend among nonhypertensive participants, U-shaped association among hypertensive participants | Yes/No | In hypertensive men, the protective effect of physical activity was eliminated with vigorous activity |
| Inverse association when adjusted only for age; null association when adjusted for cholesterol, blood pressure, BMI, diabetes, etc. | No | Follow-up report to that of Yano, Reed, McGee (1984) and Donahue et al. (1988) |
| Inverse association; RR for CHD incidence in low fitness group was 2.2 (95% CI, 1.1–4.7) compared with high fitness | NA | Similar results seen when men with electrocardiogram evidence of heart disease were excluded |
| Inverse association; point estimates and significance not reported | Yes | No adjustment for confounding variables |
| Inverse association; point estimates and significance not reported | Yes | No adjustment for confounding variables |
| Inverse association; RR for myocardial infarction and sudden death in low fit group was 1.6 relative to high fit | Yes | One of two studies to simultaneously evaluate associations of activity, fitness, and CHD |
| Inverse association; adjusted risk estimate of 3.2-fold increased risk of CHD death for a 35 beat/min increase in heart rate for stage II of exercise test | Yes | Extensive control for confounding influences |
| Inverse association; adjusted risk estimate for highest heart rate response group relative to lowest was 1.20 (95% CI, 1.10–1.26) | Yes | Risk estimate attenuated substantially after adjustment for other CHD risk factors |
| Inverse association; relative to more fit men, least fit men had an adjusted risk of 1.46 (95% CI, 0.94–2.26) | Yes | One of two studies to simultaneously evaluate activity and fitness in relation to CHD mortality |

Abbreviations: BMI = Body mass index (wt [kg] /ht [m]$^2$ ); CHD = coronary heart disease; CI = confidence interval; ICD = International Classification of Diseases (8 and 9 refer to editions); IMF = ischemic myocardial fibrosis; RR = relative risk.

*A dose-response relationship requires more than 2 levels of comparison. In this column, "NA" means that there were only 2 levels of comparison; "No" means that there were more than 2 levels but no dose-response gradient was found; "Yes" means that there were more than 2 levels and a dose-response gradient was found.

lipids in children (Lee, Lauer, Clarke 1986), and that CHD risk factor patterns persist from childhood to adulthood (Webber et al. 1991; Mahoney et al. 1991).

Recently, Armstrong and Simons-Morton (1994) reviewed the research literature on physical activity and blood lipids in children and adolescents, including over 20 observational and 8 intervention studies. They concluded that the cross-sectional observational studies did not demonstrate a relationship between physical activity level or cardiorespiratory fitness and total cholesterol, LDL-C, or HDL-C, especially when differences in body weight or fat were taken into account, suggesting that activity and body fat are not independently related to serum lipids. However, highly physically active or fit children and adolescents tended to have higher HDL-C than their inactive or unfit peers. The intervention studies generally showed favorable effects of exercise on LDL-C or HDL-C only in children and adolescents who were at high risk for CHD because of obesity, insulin-dependent diabetes mellitus, or having a parent with three or more CHD risk factors.

Alpert and Wilmore (1994) recently reviewed the research literature on physical activity and blood pressure in children and adolescents, including 18 observational and 11 intervention studies. These authors found evidence in studies of normotensive children and adolescents that higher levels of physical activity tended to be related to lower blood pressure. The associations were generally reduced in magnitude in those studies that adjusted for BMI, suggesting that lower body fat mass may at least partly explain why physical activity is related to lower blood pressure. Intervention studies tended to show that training programs lowered blood pressure by 1–6 mm Hg in normotensive children and adolescents, although the effects were inconsistent for boys and girls and for systolic and diastolic blood pressure. In hypertensive children and adolescents, physical activity interventions lowered blood pressure to a greater degree than in their normotensive peers (by approximately 10 mm Hg), although statistical significance was not always achieved because of small sample sizes.

Interpreting these studies on lipids and blood pressure in children and adolescents is hindered by several factors. Studies used a variety of physical activity categorizations, and the interventions covered a wide range of frequency, type, duration, and intensity, which were not all specified. The difficulties of assessing physical activity by self-report in children and adolescents, together with the highly self-selected population in the observational studies, may account for the less consistent findings on lipids and physical activity that were reported for children and adolescents than for adults. The relationship between dose of physical activity and amount of effect on blood pressure or serum lipids in children has not been adequately addressed.

Nonetheless, there appears to be some evidence, although not strong, of a direct relationship between physical activity and HDL-C level in children and adolescents. There is also evidence that increased physical activity can favorably influence the lipid profile in children and adolescents who are at high risk of CHD. Similarly, the evidence suggests that physical activity can lower blood pressure in children and adolescents, particularly in those who have elevated blood pressure.

## Stroke

A major cardiovascular problem in developed countries, stroke (ischemic stroke and hemorrhagic stroke) is the third leading cause of death in the United States (NCHS 1994). Atherosclerosis of the extracranial and intracranial arteries, which triggers thrombosis, is thought to be the underlying pathologic basis of ischemic stroke. Cigarette smoking and high blood pressure are major risk factors for ischemic stroke, whereas high blood pressure is the major determinant of hemorrhagic stroke. The studies cited in this section examined the association between reported level of physical activity and stroke. No published studies have examined the association between cardiorespiratory fitness and stroke.

Fourteen population-based studies (four that include women) relate physical activity to risk of all types of stroke; these closely parallel the study designs and populations previously cited for CVD and CHD (Table 4-3). Thirteen of the studies were cohort studies (follow-up range, 5–26 years). Only eight found an inverse association. As with the earlier studies on CHD, the earlier studies of stroke did not permit a dose-response evaluation. Among later studies that could do so by virtue of design, half did not find a gradient. This outcome, coupled with some suggestion of a "U-shaped" association in two studies (Menotti and Seccareccia 1985; Lindsted, Tonstad, Kuzma 1991), casts doubt on the nature of the association between physical activity and risk of both types of strokes combined.

Because of their different pathophysiologies, physical activity may not affect ischemic and hemorrhagic stroke in the same way; this issue requires more research. Only one study distinguished between ischemic and hemorrhagic stroke (Abbott et al. 1994). In this study, inactive men were more likely than active men to have a hemorrhagic stroke; physical activity was also associated with a lower risk of ischemic stroke in smokers but not in nonsmokers.

Thus the existing data do not unequivocally support an association between physical activity and risk of stroke.

## High Blood Pressure

High blood pressure is a major underlying cause of cardiovascular complications and mortality. Organ damage and complications related to elevated blood pressure include left ventricular hypertrophy (which can eventually lead to left ventricular dysfunction and congestive heart failure), hemorrhagic stroke, aortic aneurysms and dissections, renal failure, and retinopathy. Atherosclerotic complications of high blood pressure include CHD, ischemic stroke, and peripheral vascular disease. Although rates of hypertension have been declining in the United States since 1960, nearly one in four Americans can be classified as being hypertensive (DHHS 1995).

Prospective observational studies relating physical activity level or cardiorespiratory fitness to risk of hypertension are summarized in Table 4-4. Several cohort studies have followed male college alumni after graduation. One found later development of hypertension to be inversely related to the reported number of hours per week of participation in sports or exercise while in college (Paffenbarger, Thorne, Wing 1968). In a later follow-up of the same cohort, using information on physical activity during mid-life, vigorous sports were associated with a 19–30 percent reduction in risk of developing hypertension over the 14-year period (Paffenbarger et al. 1991). Follow-up of a different cohort of male college alumni similarly showed the least active men to have a 30 percent increased risk of developing hypertension (Paffenbarger et al.

1983). In a study of 55- through 69-year-old women followed for 2 years, the most active women were found to have a 30 percent reduced risk of developing hypertension (Folsom et al. 1990).

One randomized trial for the primary prevention of hypertension has been conducted. A 5-year trial of a nutrition and physical activity intervention showed that the incidence of hypertension for the intervention group was less than half that of the control group (Stamler et al. 1989). Participants in the intervention group lost more weight than those in the control group, reduced more of their sodium and alcohol intake, and were more likely to become more physically active. Although the effects of the nutritional and physical activity components of this intervention cannot be separated, the study does show that the risk for developing hypertension among persons who are at high risk for the disease can be lowered by weight loss and improvements in dietary and physical activity practices.

Like physical inactivity, low cardiorespiratory fitness in middle age is associated with increased risk for high blood pressure. After adjustment for sex, age, baseline blood pressure, and body mass index, persons with low cardiorespiratory fitness had a 52 percent higher risk of later developing high blood pressure than their fit peers (Blair et al. 1984).

Taken together, the cohort studies show that physical inactivity is associated with an increased risk of later developing hypertension among both men and women. Three of the studies had more than two categories of physical activity for comparison, and each demonstrated a dose-response gradient between amount of activity and degree of protection from hypertension. Point estimates for quantification of risk suggest that those least physically active have a 30 percent greater risk of developing hypertension than their most active counterparts. Unfortunately, none of these studies was conducted in minority populations, which have a disproportionate burden of hypertensive disease (DHHS 1995).

Several randomized controlled trials have been conducted to determine the effects of exercise on blood pressure in people with elevated blood pressure levels. The reduction of elevated blood pressure is important for preventing stroke and CHD, for which high blood pressure is a risk factor with a dose-response relationship (NIH 1992). Thirteen

**Table 4-3.** Population-based studies of association of physical activity with stroke (CVA)

| Study | Population | Definition of physical activity | Definition of stroke |
|---|---|---|---|
| Paffenbarger and Williams (1967) | > 50,000 US male college alumni aged 30–70 years | Participation in college varsity athletics (yes/no) | Hemorrhagic and ischemic stroke death (n = 171) |
| Paffenbarger (1972) | 3,991 US longshoremen aged 35 years and older; 18.5-year follow-up from 1951 | Occupational activity (cargo handler or not) | Hemorrhagic and ischemic stroke death (n = 132) |
| Kannel and Sorlie (1979) | 1,909 Framingham (MA) men aged 35–64 at 4th biennial examination; 14-year follow-up | Physical activity index based on hours per day spent at activity-specific intensity | Cerebrovascular accident (n = 87) |
| Salonen et al. (1982) | 3,829 women and 4,110 men aged 30–59 years from Eastern Finland; 7-year follow-up | Dichotomous assessment of occupational physical activity (low/high) | Cerebral stroke (ICD-8 430–437) morbidity and mortality among men (n = 71) and women (n = 56) |
| Herman et al. (1983) | 132 hospitalized Dutch stroke case-patients and 239 age- and sex-matched controls; men and women aged 40–74 years | Leisure-time physical activity (greatest portion of one's lifetime) ranging from little to regular-heavy | Rapidly developed clinical signs of focal or global disturbance of cerebral function lasting more than 24 hours or leading to death with no apparent cause other than vascular origin |
| Paffenbarger et al. (1984) | 16,936 US male college alumni who entered college between 1916 and 1950; followed from 1962–1978 | Physical activity index estimated from reports of stairs climbed, city blocks walked, and sports played each week | Death due to stroke (n = 103) |
| Menotti and Seccareccia (1985) | 99,029 Italian males railroad employees aged 40–59 years; 5-year follow-up | Classification of occupational physical activity (heavy, moderate, sedentary) | Fatal stroke (n = 187) |
| Lapidus and Bengtsson (1986) | 1,462 Swedish women aged 38–60; follow-up between 1968 and 1981 | Work and leisure physical activity assessed via 4-scales for lifetime and for the time before 1968 baseline | Fatal and nonfatal stroke (n = 13) |
| Menotti et al. (1990) | 8,287 men aged 40–59 years in six of seven countries from Seven Countries Study; 20-year follow-up | Classification of occupational physical activity (heavy, moderate, sedentary) | Fatal stroke (cohort analysis) |

| Main findings | Dose response* | Adjustment for confounders and other comments |
|---|---|---|
| Inverse association; nondecedents were 2.2 times as likely to have participated in varsity sports than were decedents; hemorrhagic strokes = 2.1, occlusive strokes = 2.5 | NA | Results adjusted for age only |
| Noncargo handlers were 1.11 times as likely as cargo handlers to die from stroke | NA | Results adjusted for age only |
| Inverse association between physical activity index and 14-year incidence of stroke | Yes | No statistical significance after controlling for several confounding variables |
| Inverse association with statistically significant RRs for men and women with low levels of physical activity at work were 1.5 (95% CI, 1.2–2.0) for men and 2.4 (95% CI, 1.5–3.7) for women | NA | Evidence for inverse association for low activity during leisure time, but no statistical significance after adjustment for other factors |
| Inverse association; relative to lowest physical activity category, risk estimates were 0.72 (95% CI, 0.37–1.42) for moderate and 0.41 (95% CI, 0.21–0.84) for high categories | Yes | Adjusted for a variety of potential confounding influences |
| Inverse association; relative to highest category of index (2,000+ kcal/week), risk estimates in next two lower categories were 1.25 and 2.71, respectively | Yes | Significant dose-response trend after adjusting for differences in age, cigarette smoking, and hypertension prevalence |
| Nonlinear "U" shape association; relative to sedentary category, men in moderate and heavy occupational activity categories had risks of 0.65 and 1.0, respectively | No | Age-adjusted only |
| Inverse association; women with low physical activity at work were 7.8 times as likely as others to have stroke (95% CI, 2.7–23.0); womenwith low physical activity leisure were 10.1 times as likely as others to have stroke (95% CI, 3.8–27.1) | NA | Age-adjusted only |
| Null association | No | No association after statistical adjustment for risk factors |

**Table 4-3.** *Continued*

| Study | Population | Definition of physical activity | Definition of stroke |
|---|---|---|---|
| Harmsen et al. (1990) | 7,495 Swedish men aged 47–55 years at baseline examination; 11.8-year average follow-up | Physical activity at work and leisure hours (low, high) | Fatal stroke (all and subtypes) (n = 230) |
| Lindsted, Tonstad, Kuzma, (1991) | 9,484 male Seventh-Day Adventists aged ≥ 30 years; 26-year follow-up | Self-report of physical activity level in 1960 (highly active, moderately active, low activity) | Fatal stroke (n = 410) |
| Wannamethee and Shaper (1992) | 7,735 British men aged 40–59 years; 8.5-year follow-up | Self-report of physical activity at baseline; 6-point scale defined on the basis of type and frequency of activity | Fatal and nonfatal stroke (n = 128) |
| Abbott et al. (1994) | 7,530 Hawaiian men of Japanese ancestry aged 45–68 years; 22-year follow-up | Self-report of 24-hour habitual physical activity in 1965–1968 (inactive, partially active, active) | Fatal and nonfatal neurologic deficit with sudden occurrence and remaining present for at least 2 weeks or until death (subtypes) (n = 537) |
| Kiely et al. (1994) | Four cohorts of Framingham (MA) men and women: cohort I—1,897 men aged 35–69 years; cohort II—2,299 women aged 35–68 years; cohort III—men aged 49–83 years; cohort IV—women aged 49–83 years; follow-up for cohorts I and II up to 32 years, for cohorts III and IV up to 18 years | Self-report of daily activity level; composite score formulated from index and categorized into high, medium, and low physical activity | Fatal and nonfatal first occurrence of atherothrombotic brain infarction, cerebral embolism, or other stroke (cohort I, n = 195; cohort II, n = 232; cohort III, n = 113; cohort IV, n = 140) |

| Main findings | Dose response* | Adjustment for confounders and other comments |
|---|---|---|
| Null association; relative to low physical activity category, slightly elevated estimates were observed for all strokes and subtypes for high activity group | No | No association after statistical adjustment for risk factors |
| Nonlinear "U" shape association; relative to low activity level, risk estimates were 0.78 (95% CI, 0.61–1.00) for moderate activity and 1.08 (95% CI, 0.58–2.01) for high activity | No | Adjusted for sociodemographic factors, BMI, and dietary pattern |
| Inverse association; statistically significant linear trend of lower risk of stroke with higher physical activity scale | Yes | Linear trend observed in men both with and without existing ischemic heart disease |
| Null association seen for all strokes and all subtypes for men aged 45–54 years | Yes, in older | No association of physical activity to risk of stroke in older smokers |
| Inverse association seen for all strokes and subtypes for men aged 55–68 years | No in younger | |
| Risk estimate relative to low physical activity group: cohort I—nonsignificant inverse association for medium group = 0.90 (0.62–1.31) and for high group = 0.84 (0.59–1.18); cohort II—nonsignificant nonlinear association for medium group = 1.21 (0.89–1.63) and for high group = 0.89 (0.60–1.31); cohort III—significant inverse association for medium group = 0.41 (0.24–0.69) and for high group = 0.53 (0.34–0.84); cohort IV—nonsignificant nonlinear association for medium group = 0.97 (0.64–1.47) and for high group = 1.21 | Yes, C I<br>Yes, C I<br>No, C II<br>No, C II<br>Yes, C III<br><br>No, C IV | Control for many confounding factors; nonlinear association in women only (cohorts III and IV); suggestion of threshold relationship (cohort III) |

Abbreviations: BMI = body mass index (wt [kg] /ht [m]$^2$); CVA = cerebrovascular accident; CI = confidence interval; ICD = International Classification of Diseases (8 and 9 refer to editions); RR = relative risk.

*A dose-response relationship requires more than 2 levels of comparison. In this column, "NA" means that there were only 2 levels of comparison; "No" means that there were more than 2 levels but no dose-response gradient was found; "Yes" means that there were more than 2 levels and a dose-response gradient was found.

Table 4-4. Population-based cohort studies of association of physical activity with hypertension

| Study | Population | Definition of physical activity | Definition of hypertension |
|---|---|---|---|
| Paffenbarger, Thorne, Wing (1968) | 7,685 men who attended the University of Pennsylvania between 1931 and 1940 and who responded to a questionnaire in 1962 | Reported hours per week of participation in sports or exercise in college | Self-reported incidence of physician-diagnosed hypertension from mail-back health questionnaire (n = 671) |
| Paffenbarger et al. (1983) | 14,998 US male college alumni who entered college between 1916 and 1950; followed from 1962–1972 (for 6–10 years) | Physical activity index (kcal/week) estimated from reports of stairs climbed, city blocks walked, and sports played each week, assessed by mail-back questionnaire in 1962 or 1966 | Self-reported incidence of physician-diagnosed hypertension from mail-back health questionnaire (n = 681) |
| Blair et al. (1984) | 4,820 US men and 1,219 US women patients of a preventive medical clinic aged 20–65 years at baseline | Maximal aerobic capacity estimated by exercise tests, categorized into "high" fitness (≥ 85th percentile) and "low" fitness | Self-reported incidence of physician-diagnosed hypertension (n = 240) |
| Stamler et al. (1989) | 201 US men and women with diastolic blood pressure 85–89 mm Hg or 80–84 mm Hg (if overweight) were randomly assigned to control or nutritional/ hygienic intervention (including exercise) | Self-report of moderate physical activity | Initiation of hypertensive therapy or sustained elevation of diastolic blood pressure ≥ 90 mm Hg |
| Folsom et al. (1990) | 41,837 Iowa women aged 55–69 years; 2-year follow-up | Self-reported frequency of leisure-time physical activity from mail-back survey | Self-reported incidence of physician-diagnosed hypertension |
| Paffenbarger et al. (1991) | 5,463 male college alumni from the University of Pennsylvania | Self-report of physical activity from mail-back questionnaire in 1962 | Self-reported incidence of physician-diagnosed hypertension from mail-back questionnaire in 1976 (n = 739) |

| Main findings | Dose response* | Adjustment for confounders and other comments |
|---|---|---|
| Inverse association; respondents who reported participation in sports or exercise fewer than 5 hours per week had a significantly increased age- and interval-adjusted risk of physician-diagnosed hypertension (RR = 1.30, p < 0.01) | NA | Adjustments for age and follow-up had little effect |
| Inverse association; alumni with < 2,000 kcal/week of energy expenditure had RR of 1.30 (95% CI, 1.09–1.55) of developing hypertension relative to others | Yes, especially in heavier men | Increased risk observed for less active alumni with stratification of student blood pressure, alumnus BMI, increase in BMI since college, and family history of hypertension |
| Patients in low fitness category were 1.52 times as likely (95% CI, 1.08–2.15) to develop hypertension as those in high fitness category | NA | Extensive control for confounding variables; no sex-specific analyses |
| Control group RR = 2.4 (90% CI, 1.2–4.8) of developing hypertension when compared with the intervention group | NA | Intervention was combined nutritional, weight loss, and physical activity |
| Inverse association; relative to women at low levels of physical activity, women at high and moderate levels had 30% and 10% lower age-adjusted risks of developing hypertension (RR high = 0.70, 95% CI, 0.6–0.9; RR moderate = 0.90, 95% CI, 0.7–1.1) | Yes | Adjustment for BMI, waist-to-hip ratio, cigarette smoking, and age eliminated the association with physical activity |
| Vigorous sports play in 1962 was associated with a 30% reduced risk of developing hypertension | Yes | Adjusted for age, BMI, weight gain since college, and parental history of hypertension |

Abbreviations: BMI = body mass index (wt [kg] /ht [m]$^2$ ); CI = confidence interval; RR = relative risk.

*A dose-response relationship requires more than 2 levels of comparison. In this column, "NA" means that there were only 2 levels of comparison; "No" means that there were more than 2 levels but no dose-response gradient was found; "Yes" means that there were more than 2 levels and a dose-response gradient was found.

controlled trials of habitual activity and blood pressure were analyzed in a meta-analysis by Arroll and Beaglehole (1992), and nine randomized controlled trials of aerobic exercise using the lower extremities (e.g., walking, jogging, cycling) and blood pressure were analyzed in a meta-analysis by Kelley and McClellan (1994). The two meta-analyses independently concluded that aerobic exercise decreases both systolic and diastolic blood pressure by approximately 6–7 mm Hg. Some of the studies were conducted with persons with defined hypertension (> 140/90 mm Hg), and others were conducted with persons with high normal blood pressure. Most of the studies tested aerobic training of 60–70 percent maximum oxygen uptake, 3–4 times/week, 30–60 minutes per session.

Three trials have specifically examined the effect of different intensities of exercise on blood pressure. Hagberg et al. (1989) randomly assigned 33 hypertensive participants to a nonexercising control group and to two groups participating in different intensities of exercise (53 percent and 73 percent of $VO_2$ max) for 9 months. Both exercise groups had comparable decreases in diastolic blood pressure (11–12 mm Hg), and the lower-intensity group had a greater decrease in systolic blood pressure than the higher-intensity group (20 mm Hg vs. 8 mm Hg). All the decreases were statistically significant when compared with the control group's blood pressure level, except the 8 mm Hg decrease in systolic blood pressure in the higher-intensity group. Matsusaki and colleagues (1992) randomly assigned 26 mildly hypertensive participants to two exercise intensities (50 percent $VO_2$ max and 75 percent $VO_2$ max) for 10 weeks. The pretest-to-posttest decreases in systolic and diastolic blood pressure in the lower-workload group were significant (9 mm Hg/6 mm Hg), but those in the higher-intensity group were not (3 mm Hg/5 mm Hg). Marceau and colleagues (1993) used a randomized crossover design to compare intensities of 50 percent and 70 percent $VO_2$ max training on 24-hour ambulatory blood pressure in persons with hypertension. A similar reduction in 24-hour blood pressure was observed for both training intensities (5 mm Hg decrease), but diurnal patterns of reduction were different.

These trials provide some evidence that moderate-intensity activity may achieve a similar, or an even greater, blood-pressure-lowering effect than vigorous-intensity activity. Because few studies have directly addressed the intensity question, however, the research base is not strong enough to draw a firm conclusion about the role of activity intensity in lowering blood pressure. It is not clear, for example, how the findings could have been affected by several issues, such as use of antihypertensive medications, changes in body weight, lack of direct intervention-control comparisons, dropout rates, and total caloric expenditure.

## Biologic Plausibility

Multiple physiological mechanisms may contribute to the protective effects of physical activity against CVDs. Postulated mechanisms involve advantageous effects on atherosclerosis, plasma lipid/lipoprotein profile, blood pressure, availability of oxygenated blood for heart muscle needs (ischemia), blood clotting (thrombosis), and heart rhythm disturbances (arrhythmias) (Haskell 1995; Leon 1991a; Gordon and Scott 1991).

Other effects of activity that may be associated with modifications of CVD risk include reduced incidence of obesity, healthier distribution of body fat, and reduced incidence of non–insulin-dependent diabetes. These other effects are discussed in later sections of this chapter.

### Atherosclerosis

Atherosclerosis begins when cholesterol is transported from the blood into the artery wall by lipoproteins, particularly LDL (Getz 1990; Yanowitz 1992). The formation of atherosclerotic plaques is increased at sites where the blood vessel lining is injured, which may occur in areas where blood flow is uneven (e.g., near the origin or branching of major vessels). An inflammatory reaction leads to the formation of atherosclerotic plaques in the wall of the artery.

In animal studies, exercise has been seen to protect against the effects of excess cholesterol and other contributors to the development of atherosclerosis (Kramsch et al. 1981). In addition, longitudinal studies of men with coronary artery disease have shown that endurance training, together with a cholesterol-lowering diet and interventions for other CVD risk factors, can help prevent the progression or reduce the severity of atherosclerosis in the coronary arteries (Ornish et al. 1990; Schuler et al. 1992; Hambrecht et al. 1993; Haskell et al. 1994). There is also an inverse relationship between cardiorespiratory fitness and ultrasound-measured severity of atherosclerosis in neck arteries to the head (carotid arteries) (Rauramaa et al. 1995).

### Plasma Lipid/Lipoprotein Profile

The relationships of physical activity to blood lipid and lipoprotein levels in men and women have been reviewed extensively (Leon 1991a; Krummel et al. 1993; Superko 1991; Durstine and Haskell 1994; Stefanick and Wood 1994). Of more than 60 studies of men and women, about half found that exercise training is associated with an increase in HDL. HDL, a lipid scavenger, helps protect against atherosclerosis by transporting cholesterol to the liver for elimination in the bile (Tall 1990). Cross-sectional studies show a dose-response relationship between the amount of regular physical activity and plasma levels of HDL (Leon 1991c). In these studies, the HDL levels of endurance-trained male and female athletes were generally 20 to 30 percent higher than those of healthy, age-matched, sedentary persons.

Moderate-intensity exercise training appears to be less likely to increase HDL levels in young to middle-aged women than men in the same age range (Leon 1991a; Kummel et al. 1993; Durstine and Haskell 1994). Moderate-intensity exercise was seen to increase HDL as much as more vigorous exercise in one randomized controlled trial of women (Duncan, Gordon, Scott 1991).

Studies have found that even a single episode of physical activity can result in an improved blood lipid profile that persists for several days (Tsopanakis et al. 1989; Durstine and Haskell 1994). Evidence also shows that exercise training increases lipoprotein lipase activity, an enzyme that removes cholesterol and fatty acids from the blood (Stefanick and Wood 1994). Exercise training also reduces elevated levels of triglycerides (Leon 1991c; Durstine and Haskell 1994), another blood lipid associated with heart disease.

### Blood Pressure

The mechanisms by which physical activity lowers blood pressure are complicated (Leon 1991a; American College of Sports Medicine [ACSM] 1993; Fagard et al. 1990) and are mentioned only briefly here (see also Chapter 3). Blood pressure is directly proportional to cardiac output and total resistance in the peripheral blood vessels. An episode of physical activity has the immediate and temporary effect of lowering blood pressure through dilating the peripheral blood vessels, and exercise training has the ongoing effect of lowering blood pressure by attenuating sympathetic nervous system activity (Leon 1991a; ACSM 1993; Fagard et al. 1990). The reduced sympathetic activity may reduce renin-angiotensin system activity, reset baroreceptors, and promote arterial vasodilatation—all of which help control blood pressure. Improved insulin sensitivity and the associated reduction in circulating insulin levels may also contribute to blood pressure reduction by decreasing insulin-mediated sodium reabsorption by the kidney (Tipton 1984).

### Ischemia

Clinical symptoms of atherosclerotic CHD occur when the heart muscle (myocardium) needs more oxygen than can be supplied from blood flowing through narrowed coronary arteries. This oxygen shortage leads to ischemia in the heart muscle—that is, to inadequate oxygenated blood for myocardial demand. Adaptations to a gradual reduction in blood flow may reduce the likelihood of myocardial ischemia. For example, new blood vessels may develop from other coronary arteries to provide an auxiliary blood supply (Cohen 1985). A person with advanced atherosclerotic CHD may remain free of symptoms at rest but may develop ischemic chest pain (angina pectoris) or electrocardiographic changes during physical exertion, which generally result from too high a myocardial oxygen demand for the blood supply available through partially occluded coronary arteries and collateral vessels (Smith and Leon 1992). Less commonly, angina pectoris may result from transient constriction (spasm) of a large coronary artery, generally at the site of an atherosclerotic plaque, or from spasm of small arterial vessels that have no evidence of plaque formation.

A recent review has summarized adaptations in the coronary circulation that are induced by endurance exercise training and that can decrease the likelihood of ischemia (Laughlin 1994). Data obtained primarily from research on animals have demonstrated that exercise leads to a greater capacity to increase coronary blood flow and an improved efficiency of oxygen exchange between blood in the capillaries and the heart muscle cells. These functional changes are the result of a remodeled vascular structure, improved control of blood flow dynamics, and promotion of biochemical pathways for oxygen transfer.

The first and most consistent structural adaptation to exercise is an increase in the interior diameter of the major coronary arteries and an associated increase in maximal coronary blood flow (Leon and Bloor 1968, 1976; Scheuer 1982; Laughlin 1994). The second vascular adaptation is the formation of new myocardial blood vessels (capillaries and coronary arterioles) (Tomanek 1994; Leon and Bloor 1968). Animal studies also have shown that exercise training alters coronary vascular reactivity and thereby improves control of blood flow and distribution (Overholser, Laughlin, Bhatte 1994; Underwood, Laughlin, Sturek 1994). This adaptation may reduce the incidence of spasms in the proximal coronary arteries and arterioles (Laughlin 1994). In addition, exercise training results in a reduced workload on the heart due to both an increase in compliance of the heart and a relative reduction in peripheral resistance; together, these reduce myocardial oxygen demand (Jorgensen et al. 1977).

### Thrombosis

An acute coronary event is usually initiated by disruption of an atherosclerotic plaque within an artery (Smith and Leon 1992). Platelet accumulation at the injury site initiates a cascade of processes leading to clot formation (thrombosis), which further reduces or completely obstructs coronary flow. A major obstruction of flow in a coronary artery may lead to the death of heart muscle (myocardial infarction) in the area served by that artery. These obstructions can, in addition, trigger potentially lethal disturbances in the rhythm of the heart (cardiac arrhythmia).

Thrombosis, usually occurring at the site of rupture or fissuring of an atherosclerotic plaque, is the precipitating event in the transition of silent or stable coronary artery disease to acute ischemic events, such as unstable angina, acute myocardial infarction, or sudden cardiac death, and in the occurrence of ischemic stroke (Davies and Thomas 1985;

Falk 1985). Endurance training reduces thrombosis by enhancing the enzymatic breakdown of blood clots (fibrinolysis) and by decreasing platelet adhesiveness and aggregation (which helps prevent clot formation) (Kramsch et al. 1981; Leon 1991b).

### Arrhythmia

Although persons with coronary artery disease have an increased risk of ventricular fibrillation (a life-threatening heart rhythm disturbance) during acute physical activity, persons with a healthy cardiovascular system do not incur this elevated risk (Siscovick et al. 1984; Mittleman et al. 1993; Willich et al. 1993; Thompson and Mitchell 1984; Thompson, Funk, et al. 1982; Haskell 1995; Dawson, Leon, Taylor 1979). Exercise training may reduce the risk of ventricular fibrillation in healthy persons and in cardiac patients by improving myocardial oxygen supply and demand and by reducing sympathetic nervous system activity (Leon 1991c). Evidence from epidemiologic studies shows that a physically active lifestyle reduces the risk of sudden cardiac death (Leon et al. 1987). A meta-analysis of studies that examined use of physical activity for cardiac rehabilitation showed that endurance exercise training reduced the overall risk of sudden cardiac death even among persons with advanced coronary atherosclerosis (O'Connor et al. 1989).

### Conclusions

The epidemiologic literature supports an inverse association and a dose-response gradient between physical activity level or cardiorespiratory fitness and both CVD in general and CHD in particular. A smaller body of research supports similar findings for hypertension. The biological mechanisms for these effects are plausible and supported by a wealth of clinical and observational studies. It is unclear whether physical activity plays a protective role against stroke.

## Cancer

Cancer, the second leading cause of death in the United States, accounts for about 25 percent of all deaths, and this percentage is increasing (NCHS 1996; American Cancer Society [ACS] 1996). The ACS has estimated that 1,359,150 new cases of cancer and 554,740 cancer-related deaths will occur among Americans during 1996 (ACS 1996). Physical inactivity has been examined as an etiologic factor for some cancers.

## Colorectal Cancer

Colorectal cancer has been the most thoroughly investigated cancer in epidemiologic studies of physical activity. To date, nearly 30 published studies have examined the association between physical activity and risk of developing colon cancer alone.

Studies that combined colon and rectal cancers as a single endpoint—colorectal cancer—are only briefly reviewed here because current research, summarized in this section, suggests that the relationship between physical activity and risk of colon cancer may be different from that for rectal cancer. Among nine studies that have examined the relationship between physical activity and colorectal cancer, one reported an inverse relationship (Wu et al. 1987), and three reported positive associations that were not statistically significant (Garfinkel and Stellman 1988; Paffenbarger, Hyde, Wing 1987 [for analysis of two cohorts]). One (Kune, Kune, Watson 1990) reported no significant associations, and in the four other studies (Albanes, Blair, Taylor 1989; Ballard-Barbash et al. 1990; Markowitz et al. 1992; Peters et al. 1989), the associations lacked consistency in subpopulations within the study, anatomic subsites of the large bowel, or measures of physical activity. Colorectal adenomas are generally thought to be precursors to colorectal cancers. A single study of colorectal adenomatous polyps has reported an inverse relationship between risk of adenomas and level of total physical activity (Sandler, Pritchard, Bangdiwala 1995). Another study of colorectal adenomas also found an inverse association, but only for running or bicycling, and only with one of two different comparison groups (Little et al. 1993).

### Colon Cancer

Of the 29 studies of colon cancer, 18 used job title as the only measure of physical activity and thus addressed only occupational physical activity. These studies are a mix of mortality and incidence studies, and few have evaluated possible confounding by socioeconomic status, diet, and other possible risk factors for colon cancer. Nonetheless, findings from these 18 studies have been remarkably consistent: 14 studies (Brownson et al. 1989; Brownson et al. 1991; Chow et al. 1993; Dosemeci et al. 1993; Fraser and Pearce 1993; Fredriksson, Bengtsson, Hardell 1989; Garabrant et al. 1984; Gerhardsson et al. 1986; Kato, Tominaga, Ikari 1990; Lynge and Thygesen 1988; Marti and Minder 1989; Peters et al. 1989; Vena et al. 1985; Vena et al. 1987) reported a statistically significant inverse relationship between estimated occupational physical activity and risk of colon cancer. Four studies (Arbman et al. 1993; Vetter et al. 1992; Vlajinac, Jarebinski, Adanja 1987; Vineis, Ciccone, Magnino 1993) found no significant relationship between occupational physical activity and risk of colon cancer. The 18 studies were conducted in a variety of study populations in China, Denmark, Japan, New Zealand, Sweden, Switzerland, Turkey, and the United States.

Eleven studies assessed the association between leisure-time or total physical activity and colon cancer risk in 13 different study populations (Table 4-5). These studies either measured physical activity and tracked participants over time to ascertain colon cancer outcomes or compared recalled histories of physical activity among colon cancer patients with those among controls. In eight study populations, an inverse association was reported between physical activity and risk of colon cancer, and results were generally consistent for men and women. The three studies that examined the effect of physical activity during early adulthood (Polednak 1976; Paffenbarger, Hyde, Wing 1987; Marcus, Newcomb, Storer 1994) found no effect, which could indicate that the earlier activity did not affect risk of colon cancer later in life. In studies that used more than two categories of physical activity, 10 potential dose-response relationships between level of physical activity or cardiorespiratory fitness and colon cancer risk were evaluated. Five of these showed a statistically significant inverse dose-response gradient, one showed an inverse dose-response gradient that was not statistically significant, three showed no gradient, and one showed a positive relationship that was not statistically significant.

Two studies of colon adenomas (Giovannucci et al. 1995; Kono et al. 1991) reported an inverse relationship between leisure-time physical activity and risk of colon adenomas.

**Table 4-5.** Epidemiologic studies of leisure-time or leisure-time plus occupational physical activity[*] and colon cancer

| Study | Population | Definition of physical activity | Definition of cancer |
|---|---|---|---|
| Polednak (1976) | Cohort of 8,393 former US college men | College athletic status; major, minor, and nonathlete | Colon cancer mortality (n = 107) |
| Paffenbarger, Hyde, Wing (1987) | Cohort of 51,977 male, 4,706 female former US college students | Sports play in college | Colon cancer incidence (n = 201) |
| | Cohort of 16,936 male US college alumni aged 35–74 years | Physical activity index (kcal/week) | Colon cancer mortality (n = 44) |
| Gerhardsson, Floderus, Norell (1988) | Cohort of 16,477 Swedish men and women twins aged 43–82 years | Categories of occupational and leisure-time activity | Colon cancer incidence |
| Slattery et al. (1988) | Cohort of Utah men (110 cases and 180 controls) and women (119 cases and 204 controls) aged 40–79 years | Occupational and leisure-time activity were both assessed by total energy expended | Colon cancer incidence |
| Severson et al. (1989) | Cohort of 7,925 Japanese men aged 46–65 years | Physical activity index from Framingham study and heart rate | Colon cancer incidence (n = 172) |
| Gerhardsson et al. (1990) | Swedish men (163 cases) and women (189 cases) and 512 controls; all ages | Categories of occupational and leisure-time activity | Colon cancer incidence |
| Whittemore et al. (1990) | North American Chinese men (179 cases and 698 controls) and women (114 cases and 494 controls) aged ≥ 20 years | Time per day spent sleeping/ reclining, sitting, in light or moderate activity, and in vigorous activity | Colon cancer incidence |
| | Asian Chinese men (95 cases and 678 controls) and women (78 cases and 618 controls) aged 20–79 years | Time per day spent sleeping/ reclining, sitting, in light or moderate activity, and in vigorous activity | Colon cancer incidence |
| Lee, Paffenbarger, Hsieh (1991) | Cohort of 7,148 male male US college alumni aged 30–79 years | Index of energy expenditure based on stair climbing, walking, and sports/recreation, assessed 2 times > 11 years apart | Colon cancer incidence |

| Main findings | Dose response[†] | Adjustment for confounders and other comments |
|---|---|---|
| No differences in mortality | No | None |
| Sports play ≥ 5 hrs/week relative to < 5 hrs/week: RR = 0.91; p = 0.60 | NA | Adjusted for age (2 levels of activity) |
| Risk increased with physical activity index: p for trend = 0.45 | No | Adjusted for age, BMI, and smoking |
| Least active relative to most active for work and leisure: RR = 3.6 (95% CI, 1.3–9.8) | NA | Adjusted for age and sex (2 levels of activity); adjustments for possible confounders said to not change results |
| High activity quartile relative to low activity quartile; men: OR total 0.70 (90% CI, 0.38–1.29); women: OR total 0.48 (90% CI, 0.27–0.87) | Yes | Adjusted for age, BMI, dietary fiber, and total energyintake; greater effect with intense activity; population-based |
| High activity tertile relative to low activity tertile: RR 0.71 (95% CI, 0.51–0.99); high heart rate relative to low: RR 1.37 (95% CI, 0.97–1.93) | No<br>Yes | Adjusted for age, BMI |
| Low activity relative to high: work and leisure, RR = 1.8 (95% CI, 1.0–3.4) | Yes | Adjusted for age, sex, BMI, dietary intake of total energy, protein, fat, fiber, and browned meat surface; population-based |
| Sedentary relative to active: RR = 1.6 (95% CI, 1.1–2.4) for men, RR = 2.0 (95% CI, 1.2–3.3) for women | NA | Adjusted for age (2 levels of activity); population-based; adjustment for diet had little effect on findings |
| Sedentary relative to active: RR = 0.85 (95% CI, 0.39–1.9) for men, RR = 2.5 (95% CI, 1.0–6.3) for women | NA | Adjusted for age (2 levels of activity); population-based; no effect of physical activity after adjustment for diet |
| Highly active relative to inactive: RR = 0.85 (90% CI, 0.6–1.1); high lifetime activity: RR = 0.5 (90% CI, 0.3–0.9) | No | Adjusted for age |

Table 4-5. *Continued*

| Study | Population | Definition of physical activity | Definition of cancer |
|---|---|---|---|
| Marcus, Newcomb, Storer (1994) | Wisconsin women aged up to 74 years, 536 cases and 2,315 controls | Total strenuous physical activity during ages 14–22 years | Colon cancer incidence |
| Giovannucci et al. (1995) | 47,723 US male health professionals aged 40–75 years | Weekly recreational physical activity index based on 8 categories of moderate and vigorous activities | Colon cancer incidence (n = 201) |
| Longnecker et al. (1995) | US men aged > 30 years, 163 cases 703 controls | Leisure-time vigorous physical activity | Right-sided colon cancer incidence |

Dietary factors may confound or modify the association between physical activity and colon cancer risk (Willett et al. 1990). Five of the studies in Table 4-5 controlled for dietary components in analyses and continued to observe a significant inverse association (Gerhardsson, Floderus, Norell 1988; Slattery et al. 1988; Gerhardsson et al. 1990; Giovannucci et al. 1995; Longnecker et al. 1995), and in one study (Whittemore et al. 1990), adjustment for dietary intakes altered findings in one study population but not in the other.

Together, the research on occupational and leisure-time or total physical activity strongly suggests that physical activity has a protective effect against the risk of developing colon cancer.

### Rectal Cancer

Many of the studies on physical activity and colon cancer risk also studied rectal cancer as a separate outcome. Of 13 studies that investigated occupational physical activity alone, 10 reported no statistically significant association with rectal cancer risk (Garabrant et al. 1984; Vena et al. 1985, 1987; Gerhardsson et al. 1986; Jarebinski, Adanja, Vlajinac 1988; Lynge and Thygesen 1988; Brownson et al. 1991; Marti and Minder 1989; Peters et al. 1989; Dosemeci et al. 1993), two reported significant inverse associations (Kato, Tominaga, Ikari 1990; Fraser and Pearce 1993), and one reported a significant

direct association (i.e., increasing risk with increasing physical activity) (Arbman et al. 1993).

Six of the studies that investigated the association between leisure-time or total physical activity and the risk of developing rectal cancer failed to find a significant association (Gerhardsson, Floderus, Norell 1988; Severson et al. 1989; Gerhardsson et al. 1990; Kune, Kune, Watson 1990; Lee, Paffenbarger, Hsieh 1991; Longnecker et al. 1995). In another study, Whittemore and colleagues (1990) observed a statistically significant inverse association in one study population and no effect in the other. Paffenbarger, Hyde, and Wing (1987) found an inverse relationship in one cohort and a direct relationship in the other.

Taken together, study results on both occupational and leisure-time or total physical activity suggest that risk of rectal cancer is unrelated to physical activity.

## Hormone-Dependent Cancers in Women

Of the epidemiologic studies examining the relationship between physical activity and hormone-dependent cancers in women, 13 have investigated the risk associated with breast cancer, two with ovarian cancer, four with uterine corpus cancer (mostly endometrial), and one with a combination of cancers. It should be noted that studies of physical activity in women have been especially prone to misclassification problems because they did not

| Main findings | Dose response[†] | Adjustment for confounders and other comments |
|---|---|---|
| Any strenuous activity relative to none: RR = 1.0 (95% CI, 0.8–1.3) | No | Adjusted for age, family history, screening sigmoidoscopy, BMI; population based |
| Most active quintile compared with least active quintile, RR = 0.53 (95% CI, 0.32–0.88) p for trend = 0.03 | Yes | Adjusted for age, BMI, parental history of colorectal cancer, history of endoscopic screening or polyp diagnosis, smoking, aspirin use, and diet |
| Vigorous activity ≥ 2 hours/week relative to none: RR = 0.6 (95% CI, 0.4–1.0) | Yes | Adjusted for BMI, family history, income, race, smoking, and intakes of alcohol, energy, fat, fiber, and calcium |

Abbreviations: BMI = body mass index (wt [kg] /ht [m]$^2$ ); CI = confidence interval; OR = odds ratio; RR = relative risk.

[*]Excludes studies where only occupational physical activity was measured.

[†]A dose-response relationship requires more than 2 levels of comparison. In this column, "NA" means that there were only 2 levels of comparison; "No" means that there were more than 2 levels but no dose-response gradient was found; "Yes" means that there were more than 2 levels and a dose-response gradient was found.

include household work and child care in their assessment. Studies of leisure-time or total physical activity and hormone-dependent cancers in women are summarized in Table 4-6.

### Breast Cancer

Four of the 13 breast cancer studies considered only occupational physical activity. Two of those studies described significant inverse associations (Vena et al. 1987; Zheng et al. 1993), and two others reported no significant association (Dosemeci et al. 1993; Pukkala et al. 1993). Only two (Dosemeci et al. 1993; Pukkala et al. 1993) adjusted for socioeconomic status, and none gathered information about reproductive factors and thus could not control for those potential confounding variables.

The epidemiologic studies of leisure-time or total physical activity and breast cancer risk have yielded inconsistent results (Table 4-6). Of these 10 studies, two reported a significant inverse association (Bernstein et al. 1994; Mittendorf et al. 1995), three reported an inverse association that was not statistically significant (Frisch et al. 1985,1987; Friedenreich and Rohan 1995), three reported no relationship (Paffenbarger, Hyde, Wing 1987; Albanes, Blair, Taylor 1989; Taioli, Barone, Wynder 1995). The other two reported a direct association,

although in one this did not reach statistical significance (Dorgan et al. 1994), and in the other it remained statistically significant (after adjustment for confounding) only for physical activity at age 30–39 years (Sternfeld et al. 1993).

Even among the studies that controlled for potential confounding by reproductive factors, findings were inconsistent (Bernstein et al. 1994; Dorgan et al. 1994; Sternfeld et al. 1993; Friedenreich and Rohan 1995; Mittendorf et al. 1995; Taioli, Barone, Wynder 1995). Results were inconsistent as well among studies that included primarily postmenopausal women (i.e., all but the study by Bernstein and colleagues [1994]).

Nonetheless, it is possible that physical activity during adolescence and young adulthood may protect against later development of breast cancer. Five of the studies cited here have examined this possibility. Among these five studies, two found a strong and statistically significant reduction in risk (Bernstein et al. 1994 [RR = 0.42]; Mittendorf et al. 1995 [RR = 0.5]), one found a nonsignificant reduction in risk (Frisch et al. 1985 [RR = 0.54]), and two found a null association (Paffenbarger, Hyde, Wing 1987; Taioli, Barone, Wynder 1995). These studies thus lend limited support to the hypothesis that physical activity during adolescence

**Table 4-6.** Epidemiologic studies of leisure-time or leisure-time plus occupational physical activity[*] and hormone-dependent cancers in women

| Study | Population | Definition of physical activity | Definition of cancer |
|---|---|---|---|
| **Breast cancer** | | | |
| Frisch et al. (1985 and 1987) | Cohort of former US college athletes and nonathletes; 5,398 women aged 21–80 years | Athletic status during college | Breast cancer prevalence (n = 69) |
| Paffenbarger, Hyde, Wing (1987) | Cohort of former US college students, 4,706 women | Sports play during college | Breast cancer incidence and mortality |
| Albanes, Blair, Taylor (1989) | NHANES cohort: 7,413 women aged 25–74 years, in US | One question on nonrecreational activity, one on recreational activity | Breast cancer incidence (n = 122) |
| Sternfeld et al. (1993) | 254 cases and 201 controls in an HMO | Age-specific recreational activity levels | Breast cancer incidence |
| Bernstein et al. (1994) | Women ≥ 40 years; 545 cases and 545 controls in California, US | Participation in several leisure-time activities after menarche | Breast cancer incidence in situ and invasive |
| Dorgan et al. (1994) | Framingham Study cohort: 2,307 women aged 35–68 years, Massachusetts, US | Physical activity index | Breast cancer incidence (n = 117) |
| Friedenreich and Rohan (1995) | Australian women aged 20–74 years; 451 cases and 451 controls (matched) | Recreational physical activity index | Breast cancer incidence |
| Mittendorf et al. (1995) | US women aged 17–74 years; 6,888 cases and 9,539 controls | Strenuous physical activity at ages 14–22 years | Breast cancer incidence |
| Taioli, Barone, Wynder (1995) | All ages in US; 617 cases; 531 controls | Leisure-time physical activity at ages 15–22 years | Breast cancer incidence |
| **Ovarian cancers** | | | |
| Mink et al. (1996) | Iowa Women's Health Study; cohort of 31,396 postmeno-pausal women | Categories of physical activity | Ovarian cancer incidence (n = 97) |

| Main findings | Dose response[†] | Adjustment for confounders and other comments |
|---|---|---|
| Nonathletes vs. athletes: RR = 1.86 (95% CI, 1.0–3.47) | NA | Adjusted for age, family history of cancer, age at menarche, number of pregnancies, oral contraceptive use, smoking, use of estrogen, leanness |
| Sports play of ≥ 5 relative to < 5 hours/week RR = 0.96 (p value = 0.92) | NA | Adjusted for age |
| Sedentary relative to most active: RR = 1.1 (95% CI, 0.6–2.0) for nonrecreational; RR = 1.0 (95% CI, 0.6–1.6) for recreational | No | Adjusted for age; adjustment for confounders had little effect on results; suggestive of variable effects by menopausal status |
| For activity from age 30–39, high activity quartile vs. low activity quartile, postmenopausal OR = 2.3 (95% CI, 1.03–5.04); premenopausal OR = 2.8 (95% CI, 0.98–5.18) | Yes (opposite direction) | Adjusted for age, menopausal status, and potential confounders |
| ≥ 3.8 hours/week relative to 0 hours of leisure-time activity, RR = 0.42 (95% CI, 0.27–0.64) | Yes | Adjusted for age, race, neighborhood, age at menarche, age at first full-term pregnancy, number of full-term pregnancies, oral contraceptive use, lactation, family history of breast cancer, Quetelet index; population-based |
| High activity quartile relative to low activity quartile: RR = 1.6 (95% CI, 0.9–2.9) | Yes (opposite direction) | Adjusted for age, menopausal status, age at first pregnancy, parity, education, occupation, and alcohol |
| > 4,000 kcal/week in physical activity relative to none: RR = 0.73 (95% CI, 0.51–1.05) | Yes | Adjusted for BMI and energy intake; effects observed for premenopausal and postmenopausal cancer and for light and vigorous activity; population-based |
| ≥ daily strenuous activity relative to none: RR = 0.5 (95% CI, 0.4–0.7) | Yes | Adjusted for age, parity, age at first birth, family history, BMI, prior breast disease, age at menopause, menopausal status, alcohol use, and menopausal status x BMI; population-based |
| > 1,750 kcal/week relative to none: RR = 1.1 (95% CI, 0.5–2.6) | No | Adjusted for age, education, BMI, age at menarche, and prior pregnancy; hospital-based |
| Most active relative to least active: RR = 1.97 (95% CI, 1.22–3.19) | Yes (opposite direction) | Adjusted for age, smoking, education, live births, hysterectomy, and family history |

**Table 4-6.** *Continued*

| Study | Population | Definition of physical activity | Definition of cancer |
|---|---|---|---|
| **Endometrial cancers** | | | |
| Levi et al. (1993) | Switzerland/Northern Italy; 274 cases and 572 controls aged 31–75 | Categories of leisure-time and occupational activity | Endometrial cancer incidence |
| Shu et al. (1993) | Women in Shanghai, China aged 18–74 years, 268 cases and 268 controls | Occupational and nonoccupational physical activity index | Endometrial cancer incidence |
| Sturgeon et al. (1993) | US women aged 20–74 years; 405 cases and 297 controls | Recreational and nonrecreational activity categories | Endometrial cancer incidence |
| **Combined set** | | | |
| Frisch et al. (1985 and 1987) | Cohort of former US college athletes and nonathletes; 5,398 women aged 21–80 years | Athletic status during college | Cervix, uterus, ovary, vagina cancer prevalence (n = 37) |

and young adulthood may be protective against later development of breast cancer.

### Other Hormone-Dependent Cancers in Women

Too little information is available to evaluate the possible effect of physical activity on risk of ovarian cancer. Zheng and colleagues (1993) found no significant associations between occupational physical activity and risk of ovarian cancer. On the other hand, data from the Iowa Women's Health Study showed that risk of ovarian cancer among women who were most active was twice the risk among sedentary women (Mink et al. 1996).

Findings are limited for uterine corpus cancers as well. Zheng et al. (1993) found no relationship between physical activity and risk of cancer of the uterine corpus. Among the endometrial cancer studies, one (Levi et al. 1993) found a decreased risk associated with nonoccupational activity, and one (Sturgeon et al. 1993) found combined recreational and nonrecreational activity to be protective. Another study (Shu et al. 1993) found no protective effect of nonoccupational activity in any age group and a possible protective effect of occupational activity among younger women but not among older women.

In Frisch and colleagues' (1985) study of the combined prevalence of cancers of the ovary, uterus, cervix, and vagina, nonathletes were 2.5 times more likely than former college athletes to have these forms of cancer at follow-up. Because these cancers have different etiologies, however, the import of this finding is difficult to determine.

Thus the data are either too limited or too inconsistent to firmly establish relationships between physical activity and hormone-dependent cancers in women. The suggestive finding that physical activity in adolescence and early adulthood may protect against later development of breast cancer deserves further study.

| Main findings | Dose response[†] | Adjustment for confounders and other comments |
|---|---|---|
| Sedentary relative to active for total activity: RR = 2.4 (95% CI, 1.0–5.8) to RR = 8.6 (95% CI, 3.0–25.3) for different ages | Yes | Adjusted for age, education, parity, menopausal status, oral contraceptive use, estrogen replacement, BMI, and caloric intake; hospital-based |
| Low average adult activity quartile relative to high quartile: occupational age ≤ 55 years RR = 2.5 (95% CI, 0.9–6.3), age > 55 years RR = 0.6 (no CI given); nonoccupational RR = 0.8 (95% CI, 0.5–1.3) | No | Adjusted for age, number of pregnancies, BMI, and caloric intake; possible modification of occupational activity by age; population-based |
| Sustained (lifetime) activity, inactive relative to active: recreational RR = 1.5 (95% CI, 0.7–3.2) nonrecreational RR = 1.6 (95% CI, 0.7–3.3) | No | Adjusted for age, study area, education, parity, oral contraceptive use, hormone replacement use, cigarette smoking, BMI, and other type of activity; recent activity also protective; population-based |
| Nonathletes vs. athletes: RR = 2.53 (95% CI, 1.17–5.47) | N/A | Adjusted for age, family history of cancer, age at menarche, number of pregnancies, oral contraceptive use, smoking, use of estrogen, leanness |

Abbreviations: BMI = body mass index (wt [kg]/ht [m]$^2$); CI = confidence interval; HMO = health maintenance organization; NHANES = National Health and Examination Survey; OR = odds ratio; RR = relative risk.

[*]Excludes studies where only occupational physical activity was measured.

[†]A dose-response relationship requires more than 2 levels of comparison. In this column, "NA" means that there were only 2 levels of comparison; "No" means that there were more than 2 levels but no dose-response gradient was found; "Yes" means that there were more than 2 levels and a dose-response gradient was found.

## Cancers in Men

### Prostate Cancer

Among epidemiologic studies of physical activity and cancer, prostate cancer is the second most commonly studied, after colorectal cancer. Results of these studies are inconsistent. Seven studies have investigated the association between occupational physical activity and prostate cancer risk or mortality. Two described significant inverse dose-response relationships (Vena et al. 1987; Brownson et al. 1991). Two showed a nonsignificant decreased risk with heavy occupational activity (Dosemeci et al. 1993; Thune and Lund 1994). In one publication that presented data from two cohorts, there was no effect in either (Paffenbarger, Hyde, Wing 1987).

The remaining study (Le Marchand, Kolonel, Yoshizawa 1991) reported inconsistent findings by age: increasing risk with increasing activity among men aged 70 years or older and no relationship among men younger than age 70.

The 10 studies of leisure-time physical activity, or total physical activity, or cardiorespiratory fitness and risk of prostate cancer have also produced inconsistent results (Table 4-7). Two of the studies described significant inverse relationships (Lee, Paffenbarger, Hsieh 1992; Oliveria et al. 1996), although one of these (Lee, Paffenbarger, Hsieh 1992) observed this relationship only among men aged 70 years or older. Four studies found inverse relationships (Albanes, Blair, Taylor 1989; Severson et al. 1989; Yu, Harris, Wynder 1988; Thune and

**Table 4-7.** Epidemiologic studies of leisure-time or total physical activity or cardiorespiratory fitness and prostate cancer

| Study | Population | Definition of physical activity or cardiorespiratory fitness | Definition of cancer |
|---|---|---|---|
| **Physical activity** | | | |
| Polednak (1976) | Cohort of 8,393 former US college men | College athletic status, major, minor, and nonathletes | Prostate cancer incidence (n = 124) |
| Paffenbarger, Hyde, Wing (1987) | Cohort of 51,977 US male former college students | Sports play | Prostate cancer incidence and mortality (n = 154 ) |
| | 16,936 US male alumni aged 35–74 years | Physical activity index | Prostate cancer mortality (n = 36) |
| Yu, Harris, Wynder (1988) | US men, all ages, 1,162 cases and 3,124 controls | Categories of leisure-time aerobic exercise | Prostate cancer incidence |
| Albanes, Blair, Taylor (1989) | NHANES cohort of 5,141 US men aged 25–74 years | Categories of recreational and nonrecreational activity | Prostate cancer incidence |
| Severson et al. (1989) | Cohort of 7,925 Japanese men in Hawaii aged 46–65 years | Physical activity index from Framingham study and heart rate | Prostate cancer incidence |
| West et al. (1991) | Utah men aged 45–74 years, 358 cases and 679 controls | Categories of energy expended | Prostate cancer incidence |
| Lee, Paffenbarger, Hsieh (1992) | Cohort of US college alumni, 17,719 men aged 30–79 years | Physical activity index based on stair climbing, walking, playing sports | Prostate cancer incidence (n = 221) |
| Thune and Lund (1994) | Cohort of Norwegian 43,685 men | Recreational and occupational activity based on questionnaire; categories of occupational and leisure-time activity | Prostate cancer incidence (n = 220) |
| **Cardiorespiratory Fitness** | | | |
| Oliveria et al. (1996) | Cohort of 12,975 Texas men aged 20–80 years | Maximal exercise test | Prostate cancer incidence or mortality (n = 94) |
| | Cohort of 7,570 Texas men | Categories of weekly energy expenditure in leisure time | Prostate cancer incidence or mortality (n = 44) |

| Main findings | Dose response[*] | Adjustment for confounders and other comments |
|---|---|---|
| Major athletes relative to nonathletes, RR = 1.64 (p < 0.05) | No | None |
| Sports play ≥ 5 relative to < 5 hours/week, RR = 1.66; (p < 0.05) | NA | Adjusted for age (2 levels of activity) |
| Comparing ≥ 2,000 with < 500 kcal/week, RR = 0.57; p = 0.33 | No | Adjusted for age, BMI, and smoking |
| Most sedentary relative to most active menduring leisure time, RR = 1.3 (95% CI, 1.0–1.6) for whites, RR = 1.4 (95% CI, 0.8–2.6) for blacks | Yes | Adjusted for age; in multivariate analysis, findings no longer significant for whites; hospital based |
| Least active relative to most active individuals, RR = 1.3 (95% CI, 0.7–2.4); for nonrecreational RR = 1.8 (95% CI, 1.0–3.3); for recreational RR = 1.8 (95% CI, 1.0–3.3) | No<br>Yes<br>No | Adjusted for age; further adjustment for confounders said to not affect results |
| Most active relative to least active men, RR = 1.05 (95% CI, 0.73–1.51); for occupation, RR = 0.77 (95% CI, 0.58–1.01); high heart rate relative to low, RR = 0.97 (95% CI, 0.69–1.36) | NA<br>No<br>NA | Adjusted for age, BMI |
| Overall no association found | | For agressive tumors, physical activity was associated with increased risk, but this was not statistically significant |
| Men aged ≥ 70 years: comparing > 4,000 with < 1,000 kcal/week; RR = 0.53 (95% CI, 0.29–0.95); men aged < 70 years, RR = 1.21 (95% CI, 0.8–0.18) | No | Adjusted for age; no effect of activity at 2,500 kcal, the level found protective for colon cancer |
| Heavy occupational activity relative to sedentary, RR = 0.81 (95% CI, 0.50–1.30); regular training in leisure time relative to sedentary, RR = 0.87 (95% CI, 0.57–1.34) | No | Adjusted for age, BMI, and geographic region |
| Among men < 60 years, most fit relative to least fit, RR = 0.26 (95% CI, 0.10–0.63); among men > 60 years, no effect, RR not given | Yes<br>No | Adjusted for age, BMI, and smoking<br>Adjusted for age, BMI, and smoking |
| ≥ 3,000 kcal/week relative to < 1,000 kcal/week, RR = 0.37 (95% CI, 0.14–0.98) | No | Adjusted for age, BMI, and smoking |

Abbreviations: BMI = body mass index (wt [kg]/ht [m]$^2$); CI = confidence interval; RR = relative risk.

[*]A dose-response relationship requires more than 2 levels of comparison. In this column, "NA" means that there were only 2 levels of comparison; "No" means that there were more than 2 levels but no dose-response gradient was found; "Yes" means that there were more than 2 levels and a dose-response gradient was found.

Lund 1994), but these were not statistically significant, and one of the four (Thune and Lund 1994) showed this relationship only for those aged 60 years or older. Two studies found that men who had been athletically active in college had significantly increased risks of later developing prostate cancer (Polednak 1976; Paffenbarger, Hyde, Wing 1987). One study found no overall association between physical activity and prostate cancer risk but found a higher risk (although not statistically significant) of more aggressive prostate cancer (West et al. 1991).

The two studies of the association of cardiorespiratory fitness with prostate cancer incidence were also inconsistent. Severson and colleagues (1989) found no association between resting pulse rate and subsequent risk of prostate cancer. Oliveria and colleagues (1996) found a strong inverse dose-response relationship between fitness assessed by time on a treadmill and subsequent risk of prostate cancer.

Thus the body of research conducted to date shows no consistent relationship between prostate cancer and physical activity.

### Testicular Cancer

Two studies investigated physical activity and risk of developing testicular cancer; again, results are inconsistent. A case-control study in England found that men who spent at least 15 hours per week in recreational physical activity had approximately half the risk of sedentary men, and a significant trend was reported over six categories of total time spent exercising (United Kingdom Testicular Cancer Study Group 1994). A cohort study in Norway (Thune and Lund 1994) was limited by few cases. It showed no association between leisure-time physical activity and risk of testicular cancer, but heavy manual occupational activity was associated with an approximately twofold increase in risk, although this result was not statistically significant. Thus no meaningful conclusions about a relationship between physical activity and testicular cancer can be drawn.

## Other Site-Specific Cancers

Few epidemiologic studies have examined the association of physical activity with other site-specific cancers (Lee 1994). The totality of evidence provides little basis for a suggestion of a relationship.

### Biologic Plausibility

Because the data presented in this section demonstrate a clear association only between physical activity and colon cancer, the biologic plausibility of this relationship is the focus of this section. The alteration of local prostaglandin synthesis may serve as a mechanism through which physical activity may confer protection against colon cancer (Shephard et al. 1991; Lee 1994; Cordain, Latin, Behnke 1986). Strenuous physical activity increases prostaglandin $F_2$ alpha, which strongly increases intestinal motility, and may suppress prostaglandin $E_2$, which reduces intestinal motility and, released in greater quantities by colon tumor cells than normal cells, accelerates the rate of colon cell proliferation (Thor et al. 1985; Tutton and Barkla 1980). It has been hypothesized that physical activity decreases gastrointestinal transit time, which in turn decreases the length of contact between the colon mucosa and potential carcinogens, cocarcinogens, or promoters contained in the fecal stream (Shephard 1993; Lee 1994). This hypothesis could partly explain why physical activity has been associated with reduced cancer risk in the colon but not in the rectum. Physical activity may shorten transit time within segments of the colon without affecting transit time in the rectum. Further, the rectum is only intermittently filled with fecal material before evacuation. Despite these hypothetical mechanisms, studies on the effects of physical activity on gastrointestinal transit time in humans have yielded inconsistent results (Shephard 1993; Lee 1994).

### Conclusions

The relative consistency of findings in epidemiologic studies indicates that physical activity is associated with a reduced risk of colon cancer, and biologically plausible mechanisms underlying this association have been described. The data consistently show no association between physical activity and rectal cancer. Data regarding a relationship between physical activity and breast, endometrial, ovarian, prostate, and testicular cancers are too limited or too inconsistent to support any firm conclusions. The suggestion that physical activity in adolescence and early adulthood may protect against later development of breast cancer clearly deserves further study.

# Non–Insulin-Dependent Diabetes Mellitus

An estimated 8 million Americans (about 3 percent of the U.S. population) have been diagnosed with diabetes mellitus, and it is estimated that twice that many have diabetes but do not know it (Harris 1995). More than 169,000 deaths per year are attributed to diabetes as the underlying cause, making it the seventh leading cause of mortality in the United States (NCHS 1994). This figure, however, underestimates the actual death toll: in 1993, more than twice this number of deaths occurred among persons for whom diabetes was listed as a secondary diagnosis on the death certificate. Many of these deaths were the result of complications of diabetes, particularly CVDs, including CHD, stroke, peripheral vascular disease, and congestive heart failure. Diabetes accounts for at least 10 percent of all acute hospital days and in 1992 accounted for an estimated $92 billion in direct and indirect medical costs (Rubin et al. 1993). In addition, by age 65 years, about 40 percent of the general population has impaired glucose tolerance, which increases the risk of CVD (Harris et al. 1987).

Diabetes is a heterogeneous group of metabolic disorders that have in common elevated blood glucose and associated metabolic derangements. Insulin-dependent diabetes mellitus (IDDM, or type I) is characterized by an absolute deficiency of circulating insulin caused by destruction of pancreatic beta islet cells, thought to have occurred by an autoimmune process. Non–insulin-dependent diabetes mellitus (NIDDM, or type II) is characterized either by elevated insulin levels that are ineffective in normalizing blood glucose levels because of insulin resistance (decreased sensitivity to insulin), largely in skeletal muscle, or by impaired insulin secretion. More than 90 percent of persons with diabetes have NIDDM (Krall and Beaser 1989).

Nonmodifiable biologic factors implicated in the etiology of NIDDM include a strong genetic influence and advanced age, but the development of insulin resistance, hyperinsulinemia, and glucose intolerance are related to a modifiable factor: weight gain in adults, particularly in those persons in whom fat accumulates around the waist, abdomen, and upper body and within the abdominal cavity (this is also called the android or central distribution pattern) (Harris et al. 1987).

## Physical Activity and NIDDM

Considerable evidence supports a relationship between physical inactivity and NIDDM (Kriska, Blair, Pereira 1994; Zimmet 1992; King and Kriska 1992; Kriska and Bennett 1992). Early suggestions of a relationship emerged from the observation that societies that had discontinued their traditional lifestyles (which presumably included large amounts of regular physical activity) experienced major increases in the prevalence of NIDDM (West 1978). Additional evidence for the importance of lifestyle was provided by comparison studies demonstrating that groups of people who migrated to a more technologically advanced environment had higher prevalences of NIDDM than their ethnic counterparts who remained in their native land (Hara et al. 1983; Kawate et al. 1979; Ravussin et al. 1994) and that rural dwellers had a lower prevalence of diabetes than their urban counterparts (Cruz-Vidal et al. 1979; Zimmet 1981; Taylor et al. 1983; King, Taylor, Zimmet, et al. 1984).

Many cross-sectional studies have found physical inactivity to be significantly associated with NIDDM (Taylor et al. 1983; Taylor et al. 1984; King, Taylor, Zimmet, et al. 1984; Dowse et al. 1991; Ramaiya et al. 1991; Kriska, Gregg, et al. 1993; Chen and Lowenstein 1986; Frish et al. 1986; Holbrook, Barrett-Connor, Wingard 1989). Cross-sectional studies that have examined the relationship between physical activity and glucose intolerance in persons without diabetes have generally found that after a meal, glucose levels (Lindgärde and Saltin 1981; Cederholm and Wibell 1985; Wang et al. 1989; Schranz et al. 1991; Dowse et al. 1991; Kriska, LaPorte, et al. 1993) and insulin values (Lindgärde and Saltin 1981; Wang et al. 1989; McKeigue et al. 1992; Feskens, Loeber, Kromhout 1994; Regensteiner et al. 1995) were significantly higher in less active than in more active persons. However, some cross-sectional studies did not find that physical inactivity was consistently associated with NIDDM in either the entire population or in all subgroups (King, Taylor, Zimmet, et al. 1984; Dowse et al. 1991; Kriska, Gregg, et al. 1993; Montoye et al. 1977; Taylor et al. 1983; Fisch et al. 1987; Jarrett, Shipley, Hunt 1986; Levitt et al. 1993; Harris 1991). For example, the Second National Health and Nutrition Examination Survey and the Hispanic Health and Nutrition Examination Survey found that higher levels of occupational physical activity among Mexican Americans were associated with less NIDDM (Harris 1991). However, in contrast to findings from the First National Health and Nutrition Examination Survey (Chen and Lewenstein 1986), this association was not found for either occupational or leisure-time physical activity among blacks or whites.

Two case-control studies have found physical inactivity to be significantly associated with NIDDM (Kaye et al. 1991; Uusitupa et al. 1985). One was a population-based nested case-control study, in which women aged 55–69 years who had high levels of physical activity were found to be half as likely to develop NIDDM as were same-aged women with low levels of physical activity (age-adjusted OR = 0.5; 95% CI, 0.4–0.7) (Kaye et al. 1991). Moderately active women had an intermediate risk (OR = 0.7; 95% CI, 0.5–0.9).

Prospective cohort studies of college alumni, female registered nurses, and male physicians have demonstrated that physical activity protects against the development of NIDDM (Table 4-8). A study of male university alumni (Helmrich et al. 1991) demonstrated that physical activity was inversely related to the incidence of NIDDM, a relationship that was particularly evident in men at high risk for developing diabetes (defined as those with a high BMI, a history of high blood pressure, or a parental history of diabetes). Each 500 kilocalories of additional leisure-time physical activity per week was associated with a 6 percent decrease in risk (adjusted for age, BMI, history of high blood pressure, and parental history of diabetes) of developing NIDDM. This study showed a more pronounced benefit from vigorous sports than from stair climbing or walking. In a study of female registered nurses aged 34–59 years, women who reported engaging in vigorous physical activity at least once a week had a 16 percent lower adjusted relative risk of self-reported NIDDM during the 8 years of follow-up than women who reported no vigorous physical activity (Manson et al. 1991). Similar findings were observed between physical activity and incidence of NIDDM in a 5-year prospective study of male physicians 40–84 years of age

Table 4-8. Cohort studies of association of physical activity with non–insulin-dependent diabetes mellitus (NIDDM)

| Study | Population | Definition of physical activity | Definition of NIDDM |
|---|---|---|---|
| Helmrich et al. (1991) | Male college alumni | Leisure-time physical activity (walking, stair climbing, and sports) | Self-reported physician-diagnosed diabetes |
| Manson et al. (1991) | Female nurses | Single questions regarding number of times per week of vigorous activity | Self-reported diagnosed diabetes, confirmed by classic symptoms plus fasting plasma glucose $\geq 140$ mg/dl; two elevated plasma glucose levels on two different occasions; hypoglycemic medication use |
| Manson et al. (1992) | Male physicians | Single questions regarding number of times per week of vigorous activity | Self-reported physician-diagnosed diabetes |

126

(Manson et al. 1992). Although the incidence of diabetes was self-reported in these cohorts, concerns about accuracy are somewhat mitigated by the fact that these were studies of health professionals and college-educated persons. In these three cohort studies, two found an inverse dose-response gradient of physical activity and the development of NIDDM (Helmrich et al. 1991; Manson et al. 1992).

In a feasibility study in Malmo, Sweden, physical activity was included as part of an intervention strategy to prevent diabetes among persons with impaired glucose tolerance (Eriksson and Lindgärde 1991). At the end of 5 years of follow-up, twice as many in the control group as in the intervention group had developed diabetes. The lack of random assignment of participants, however, limits the generalizability of this finding. A study conducted in Daqing, China, also included physical activity as an intervention to prevent diabetes among persons with impaired glucose tolerance (Pan, Li, Hu 1995). After 6 years of follow-up, 8.3 cases per 100 person-years occurred in the exercise intervention group and 15.7 cases per 100 person-years in the control group.

It has been recommended that an appropriate exercise program may be added to diet or drug therapy to improve blood glucose control and reduce certain cardiovascular risk factors among persons with diabetes (American Diabetes Association 1990). Diet and exercise have been found to be most effective for controlling NIDDM in persons who have mild disease and are not taking medications (Barnard, Jung, Inkeles 1994). However, excessive physical activity can sometimes cause persons with diabetes (particularly those who take insulin for blood glucose control) to experience detrimental effects, such as worsening of hyperglycemia and ketosis from poorly controlled diabetes, hypoglycemia (insulin-reaction) either during vigorous physical activity or—more commonly—several hours after prolonged physical activity, complications from proliferative retinopathy (e.g., detached retina), complications from superficial foot injuries, and a risk of myocardial infarction and sudden death, particularly among older people with NIDDM and advanced, but silent, coronary atherosclerosis. These risks can be minimized by a preexercise medical evaluation and by taking proper precautions (Leon 1989, 1992). To

| Main findings | Dose response[*] | Adjustment for confounder and other comments |
|---|---|---|
| 0.94 (95% CI, 0.90–0.98) or 6% decrease in NIDDM for each 500 kcal increment | Yes | Adjusted for age, BMI, hypertension history, parental history of diabetes |
| 0.84 (95% CI, 0.75–0.94) for ≥ 1 time per week vs. < 1 time per week vigorous activity | No | Adjusted for age, BMI, family history of diabetes, smoking, alcohol consumption, hypertension history, cholesterol history, family of history coronary heart disease |
| 0.71 (95% CI, 0.54–0.94) for ≥ 1 time per week vs. < 1 time per week vigorous activity | Yes | Adjusted for age, BMI, smoking, alcohol consumption, reported blood pressure, hypertension history, cholesterol history, parental history of myocardial infarction |

Abbreviations: BMI = body mass index (wt [kg]/ht [m]$^2$ ); CI = confidence interval.

[*]A dose-response relationship requires more than 2 levels of comparison. In this column, "NA" means that there were only 2 levels of comparison; "No" means that there were more than 2 levels but no dose-response gradient was found; "Yes" means that there were more than 2 levels and a dose-response gradient was found.

reduce risk of hypoglycemic episodes, persons with diabetes who take insulin or oral hypoglycemic drugs must closely monitor their blood glucose levels and make appropriate adjustments in insulin or oral hypoglycemic drug dosage, food intake, and timing of physical activity sessions.

## Biologic Plausibility

Numerous reviews of the short- and long-term effects of physical activity on carbohydrate metabolism and glucose tolerance describe the physiological basis for a relationship (Björntorp and Krotkiewski 1985; Koivisto, Yki-Järvinen, DeFronzo 1986; Lampman and Schteingart 1991; Horton 1991; Wallberg-Henriksson 1992; Leon 1992; Richter, Ruderman, Schneider 1981; Harris et al. 1987). During a single prolonged session of physical activity, contracting skeletal muscle appears to have a synergistic effect with insulin in enhancing glucose uptake into the cells. This effect appears to be related to both increased blood flow in the muscle and enhanced glucose transport into the muscle cell. This enhancement persists for 24 hours or more as glycogen levels in the muscle are being replenished. Such observations suggest that many of the effects of regular physical activity are due to the overlapping effects of individual physical activity sessions and are thus independent of long-term adaptations to exercise training or changes in body composition (Harris et al. 1987).

In general, studies of exercise training have suggested that physical activity helps prevent NIDDM by increasing sensitivity to insulin (Saltin et al. 1979; Lindgärde, Malmquist, Balke 1983; Krotkiewski 1983; Trovati et al. 1984; Schneider et al. 1984; Rönnemaa et al. 1986). These studies suggest that physical activity is more likely to improve abnormal glucose tolerance when the abnormality is primarily caused by insulin resistance than when it is caused by deficient amounts of circulating insulin (Holloszy et al. 1986). Thus, physical activity is likely to be most beneficial in preventing the progression of NIDDM during the earlier stages of the disease process, before insulin therapy is required. Evidence supporting this theory includes intervention programs that promote physical activity together with a low-fat diet high in complex carbohydrates (Barnard, Jung, Inkeles 1994) or programs that promote diet alone (Nagulesparan et al. 1981). These studies have shown that diet and physical activity interventions are much less beneficial for persons with NIDDM who require insulin therapy than for those who do not yet take any medication or those who take only oral medications for blood glucose control.

Cross-sectional studies also show that, compared with their sedentary counterparts, endurance athletes and exercise-trained animals have greater insulin sensitivity, as evidenced by a lower plasma insulin concentration at a similar plasma glucose concentration, and increased [121]I-insulin binding to white blood cells and adipocytes (Koivisto et al. 1979). Insulin sensitivity and rate of glucose disposal are related to cardiorespiratory fitness even in older persons (Hollenbeck et al. 1984). Resistance or strength-training exercise has also been reported to have beneficial effects on glucose-insulin dynamics in some, but not all, studies involving persons who do not have diabetes (Goldberg 1989; Kokkinos et al. 1988). Much of the effect of physical activity appears to be due to the metabolic adaptation of skeletal muscle. However, exercise training may contribute to improved glucose disposal and glucose-insulin dynamics in both adipose tissue and working skeletal muscles (Leon 1989, 1992; Gudat, Berger, Lefèbvre 1994; Horton 1991).

In addition, exercise training may reduce other risk factors for atherosclerosis (e.g., blood lipid abnormalities and elevated blood pressure levels), as discussed previously in this chapter, and thereby decrease the risk of macrovascular or atherosclerotic complications of diabetes (Leon 1991a).

Lastly, physical activity may prevent or delay the onset of NIDDM by reducing total body fat or specifically intra-abdominal fat, a known risk factor for insulin resistance. As discussed later in this chapter, physical activity is inversely associated with obesity and intra-abdominal fat distribution, and recent studies have demonstrated that physical training can reduce these body fat stores (Björntorp, Sjöström, Sullivan 1979; Brownell and Stunkard 1980; Després et al. 1988; Krotkiewski 1988).

## Conclusions

The epidemiologic literature strongly supports a protective effect of physical activity on the likelihood of developing NIDDM in the populations studied. Several plausible biologic mechanisms exist to explain this effect. Physical activity may also reduce the risk of developing NIDDM in groups of people with impaired glucose tolerance, but this topic needs further study.

# Osteoarthritis

Osteoarthritis, the most common form of arthritis, is characterized by both degeneration of cartilage and new growth of bone around the joint. Because its prevalence increases with age, osteoarthritis is the leading cause of activity limitation among older persons. The etiology of osteoarthritis is unknown, and the risk factors and pathogenesis of osteoarthritis differ for each joint group.

Whether an active lifestyle offers protection against the development of osteoarthritis is not known, but studies have examined the risk of developing it in relation to specific athletic pursuits. Cross-sectional studies have associated competitive—as opposed to recreational—running at high levels and for long periods with the development of osteoarthritis seen on x-rays (Marti and Minder 1989; Kujala, Kaprio, Sarna 1994; Kujala et al. 1995). On the other hand, both cross-sectional and cohort studies have suggested that persons who engage in recreational running over long periods of time have no more risk of developing osteoarthritis of the knee or hip than sedentary persons (Lane 1995; Lane et al. 1986, 1993; Panush et al. 1995; Panush et al. 1986; Panush and Lane 1994). There is also currently no evidence that persons with normal joints increase their risk of osteoarthritis by walking.

Studies of competitive athletes suggest that some sports—specifically soccer, football, and weight lifting—are associated with developing osteoarthritis of the joints of the lower extremity (Kujala, Kaprio, Sarna 1994; Kujala et al. 1995; Rall, McElroy, Keats 1964; Vincelette, Laurin, Lévesque 1972; Lindberg, Roos, Gårdsell 1993). Other competitive sports activities in which specific joints are used excessively have also been associated with the development of osteoarthritis. For example, baseball pitchers are reported to have an increased prevalence of osteoarthritis in the elbow and shoulder joint (Adams 1965; Bennett 1941). These studies are limited because they involve small sample sizes. Further confounding these studies is the high incidence of fractures, ligamentous and cartilage injuries, and other injuries to joints that occur with greater-than-average frequency among competitive participants in these sports. Because joint injury is a strong risk factor for the development of osteoarthritis, it may not be the physical activity but rather the associated injuries that cause osteoarthritis in these competitive athletes. In a study by Roos and colleagues (1994), soccer players who had not suffered knee injuries had no greater prevalence of osteoarthritis than did sedentary controls. Regular noncompetitive physical activity of the amount and intensity recommended for improving health thus does not appear harmful to joints that have no existing injury.

## Physical Activity in Persons with Arthritis

Given the high prevalence of osteoarthritis among older people, it is important to determine whether persons with arthritis can safely exercise and be physically active. Experimental work with animals shows that use of injured joints inhibits tissue repair (Buckwalter 1995). More specifically, several studies have indicated that running accelerates joint damage in animal models where osteoarthritis has been experimentally induced (Armstrong et al. 1993).

In contrast, several short-term studies of human subjects have indicated that regular moderate-exercise programs, whether including aerobic or resistance training, relieve symptoms and improve function among people with both osteoarthritis and rheumatoid arthritis (Ettinger and Afable 1994; Allegrante et al. 1993; Fisher et al. 1991; Fisher et al. 1994; Fisher and Pendergast 1994; Puett and Griffin 1994). For example, it has been shown that after regular physical activity, persons with arthritis have a significant reduction in joint swelling (Minor et al. 1988). In other studies of persons with osteoarthritis, increased levels of physical activity were associated with improved psychosocial status, functional status, and physical fitness (Minor 1991; Minor and Brown 1993). Furthermore, regular physical activity of moderate intensity has been found to raise the pain threshold, improve energy level, and improve self-efficacy among persons with osteoarthritis (Minor et al. 1989; Chow et al. 1986; Holman, Mazonson, Lorig 1989).

## Biologic Plausibility

The biologic effects of physical activity on the health and function of joints have not been extensively investigated, but some level of physical activity is necessary to preserve joint function. Because hyaline cartilage has no blood vessels or nerves, mature cartilage cells (chondrocytes) receive nourishment only from the diffusion of substances through the cartilage matrix from joint fluid. Physical activity enhances this process. In the laboratory, putting pressure on cartilage deforms the tissue, creating pressure gradients that cause fluid to flow and alter osmotic pressures within the cartilage matrix (Hall, Urban, Gehl 1991). The effect of such loading on the metabolism of chondrocytes is not well described, but when loading is performed within the physiologic range, chondrocytes increase proteoglycan synthesis (Grodzinsky 1993). In contrast, high-intensity loading and repetitive high-impact loads disrupt the cartilage matrix and inhibit proteoglycan synthesis (Lammi 1993).

The role of normal loading is confirmed by the effect of inactivity on articular cartilage. Immobility leads to decreased cartilage proteoglycan synthesis, increased water content, and decreased cartilage stiffness and thickness. Disuse may make the cartilage more vulnerable to injury, and prolonged disuse causes loss of normal joint function as the joint cavity is obliterated by fibrous tissue.

Studies of running on joint function in dogs with normal joints have confirmed that running does affect the proteoglycan and water content of cartilage and does not lead to degeneration of articular surfaces or to degenerative joint disease (Arokoski et al. 1993). In contrast, in dogs with injured joints, running has been shown to cause arthritis (Buckwalter 1995).

## Conclusions

Physical activity is essential for maintaining the health of joints and appears to be beneficial for control of symptoms among people with osteoarthritis. Although there is no evidence that physical activity itself causes osteoarthritis, injuries sustained during competitive sports have been shown to increase the risk of developing osteoarthritis.

## Osteoporosis

Osteoporosis is characterized by decreased bone mass and structural deterioration of bone tissue, leading to bone fragility and increased susceptibility to fractures. Because bone mass and strength progressively decline with advancing age, this disease primarily affects older persons (Cummings et al. 1985). Osteoporosis is more common among women than among men, for at least three reasons: women have lower peak bone mass than men, women lose bone mass at an accelerated rate after menopause when estrogen levels decline, and women have a longer life span than men.

The most common potential fracture sites are vertebrae of the chest and lower back, the distal radius (or wrist), the hips, and the proximal humerus (NIH 1984). Vertebral fractures can occur spontaneously or with minimal trauma (e.g., bending forward or coughing); once deformed, the vertebrae never return to their normal shape. These fractures may be asymptomatic and discovered only incidentally on a chest or spine x-ray. Accumulation of such vertebral fractures causes a bent-over or hunchbacked posture that is generally associated with chronic back pain and often with gastrointestinal and abdominal problems related to a lowering of the rib cage.

In the United States, fractures of the hip account for 250,000 of the 1.5 million fractures that are attributed each year to osteoporosis. Hip fractures are associated with more deaths (a 15–20 percent 1-year mortality rate), permanent disability, and medical and institutional care costs than all other osteoporotic fractures combined (Cummings et al. 1985; Rankin 1993). By age 90, about one-third of women and about one-sixth of men will have sustained a hip fracture.

In both men and women, the development of osteoporosis may be related to three factors: a deficient level of peak bone mass at physical maturity, failure to maintain this peak bone mass during the third and fourth decades of life, and the bone loss that begins during the fourth or fifth decade of life. Physical activity may positively affect all three of these factors.

Physical activity may play a substantial role in the development of bone mass during childhood and adolescence and in the maintenance of skeletal mass as a young adult. This inference is partly based on findings that athletic young adults have a higher density of bone mineral than sedentary young adults (Kirchner, Lewis, O'Connor 1996; Grimston, Willows, Hanley 1993; Conroy et al. 1993; Nichols et al. 1994; Rubin et al. 1993), on reports that athletes have a differential density of bones according to the sport they train for (Robinson et al. 1995; Heinonen et al. 1995), and on evidence that increase in bone mass in university students is related to higher levels of physical activity (Recker et al. 1992).

Beyond this hypothesized function in youth, physical activity plays a well-established role throughout the life span in maintaining the normal structure and functional strength of bone. Prolonged bed rest or immobility causes rapid and marked reduction in bone mineral density (Krølner et al. 1983; Chesnut 1993; Donaldson et al. 1970). Of particular public health interest is the degree to which physical activity can prevent or slow the bone loss that begins occurring in women as a normal process after menopause. Cross-sectional studies of postmenopausal women have shown that bone mineral density is correlated with muscle strength (Sinaki et al. 1986; Sinaki and Offord 1988), physical activity (Sinaki and Offord 1988; Shimegi et al 1994; Jacobson et al. 1984; Talmage et al. 1986), and cardiorespiratory fitness (Pocock et al. 1986; Chow et al. 1986). Longitudinal studies of postmenopausal women have attributed increases in both cardiorespiratory fitness and bone mass to physical activity (Chow et al. 1987; Dalsky et al. 1988). There is some evidence that through physical activity, osteoporotic women can minimize bone loss or facilitate some gain in bone mineral content (Krølner et al. 1983; Kohrt et al. 1995). However, other studies have failed to show such benefits (Nelson et al. 1991; Sandler et al. 1989; Cavanaugh and Cann 1988). The intensity of the physical activity and the degree to which it stresses the bones may be crucial factors in determining whether bone mass is maintained. Thus it is likely that resistance exercise may have more pronounced effects than endurance exercise, although this has not yet been unequivocally established.

Several investigators have found that the positive effect of physical activity on the bones of both premenopausal and postmenopausal women depends on the presence of estrogen. In postmenopausal women, greater gain in bone density accrues when physical activity and estrogen replacement therapy occur simultaneously (Prince et al. 1991; Kohrt et al. 1995). In young, premenopausal women, however, excessive amounts of vigorous training may lead to a low estrogen level and secondary amenorrhea, with subsequent decreased bone mass and increased risk of stress fractures (Marcus et al. 1985; Drinkwater et al. 1984; Allen 1994).

The exercise-associated changes in bone mineral density observed over time among both premenopausal and postmenopausal women are much less pronounced than those differences observed cross-sectionally between active and sedentary persons (Drinkwater 1993). Cross-sectional studies demonstrate differences of 10–15 percent in bone mineral density at various sites (Aloia et al. 1988; Lane et al. 1986; Michel, Bloch, Fries 1989; Recker et al. 1992), whereas intervention studies show smaller gains of 1–5 percent (Krølner et al. 1983; Dalsky et al. 1988; Nelson et al. 1991; Pruitt et al. 1992; Drinkwater 1993). These differences may be due to differences in comparison groups, to follow-up duration insufficient to show large changes in bone mineral density, or to measurement at different skeletal sites. Still to be conducted are well-designed randomized clinical trials that are of sufficient size and duration to determine definitively the longitudinal effects of physical activity change or the differential effects of resistance and endurance activity on bone mineral density.

## Biologic Plausibility

Bone is a dynamic tissue that is constantly remodeling its structure by resorption and formation. Physical activity, through its load-bearing effect on the skeleton, is likely the single most important influence on bone density and architecture (Lanyon 1996). Bone cells respond to mechanical loading by improving the balance between bone formation and bone resorption, which in turn builds greater bone mass (Lanyon 1987, 1993). The higher the load, the greater the bone mass; conversely, when the skeleton is unloaded (as with inactivity), bone mass declines. Glucose-6-phosphate, prostaglandins, and nitric oxide play a role in mediating the mechanical loading effect on bone (Pitsillides et al. 1995; Turner et al. 1995; Tang et al. 1995). Because it is muscle that exerts the largest forces on bone during physical activity, the role of muscle mass and strength in maintaining skeletal integrity should be explored more fully.

Nonmechanical factors, such as age, hormonal milieu, nutritional intake, and medications, are increasingly being recognized as important determinants of the bone's response to mechanical loading (Lanyon 1996). The relative contributions of each of these factors are currently under study and are not yet clearly delineated. Animal studies confirm a difference in bone response to mechanical loading with age and by estrogen status (Turner, Takano, Owan 1995). The potential clinical relevance of this research is to better define the optimal amount and type of exercise for maintaining or increasing bone mass, particularly with aging or in the absence of estrogen replacement therapy after menopause.

## Physical Activity and the Prevention of Fractures and Falling

Studies of physical activity in relation to hip fracture in women have generally found a lower risk of hip fracture among those who were more active. Three cohort studies have reported such a protective effect. One showed a statistically significant protective effect among those reporting the most recreational activity at baseline (Farmer et al. 1989), one showed inverse but not statistically significant associations for both work and leisure-time physical activity (Meyer, Tverdal, Falch 1993), and one showed a significant protective effect of walking for exercise (Cummings et al. 1995). Case-control studies have been more equivocal. One such study found a significant protective effect for two levels of past activity, but for recent activity only moderate amounts of activity showed a significant protective effect (Jaglal, Kreiger, Darlington 1993). Another case-control study showed inconsistent effects across a variety of physical activity classifications (Cumming and Klineberg 1994).

Nonskeletal factors that increase the risk of fractures due to falls include limitations in activities of daily living (e.g., dressing and feeding oneself); compromised gait, balance, reaction time,

and muscle strength; impaired vision; medication use; and environmental hazards (Dunn et al. 1992; Gilligan, Checovich, Smith 1993; Tinetti, Speechley, Ginter 1988; Cummings et al. 1995). Various exercises may help prevent falls by improving muscle strength, functional capacity, gait, balance, and reaction time. Tinetti and colleagues (1994) showed a significant decrease in falls in the elderly concomitant with an improvement in balance and gait achieved through exercise. Province and colleagues (1995) demonstrated a protective effect against falls through general exercise and exercises designed to improve balance. Moreover, Fiatarone and colleagues (1994) have shown that even frail elderly persons who have multiple chronic diseases benefit substantially from resistance training. This well-controlled randomized trial demonstrated the importance of strength training in improving stair-climbing power, gait, and other measures of physical function. Moderate exercise-training techniques, such as tai chi chuan, have also been shown to decrease falling and to improve function in older adults by increasing or maintaining aerobic power, strength, and balance (Lai et al. 1995; Wolf et al. 1996; Wolfson et al. 1996).

## Conclusions

Physical activity appears to build greater bone mass in childhood and early adolescence and to help maintain peak bone mass in adulthood. Among women after menopause, physical activity may protect against the rapid decline in bone mass, but findings are inconsistent in this regard, and it is unclear whether muscle-strengthening (resistance) activity may be more effective than endurance activity for this purpose. Estrogen replacement therapy has been shown conclusively to decrease bone loss after menopause, and there is evidence that this effect is enhanced with physical activity. However, it is not clear whether physical activity alone, in the absence of estrogen replacement therapy, can prevent bone loss.

Physical activity, including muscle-strengthening (resistance) exercise, appears to be protective against falling and fractures among the elderly, probably by increasing muscle strength and balance.

# Obesity

Obesity, a major public health problem in the United States, plays a central role in the development of diabetes mellitus (West 1978) and confers an increased risk for CHD, high blood pressure, osteoarthritis, dyslipoproteinemia, various cancers, and all-cause mortality (Hubert et al. 1983; Bray 1985; Albanes 1987; Lee et al. 1993; Manson et al. 1995). The progressive weight gain often observed between the third and sixth decades of life may be partly explained by age-related changes: although energy intake tends to decline after the second decade of life, this decrease is insufficient to offset the greater decline in the amount of energy that most people expend throughout their adult years (Bray 1983; Federation of American Societies for Experimental Biology 1995). In addition to these age trends, population surveys indicate that the age-adjusted prevalence of overweight among adults in the United States has increased from about 25 percent in the 1970s to 33 percent in 1988–1991 (Kuczmarski et al. 1994). The increase is evident for all race and sex groups. This phenomenon is believed to be due to high rates of inactivity combined with easy access to energy-dense food (Blackburn and Prineas 1983).

Obesity, defined as an excess of adipose tissue, is difficult to measure in population-based studies. Most investigations have therefore either used a relative weight index, such as percent desirable weight (Metropolitan Life Insurance Company 1959), or have used BMI (defined by a ratio of weight to height) as a surrogate measure. Quetelet's index (weight [kg]/height[m]$^2$) has been the most frequently used BMI. Although these weight-height indices are strongly correlated with more direct measures of adiposity, such as underwater weighing, they have limitations: fatty tissue cannot be distinguished from muscle mass or edema, and associations between weight-height indices and adiposity may be nonlinear or may differ by age or ethnic group (Harrison et al. 1985; Garn, Leonard, Hawthorne 1986; Lillioja and Bogardus 1988). Despite these limitations, BMI has shown a monotonic association with mortality in several recent cohort studies (Lee et al. 1993; Manson et al. 1995; Willett et al. 1995).

Using nationally representative data, the CDC has defined overweight as a Quetelet's index at or above the 85th percentile for 20- to 29-year-olds

($\geq$ 27.3 kg/m$^2$ for women, $\geq$ 27.8 kg/m$^2$ for men), corresponding to 120–125 percent of desirable weight (NIH 1985; Kuczmarkski 1992; Kuczmarkski et al. 1994). The 95th percentile of Quetelet's index (32.3 kg/m$^2$ for women, 31.1 kg/m$^2$ for men), equivalent to a relative weight of approximately 145 percent, has been used to classify persons as severely overweight. Between 1976 and 1991, the mean weight of U.S. adults increased by 3.6 kg (almost 8 pounds), and 58 million American adults (33 percent) are now considered to be overweight (Kuczmarski et al. 1994).

Because substantial weight loss in adults is difficult to achieve and maintain (Dyer 1994), childhood obesity and its prevention have received increased attention. Overweight children are likely to remain overweight as adolescents and adults (Johnston 1985) and are subsequently at increased risk for high blood pressure, diabetes, CHD, and all-cause mortality (Abraham, Collins, Nordsieck 1971; Nieto, Szklo, Comstock 1992; Must et al. 1992). Moreover, paralleling the trend seen among adults, the prevalence of overweight among U.S. children and adolescents has increased substantially over the past decade (Shear et al. 1988; Troiano et al. 1995).

## Physical Activity and Obesity

It is commonly believed that physically active people are less likely to gain weight over the course of their lives and are thus more likely to have a lower prevalence of obesity than inactive people; accordingly, it is also commonly believed that low levels of physical activity are a cause of obesity. Few data, however, exist to evaluate the truth of these suppositions.

Several cross-sectional studies report lower weight, BMI, or skinfold measures among people with higher levels of self-reported physical activity or fitness (DiPietro 1995; Ching et al. 1996; Williamson et al. 1993; French et al. 1994; Folsom et al. 1985; Dannenberg et al. 1989; Slattery et al. 1992; Gibbons et al. 1983; Voorrips et al. 1992). Prospective studies have shown less consistent results. French and colleagues (1994) reported an inverse association between leisure-time physical activity (either walking or engaging in high-intensity activity) and later weight gain, and Ching and colleagues (1996) found that physical activity was inversely related to the risk of becoming overweight. Klesges and colleagues (1992) reported that weight gain was inversely associated with leisure-time physical activity among women but not among men. Williamson and colleagues (1993), however, found no association between physical activity and subsequent weight change. Williamson and colleagues (1993) and Voorrips and colleagues (1992) proposed that decreases in physical activity may be both a cause and a consequence of weight gain over a lifetime and that multiple measurements over time may be necessary to characterize the interrelationship. One cohort study that assessed changes in physical activity reported that among women, decreased physical activity performed as work was related to weight gain; no associations were found among men (Klesges et al. 1992).

The relationship between physical activity and obesity in children is still under investigation. Some studies comparing obese and nonobese children have shown higher physical activity levels in nonobese children (Johnson, Burke, Mayer 1956; Bullen, Reed, Mayer 1964); others have shown little or no relationship (Stefanik, Heald, Mayer 1959; Bradfield, Paulos, Grossman 1971). Somewhat inconsistent results have also been seen in cross-sectional studies, with several finding lower BMIs or skinfold measures among children with higher levels of physical activity or fitness (Wolf et al. 1993; Obarzanek et al. 1994; Strazzullo et al. 1988; Tell and Vellar 1988) and some smaller studies finding no association (Sallis et al. 1988; LaPorte et al. 1982). More recently, two longitudinal studies have reported inverse relationships between physical activity and triceps skinfold measures (Moore et al. 1995) and BMI (Klesges et al. 1995) in young children. A third longitudinal study (Ku et al. 1981) found a significant negative association between physical activity and percentage of body fat in boys but not in girls. Additional longitudinal studies of children, including measurement of changes in physical activity, will help clarify whether physical activity prevents the development of obesity.

Over the past two decades, several comprehensive review articles (Oscai 1973; Stefanick 1993; Thompson, Jarvie, et al. 1982; Wilmore 1983), as well as two meta-analyses (Ballor and Keesey 1991; Epstein and Wing 1980), have examined the impact of exercise training on body weight and obesity. These reviews conclude that 1) physical activity generally affects body composition and weight favorably by promoting fat loss while preserving or increasing lean mass; 2) the rate of weight loss is positively related, in a dose-response manner, to the frequency and duration of the physical activity session, as well as to the duration (e.g., months, years) of the physical activity program; and 3) although the rate of weight loss resulting from increased physical activity without caloric restriction is relatively slow, the combination of increased physical activity and dieting appears to be more effective for long-term weight regulation than is dieting alone (Brownell and Stunkard 1980; Kayman, Bruvold, Stern 1990).

Independent of its effect on body weight and total adiposity, physical activity may favorably affect fat distribution. Several large cross-sectional studies in Europe (Seidell et al. 1991), Canada (Tremblay et al. 1990), and the United States (Kaye et al. 1990; Slattery et al. 1992; Troisi et al. 1991; Wing et al. 1991) report an inverse association between energy expenditure from physical activity and several indicators of central body fat distribution, such as the waist-to-hip ratio or the waist-to-thigh-circumference ratio.

## Biologic Plausibility

Increase in fat mass and the development of obesity occur when energy intake exceeds total daily energy expenditure for a prolonged period (Bray 1983; Leibel, Rosenbaum, Hirsch 1995). Total energy expenditure represents the sum of 1) resting energy expenditure for maintaining basic body functions (approximately 60 percent of total energy requirements); 2) the thermic effect of eating for digestion, absorption, transport, and deposition of nutrients (about 10 percent); and 3) nonresting energy expenditure, primarily in the form of physical activity (about 30 percent) (Leibel, Rosenbaum, Hirsch 1995). This third component, nonresting energy expenditure, is the most variable. Energy balance tilts to weight gain when disproportionately more energy is taken in; theoretically, about one pound (or 0.45 kg) of fat energy is stored for each 3,500 kilocalories of excess energy intake. By increasing nonresting energy expenditure, regular physical activity contributes to weight maintenance and weight reduction. Evidence supports the metabolic and physiological benefits of incorporating physical activity into programs that prevent or manage obesity (Pi-Sunyer 1988; Leon 1989; Bouchard, Després, Tremblay 1993; DiPietro 1995; Ewbank, Darga, Lucas 1995).

Controversy exists over whether physical activity following a meal increases the thermic effect of food ingestion and whether physical activity before a meal reduces appetite. The evidence suggests that physical activity programs do not necessarily produce a compensatory increase in food intake in obese individuals (Woo, Garrow, Pi-Sunyer 1982a, 1982b). Moreover, daily physical activity may further assist in weight loss by partially reducing the decline in resting energy expenditure that occurs during dieting and associated weight loss (Lennon et al. 1985). This effect is plausible because endurance exercise and strength training may help preserve, to some degree, metabolically active, lean body mass, whereas caloric restriction does not (Hill, Drougas, Peters 1994; Ballor and Keesy 1991).

Because abdominal fat is more responsive than gluteal or lower-body fat to epinephrine stimulation (Wahrenberg, Bolinder, Arner 1991), physical activity may result in a more beneficial redistribution of body fat in both sexes (Bouchard, Després, Tremblay 1993). Further investigation, however, is needed to clarify the associations between gonadal hormone levels, baseline regional fat distribution, and exercise-related changes in weight and body fat distribution.

## Conclusions

Physical activity is important for weight control. By using energy and maintaining muscle mass, physical activity is a useful and effective adjunct to dietary management for avoiding weight gain or losing weight. Physical activity appears to favorably affect distribution of body fat.

# Mental Health

Mental disorders pose a significant public health burden in the United States. Some disorders, such as depression, are associated with suicide, which is currently the ninth leading cause of death among Americans (NCHS 1996). A major cause of hospitalization and disability, mental disorders cost $148 billion per year, about half of which is due to severe mental illness (National Advisory Mental Health Council 1993).

The annual prevalence of mental disorders in the United States population is high. Nearly three out of 10 persons 15–54 years of age who live in households report having had a mental disorder during the previous year (Regier et al. 1993; Kessler et al. 1994). The most frequently reported disorders are affective (mood) and anxiety disorders. More than one out of 10 adults suffers from a depressive disorder in any given year; between 13 and 17 percent suffer from an anxiety disorder. Women report a higher prevalence of affective and anxiety disorders than do men. Most people with mental disorders do not obtain any professional treatment; only one in five people with a disorder during the previous year has received help from a health service provider.

Mental disorders, mental illnesses, mental health, and psychological well-being relate to such factors as mood or affect, personality, cognition, and perception. Psychological constructs about these factors are interrelated with a person's physical health status and quality of life. In studies of the effects of physical activity on mental health, the most frequently studied outcomes include mood (anxiety, depression, negative affect, and to a lesser extent, positive affect), self-esteem, self-efficacy, and cognitive functioning. The general hypothesis is that people who are physically active or have higher levels of cardiorespiratory fitness have enhanced mood (less negative and greater positive affect), higher self-esteem, greater confidence in their ability to perform tasks requiring physical activity (i.e., greater self-efficacy), and better cognitive functioning than sedentary persons or those who are less physically fit. One National Institutes of Mental Health workshop (Morgan and Goldston 1987) and numerous recent reviews have been devoted to this literature (Brown 1990; LaFontaine et al. 1992; Landers and Petruzzello 1994; Martinsen and Stephens 1994; McAuley 1994; McDonald and Hodgdon 1991; Morgan 1994; North, McCullagh, Tran 1990; Plante and Rodin 1990; Raglin 1990; Sime 1990). The effects of physical activity on most mental disorders—including sleep and eating disorders, schizophrenia, dementia, personality disorders, and substance-related disorders—are not as well studied

(Dishman 1986; Taylor, Sallis, Needle 1985; Martinsen and Stephens 1994).

This section focuses primarily on the association of physical activity with anxiety and depression. Evidence related to other psychological factors, such as positive affect, self-esteem, self-efficacy, and cognitive functioning, is discussed later in this chapter in the "Health-Related Quality of Life" section.

## Physical Activity and Mental Health

Epidemiologic research among men and women suggests that physical activity may be associated with reduced symptoms of depression (Ross and Hayes 1988; Stephens 1988; Stephens and Craig 1990; Farmer et al. 1988; Camacho et al. 1991), clinical depression (Weyerer 1992), symptoms of anxiety (Ross and Hayes 1988; Stephens 1988), and improvements in positive affect (Stephens 1988; Stephens and Craig 1990) and general well-being (Stephens 1988). In general, persons who are inactive are twice as likely to have symptoms of depression than are more active persons.

Most epidemiologic and intervention studies on the relationship of physical activity and mental health have used self-report questionnaires to assess symptoms of anxiety and depression among persons from the general population, although some studies have focused on patients diagnosed by clinicians. These questionnaires are useful for identifying persons experiencing mental distress (i.e., symptoms of anxiety or depression), but such identifications do not necessarily correspond to diagnoses of anxiety or depression by clinicians using standard interview criteria (Fechner-Bates, Coyne, Schwenk 1994).

The literature suggests that physical activity helps improve the mental health of both clinical and nonclinical populations. Physical activity interventions have benefited persons from the general population who report mood disturbance (Simons and Birkimer 1988; Wilfley and Kunce 1986), including symptoms of anxiety (Steptoe et al. 1989) and depression (Morgan et al. 1970), as well as patients who have been diagnosed with nonbipolar, nonpsychotic depression (Doyne et al. 1987; Klein et al. 1985; Martinsen, Medhus, Sandvik 1985). These findings are supported by a limited number of intervention studies conducted in community and laboratory settings (Brown 1990; Landers and Petruzzello

1994; Martinsen and Stephens 1994; McAuley 1994; Morgan 1994; Plante and Rodin 1990; Sime 1990). Intervention studies have primarily evaluated the effects of aerobic physical activities, such as brisk walking and running, on mental health; how other forms of physical activity, such as strength training, affect mental health requires further study.

The psychological benefits of regular physical activity for persons who have relatively good physical and mental health are less clear. Some intervention studies have found that physical activity provides mental health benefits to persons recruited from the community who are without serious psychological problems. These benefits included increases in general well-being (Cramer, Nieman, Lee 1991) and reductions in tension, confusion (Moses et al. 1989), and perceived stress and anxiety (King, Taylor, Haskell 1993). Other researchers have found that few (Brown et al. 1995; Blumenthal et al. 1989; King, Taylor, Haskell 1989) or no mental health benefits (Hughes, Casal, Leon 1986; Lennox, Bedell, Stone 1990) occurred among people without mental disorders who participated in physical activity interventions.

Most of these studies involved relatively small sample sizes. Furthermore, the participants had little opportunity to show improvement on objective and standardized mental health measures, since their baseline scores were already in the normal range or lower on measures of negative affect and were in the normal range or higher for positive affect. Even when no change was observed on objective measures, in some of these studies, participants reported feeling a subjective sensation of improved physical, psychological, or social well-being after participating in regular physical activity (Blumenthal et al. 1989; King, Taylor, Haskell 1993).

Psychological assessments that have been used in physical activity research have included state and trait measures. State measures, which reflect how a person feels "right now," are particularly useful in assessing changes in mood that occur before and after an intervention, such as a single episode of physical activity. Trait measures, which evaluate how a person "generally" feels, focus on personality characteristics that tend to be stable or sustained across the life span. Although physical activity training programs can result in sustained psychological benefits, many people after a single session of physical activity report improvements in transient moods, such as reduced anxiety (Morgan 1979a; Roth 1989), and have temporary reductions in muscular tension (DeVries 1981; DeVries and Adams 1972). The reduction in anxiety may persist for 2 to 6 hours following a session of physical activity (Landers and Petruzzello 1994; Raglin and Morgan 1987). Regular daily physical activity is required to experience this calming effect on an ongoing basis. Some researchers have thus proposed that the episodic mental health benefits associated with physical activity may act as an important preventive measure that could lead to the maintenance of mental health over time (Morgan 1981; Morgan et al. 1980; Raglin 1990).

A number of epidemiologic studies of noninstitutionalized populations have evaluated the associations between self-reported levels of physical activity and mental health. These studies typically assessed retrospective self-reports of leisure-time physical activity during the previous several weeks or more. How these assessments relate to changes in cardiorespiratory fitness is unknown. The available evidence indicates, however, that increases in cardiorespiratory fitness are not necessary for psychological benefits to occur (Brown and Wang 1992; King, Taylor, Haskell 1989; Landers and Petruzzello 1994; Martinsen and Stephens 1994).

Cross-sectional epidemiologic or community population studies support an association between physical activity and psychological well-being in the general population. For example, in one cross-sectional study using data generated from a state telephone survey, researchers determined that adults (n = 401) who spent more time participating in regular exercise, sports, or other physical activities had fewer symptoms of depression and anxiety than persons reporting no physical activity or low levels of participation (Ross and Hayes 1988). These associations were similar for men and women and for older and younger adults. The cause-and-effect relationship, however, cannot be determined because physical activity and mood were measured at the same time.

In another cross-sectional study (Stephens 1988), secondary analyses of two Canadian surveys (n = 23,791 and 22,250 young people and adults) and two U.S. surveys (n = 3,025 and 6,913 adults) conducted

between 1971 and 1981 associated physical activity with fewer symptoms of anxiety and depression and with higher positive mood and general well-being. These associations were observed in all four surveys, even though they used different measures of physical activity and mental health, and were strongest among women and among persons aged 40 years or older. However, one of the Canadian surveys found that women manifested higher positive affect when their energy expenditure scores were based on recreational activities only, rather than on a combination of recreational and household activities. Hence, mental health outcomes may depend on the type of physical activities being performed and perhaps on the setting in which they occur. This finding is important in that investigators have typically evaluated the mental health effects of recreational aerobic activities, such as running, rather than occupational and household activities.

A subsequent nationwide Canadian survey (Stephens and Craig 1990) of approximately 4,000 respondents aged 10 years and older found that persons who reported higher levels of total daily leisure-time energy expenditure had a more positive mood than persons reporting lower levels of expenditure. Persons aged 25 years and older demonstrated an inverse relationship between physical activity and symptoms of depression.

Although many cross-sectional studies suggest a positive association between physical activity and mental health, they do not necessarily indicate a cause-and-effect relationship. Persons who have good mental health may simply be more likely to be active. Another possibility is that physical activity and mental health vary together, in which case a third variable, such as chronic health conditions, would mediate this relationship.

Cohort studies provide additional insights into whether physical activity contributes to the primary prevention of mental health problems (Table 4-9). In one cohort study of 1,900 U.S. adults, a cross-sectional analysis of the baseline data revealed an association between depressive symptoms and little or no involvement in physical activity (Farmer et al. 1988). At 8-year follow-up, little or no recreational physical activity was found to be a significant predictor of increased depressive symptoms among white women who had reported few depressive symptoms

**Table 4-9. Longitudinal population-based studies of physical activity as related to depressive symptoms**

| Study | Population | Definition of physical activity | Definition of cancer |
|---|---|---|---|
| Farmer et al. (1988) | NHANES I Follow-up Study participants, white adults, aged 25–77 years, 1975 baseline | Little or no exercise done for recreation at baseline | Depressive symptoms scores of (a) < 16 and (b) ≥ 16 at baseline |
| Camacho et al. (1991) | Alameda County, CA population study participants aged ≥ 20 years; or ever married, 1965 baseline | Self-reported frequency of involvement in active sports, swimming or walking, daily exercise, and gardening; (low = 0–4, moderate = 5–8, high = 9–14) | Depressive symptoms at 1974 follow-up |
| Weyerer (1992) | German population study participants aged ≥ 16 years at 1975–1979 baseline | Regular, occasional, or no exercise at baseline based on single question: How often do you currently exercise for sports? | Psychiatric interview assessed depression at follow-up (1980–1984) |
| Paffenbarger, Lee, Leung (1994) | Harvard alumni study participants, men aged 35–74 years, 1962 or 1966 baseline | (a) ≤ 1 hour, 1–2 hours, 3+ hours of sports play/week at baseline<br><br>(b) < 1,000 kcal, 1,000–2,499 kcal, or 2,500+ kcal/week at baseline | Physician-diagnosed depression at 1988 follow-up |

| Main findings | Dose response[*] | Adjustment for confounders and other comments |
|---|---|---|
| (a) Men: 1.3 (95% CI, 0.5–3.1)<br>Women: 1.9 (95% CI, 1.1–3.2)<br>(b) Men: 12.9 (95% CI, 1.7–98.9)<br>Women: 2.0 (95% CI, 0.8–14.5) | NA | Odds ratio adjusted for age, education, chronic conditions, employment status, household income, physical activity apart from recreation at baseline, length of follow-up |
| Relative to high active,<br>low active men: | | Odds ratio adjusted for age, income, race, smoking status, alcohol consumption, |
| 1.76 (95% CI, 1.06–2.92) | Yes | relative weight for height, education, chronic |
| moderate active men: | | conditions, physical symptoms/disability, |
| 1.46 (95% CI, 0.91–2.34) | No | stress events, isolation, feelings of anomie |
| low active women: | | |
| 1.70 (95% CI, 1.06–2.70) | NA | |
| moderate active women: | | |
| 1.00 (95% CI, 0.63–1.59) | NA | |
| Relative to regular exercise,<br>men/no exercise: | | Odds ratio adjusted for age, social class, and physical health |
| 1.15 (95% CI, 0.30–4.36) | NA | |
| men/occasional exercise: | | |
| 0.27 (95% CI, 0.03–2.35) | No | |
| women/no exercise: | | |
| 0.70 (95% CI, 0.30–1.62) | NA | |
| women/occasional exercise: | | |
| 0.65 (95% CI, 0.26–1.61) | No | |
| Total/no exercise: | | |
| 0.88 (95% CI, 0.44–1.77) | NA | |
| Total/occasional exercise: | | |
| 0.70 (95% CI, 0.30–1.50) | No | |
| Relative to ≤ 1 hour of sports play/week,<br>RR for 1–2 hours = 0.96,<br>RR for 3+ hours = 0.73 | Yes | Adjusted for age |
| Relative to < 1,000 kcal/week,<br>RR for 1,000–2,499 kcal/week = 0.83<br>RR for 2,500 kcal/week = 0.72 | Yes | |

Abbreviations: CI = confidence interval; NA = not available; NHANES = National Health and Nutrition Examination Survey; RR = relative risk.

[*] A dose-response relationship requires more than 2 levels of comparison. In this column, "NA" means that there were only 2 levels of comparison; "No" means that there were more than 2 levels but no dose-response gradient was found; "Yes" means that there were more than 2 levels and a dose-response gradient was found.

at baseline. Among white men who had excessive depressive symptoms at baseline, low levels of recreational activity predicted continued depressive symptoms at follow-up.

A cross-sectional analysis (Camacho et al. 1991) of 1965 baseline data on 6,928 U.S. residents revealed an inverse association between physical activity (low, moderate, and high levels of participation in active sports, swimming or walking, doing exercises, or gardening) and depressive symptoms. Follow-up study of the men and women who had few depressive symptoms in 1965 showed that those who had low levels of physical activity were at greater risk than their highly active counterparts for having a high number of depressive symptoms in 1974.

A 23- through 27-year follow-up study of 10,201 Harvard alumni men revealed that level of physical activity reported at an initial interview in 1962 or 1966 was inversely related to self-reported physician-diagnosed depression in 1988 (Paffenbarger, Lee, Leung 1994). Physical activity in 1962 and 1966 was defined as the number of hours per week spent doing physical activities (e.g., golf, gardening, carpentry, tennis, swimming, brisk walking, jogging, or running); from this information, a physical activity index was computed as kilocalories of energy expended per week. In 1988, respondents were asked whether they had ever been told by a physician that they had health problems (e.g., CHD, emphysema), including depression, and to list the year of onset. Incidence of depression was determined by an attack first experienced (at a known age of the respondent) during the follow-up period. This study was unique in that the relationship between physical activity and deaths due to suicides was also evaluated. The incidence of suicide (as identified on death certificates) was largely unrelated to the 1962 or 1966 physical activity history of the college alumni. However, the relative risk of depression was 27 percent lower for men who had reported playing 3 or more hours of sports each week than for men who had reported playing none. In addition, men who had expended 1,000 to 2,499 kilocalories per week and those who had expended 2,500 kilocalories or more per week were at 17 percent and 28 percent less risk for depression, respectively, than men who had expended fewer than 1,000 kilocalories per week.

In a study of rural Europeans (n = 1,536), a cross-sectional association was observed between inactivity (no physical exercise or sports participation) and depression (diagnosed by research psychiatrists) (Weyerer 1992). However, low levels of physical activity at baseline were not a risk factor for depression at 5-year follow-up for men or women in this study.

Two of the epidemiologic studies reviewed above examined a possible dose-response relationship. In one study (Camacho et al. 1991), the baseline prevalence of symptoms of depression was higher for persons reporting low levels of physical activity than for highly active persons; the risk was intermediate for the moderately active group. At follow-up, the incidence of depressive symptoms revealed a significant difference only between persons in the lowest and highest activity groups. In the second study (Paffenbarger, Lee, Leung 1994), an inverse dose-response gradient was found between the baseline self-reported amount of physical activity calculated as kilocalories per week (< 1,000, 1,000–2,499, ≥ 2,500) and the follow-up incidence of physician-diagnosed depression. Men who at baseline had reported no hours of sports play per week had a similar follow-up incidence of depression as men who reported 1 to 2 hours of weekly play; but men who had participated in 3 or more hours of weekly play had a 27 percent lower risk for developing depression than the least active group.

The findings from these two studies provide limited support for a dose-response relationship between levels of physical activity and measures of depressive symptoms or depression. However, among some endurance athletes, mood disturbances (decreased vigor and increased fatigue, anxiety, and symptoms of depression) have been observed with overtraining; mood improved after training was tapered (Morgan et al. 1987). It is therefore conceivable that for the general population, too strenuous a physical activity regimen may lead to deleterious effects on mental health (Morgan 1979b, 1994; Polivy 1994; Raglin 1990). To date, research has not identified a threshold or an optimal frequency, duration, or intensity of physical activity necessary to improve mental health status.

## Biologic Plausibility

Some researchers have proposed that exercise-induced changes in brain neuroreceptor concentrations of monoamines (norepinephrine, dopamine, or serotonin) (Ransford 1982) or endogenous opiates (endorphins and enkephalins) (Moore 1982) may help to favorably alter mood. The increased core body temperature that occurs from physical activity may also decrease muscle tension (DeVries 1981). Other hypothalamic, metabolic, hormonal, or cardiorespiratory changes that result from training may eventually be linked to enhanced mental health.

Psychosocial aspects of physical activity, such as having the opportunity for social interaction and support (Hughes, Casal, Leon 1986), experiencing increased feelings of self-mastery and self-efficacy (Simons et al. 1985; Hughes, Casal, Leon 1986), and experiencing relief from daily stressors (Bahrke and Morgan 1978), may improve mental health status in some people.

## Conclusions

The literature reported here supports a beneficial effect of physical activity on relieving symptoms of depression and anxiety and on improving mood. There is some evidence that physical activity may protect against the development of depression, although further research is needed to confirm these findings.

# Health-Related Quality of Life

For several decades, it has been recognized that health should not be defined simply as the absence of disease and disability; rather, health is now conceptualized by the World Health Organization as a positive state of physical, mental, and social well-being (World Health Organization 1947). This recognition has resulted in an increasing clinical, scientific, and public interest in the assessment and promotion of health-related quality of life (HRQL).

Kaplan and Bush (1982) introduced the term HRQL to capture the influence that health status and health care have on the quality of day-to-day life. Viewed as a multidimensional construct that represents a person's overall satisfaction with life, HRQL includes the following dimensions: cognitive, social, physical, and emotional functioning; personal productivity; and intimacy (Shumaker, Anderson, Czajkowski 1990). Rejeski, Brawley, and Shumaker (1996) have shown that physical activity has significant potential to influence HRQL. The most direct effects are likely in the areas of psychological well-being (e.g., self-concept, self-esteem, mood, and affect), perceived physical function (e.g., perceived ability to perform activities of daily living), physical well-being (e.g., perceived symptoms and perceived physical states, such as dyspnea, pain, fatigue, and energy), and, to a limited extent, cognitive function.

In a recent review, McAuley (1994) concluded that a positive association exists between physical activity habits and self-esteem in both young adults and children. The strength of this relationship increases when physical activity is personally valued and when measures of psychological well-being are specific rather than general. Among nonclinical and clinical samples of men and women, this association is observed both with the long-term effects of exercise training and with the immediate, short-term effects of a single episode of activity.

In a review of studies of middle-aged participants (mean age, 56.7 years), McAuley and Rudolph (1995) found correlations between involvement in physical activity and psychological well-being that were similar to those patterns observed among younger persons. Further, the strength of these relationships was directly related to the length of time that the participants had been involved in physical activity programs. This moderating effect requires cautious interpretation because of the possibility of selective adherence. There was little evidence that the relationship between physical activity and psychological well-being was affected by either sex or age. Finally, although a number of studies noted improvements in both the cardiorespiratory fitness and the psychological well-being of older adults, these improvements were not necessarily correlated (McAuley and Rudolph 1995). Involvement in physical activity may thus increase the psychological well-being of older adults independently of cardiorespiratory fitness (Brown and Wang 1992; King, Taylor, Haskell 1989; Landers and Petruzzello 1994; Martinsen and Stephens 1994; McAuley and Rudolph 1995).

Other data suggest that physical activity is related to perceived improvement in physical function in activities of daily living. However, there is a limit to this effect, since sedentary people can usually do their daily tasks. Most research on this aspect of HRQL is thus confined to populations of people who, because of health problems, have restrictions in their activities of daily living. The growing body of literature on this topic indicates that patients whose physical function is compromised by heart disease (Ewart 1989) or arthritis (Fisher et al. 1993) experience improved daily function from increases in physical activity.

HRQL requires a number of different types of measurements; however, few studies on physical activity have used a multidimensional measurement scheme. Exceptions include a randomized clinical trial involving healthy elderly persons (Stewart, King, Haskell 1993) and a 2-year observational study of persons with chronic disease (Stewart et al. 1994). In the clinical trial, healthy persons who were assigned to endurance exercise had better self-reported ratings of their physical functioning and health (e.g., physical and role function, experiencing of pain, perception of health status) than control participants, yet endurance training brought no changes in self-reported energy/fatigue, psychological distress, or psychological well-being. By contrast, among persons with chronic diseases, physical activity was associated with improvement in both psychological well-being and physical function; however, the magnitude of these effects was highly dependent on the status of the patient's chronic disease. Participants who have lower levels of mental or physical health may have the most to gain from physical activity (Lennox, Bedell, Stone 1990; Morgan et al. 1970; Simons and Birkimer 1988; Rejeski et al. 1995), since they have more room to improve their health status than people already possessing good health.

A relatively small number of cross-sectional studies have shown a strong positive association between regular physical activity and cognitive and neuropsychological performance on tasks such as math, acuity, and reaction time (Dustman, Emmerson, Shearer 1994; Thomas et al. 1994). However, longer-term training studies (2 or more years) are required to confirm whether aerobic exercise has a pronounced effect on cognitive function. Also unclear are whether the effects of low-intensity physical activity are similar to those of aerobic exercise and whether objective measures of cognitive function can elucidate the perceived cognitive function of participants (Dustman, Emmerson, Shearer 1994).

## Conclusions
Physical activity appears to improve psychological well-being. Among people compromised by ill health, physical activity appears to improve their ability to perform activities of daily living.

# Adverse Effects of Physical Activity
Although physical activity has numerous health benefits, its potential adverse effects must also be considered. Listing the potential risks associated with physical activity is a straightforward matter. It is much more difficult to determine how commonly they occur among people who are physically active.

## Types of Adverse Effects
### Musculoskeletal Injuries
Acute stress from sudden forceful movement can cause strains, tears, and even fractures. For example, a vigorous swing of a baseball bat can lead to a dislocated shoulder. An attempt to accelerate forward in tennis can tear an Achilles tendon. Bending to retrieve an object can rupture an intervertebral disc. Injuries like these can result from any activity, exercise, or sport that features sudden movements, such as those that can occur in professional or amateur track and field, racquet sports, basketball, baseball, football, soccer, and golf. Collisions with equipment, other participants, and surfaces can also produce severe injury. Children and adolescents with developing bodies are at special risk of permanent physical damage if injury occurs to the growth plates of long bones or to other bone or connective tissue structures.

Activities that involve repetitive motions, sometimes with traumatic contact with a ground surface or ball, are associated with other musculoskeletal injuries. An extensive literature describes injuries related to jogging and running (Hoeberigs 1992; Rolf 1995; Van Mechelen 1992). Lower-extremity injuries appear to be the most common; of these, the knee, ankle, and foot have the highest proportions of injuries (e.g., torn cartilage, tendinitis, plantar fasciitis, neuromas, and shinsplints). Injuries are also seen in excessive bicycling (e.g., ulnar nerve palsies, ischial bursitis [Cohen 1993; Mellion 1991; Pfeiffer and Kronisch 1995]), swimming (e.g., shoulder pain [Allegrucci, Whitney, Irrgang 1994; Johnson, Sim, Scott 1987]), racquet sports (e.g., epicondylitis [Kamien 1990]), aerobic dancing (e.g., shin pain and plantar fasciitis [Richie, Kelso, Bellucci 1985]), and rowing (e.g., back and knee injuries [Howell 1984]).

## Metabolic Abnormalities

Severe exertion, particularly of prolonged duration and under hot or humid conditions, can lead to hyperthermia, electrolyte imbalance, and dehydration (England et al. 1982; Frizzell et al. 1986; Surgenor and Uphold 1994). Timely fluid intake and replacement, with proper electrolyte and caloric composition, can prevent or ameliorate such metabolic upsets. Hypothermia is a risk in many water sports and for any activities undertaken in cold weather (or even cool weather if inadequate clothing is worn). Extreme endurance training regimens can lead to endocrine system alterations, sometimes resulting in anovulation and amenorrhea in females, in association with a decrease in body weight below a critical lean mass, as well as with a decrease in bone mass (Shangold 1984). Hypoglycemia can occur in people with diabetes if they do not develop a routine of regular activity in conjunction with regular monitoring of their blood sugar (and adjustment of their medication accordingly).

## Hematologic and Body Organ Abnormalities

Anemia is reported in athletes vigorously engaged in sports such as long-distance running; hemoglobinuria can occur secondary to breakage of red blood cells during the repetitive impact of distance running, and hematuria can occur when distance running traumatizes the bladder or other structures in the genitourinary system. Rhabdomyolysis, the leakage of contents of muscle cells, can occur as a result of strenuous activity, such as weight lifting or military basic training, and can lead to renal failure (Kuipers 1994; Sinert et al. 1994).

## Hazards

Cyclists, runners, and walkers often face risks associated with travel on roadways—collisions with motor vehicles, injuries from falls secondary to uneven surfaces, and attacks by animals or humans. Skiers and skaters must contend with falls at high velocities. Baseball players may be struck by a thrown or batted ball or injured by a spike-soled shoe. Basketball and soccer entail collisions with other players and frequent falls to hard surfaces. Football, hockey, and boxing, by their very nature, are sports where sanctioned and moderately controlled interpersonal violence often leads to contusions, lacerations, musculoskeletal injury, and fractures, as well as to concussions and chronic disability (Kraus and Conroy 1984).

## Infectious, Allergic, and Inflammatory Conditions

Swimming increases the risk of otitis externa ("swimmer's ear"). Overtrained athletes may have an increased risk of infections from immunosuppression (Newsholme and Parry-Billings 1994). Exertion may provoke asthmatic attacks, usually occurring after exercise in susceptible individuals (Anderson, Daviskas, Smith 1989).

## Cardiac Events

As was discussed earlier in this chapter, regular physical activity improves cardiorespiratory fitness and reduces the risk of CVD mortality over the long term, although it can acutely increase risk for untoward cardiac events in the short term. Persons with compromised coronary circulation may develop angina or acute myocardial infarction during vigorous activity (Mittleman et al. 1993; Willich et al. 1993). Arrythmias may be precipitated by a combination of exertion and underlying heart disease, and some can lead to sudden death (Kohl et al. 1992; Koplan 1979; Siscovick et al. 1984; Thompson, Funk, et al. 1982). Compared with sedentary people who suddenly begin exercising vigorously, persons who exercise regularly have a lower risk of exercise-related sudden death, although even this group has a transient elevation of risk during and immediately after vigorous exercise (Kohl et al. 1992; Siscovick et al. 1984). Nonetheless, the net effect of regular physical activity is to decrease the risk of cardiac death.

## Occurrence of Adverse Effects

Determining the incidence or prevalence of adverse effects of physical activity, or factors that influence the likelihood of their occurrence, is hampered by not knowing how many people have similar physical activity patterns and are thus similarly at risk of an adverse event, or how many inactive people sustain similar injuries. Nevertheless, a few studies have provided some insight into the occurrence of adverse events. Of the activities that are common in the United States, including jogging/running, walking, gardening, bicycling, swimming, aerobic dance, and softball, running has received the most attention by researchers.

Injuries among runners are common, ranging from 25 through 65 percent (Jones, Cowan, Knapik 1994). Most running-related injuries involve the leg and foot and are usually self-correcting in a relatively short time. Studies of such injuries have generally shown that occurrence of musculoskeletal injury is directly related to mileage run (Blair, Kohl, Goodyear 1987; Hoeberigs 1992; Koplan et al. 1982; Macera 1992; Macera et al. 1989; Marti 1988; Marti et al. 1988; Walter et al. 1989) or to frequency or duration of running (Pollock et al. 1977). Previous injury appears to be a risk factor for subsequent injury. In one small study of people aged 70–79 years, the injury rate was lower for walking than jogging (5 percent vs. 57 percent) (Pollock et al. 1991). Whether this finding is true only among the elderly or is characteristic of these activities at all ages remains to be determined.

Although few studies of aerobic dance have been conducted, the injury rate appears to be higher among those taking more than 4 classes per week (Richie, Kelso, Bellucci 1985).

## Conclusions

A wide spectrum of adverse events can occur with physical activity, ranging from those that cause minor inconvenience to those that are life-threatening. At least some of the musculoskeletal injuries are likely to be preventable if people gradually work up to a physical activity goal and avoid excessive amounts of physical activity or excessively high levels of intensity. Although adverse cardiac events are more likely to occur with physical exertion, the net effect

of regular physical activity is a lower CVD mortality rate among active than inactive people (see earlier sections of this chapter).

People should be advised not to undertake physical activities well beyond their normal level of exertion. Inactive people wishing to begin a new program of moderate activity should begin with short durations and gradually lengthen them toward their target. Men over age 40 and women over age 50 who wish to begin a new program involving vigorous-intensity activity, people who have preexisting health problems, and people who are at high risk of CVD should consult a physician before embarking on a program of physical activity to which they are unaccustomed (ACSM 1991).

# Nature of the Activity/Health Relationship

## Causality

The studies reviewed in this chapter indicate that physical activity is associated with a reduction in risk of all-cause mortality, all CVDs combined, CHD, hypertension, colon cancer, and NIDDM. To evaluate whether the information presented is sufficient to infer that these associations are causal in nature, it is useful to review the evidence according to Hill's classic criteria for causality (Hill 1965; Paffenbarger 1988).

*Strength of Association.* The numerous estimated measures of association for cardiovascular outcomes presented in this chapter generally fall within the range of a 1.5- to 2.0-fold increase in risk of adverse health outcomes associated with inactivity. This range represents a moderately strong association, similar in magnitude to the relationship between CHD and smoking, hypertension, or elevated cholesterol. The associations with NIDDM, hypertension, and colon cancer have been somewhat smaller in magnitude. The difficulty in measuring physical activity may lead to substantial misclassification, which in turn would bias studies toward finding less of an effect of activity than may actually exist. On the other hand, not controlling for all potential confounders could bias studies toward finding more of an effect than may actually exist. Efforts to stratify studies of physical activity and CHD by the quality of measurement have found that the methodologically better studies showed larger associations than those with lower quality scores (Powell et al. 1987; Berlin and Colditz 1990). In addition, cardiorespiratory fitness, which is more objectively and precisely measured than the reported level of physical activity, often is also more strongly related to CVD and mortality. Measures of association between physical activity and health outcomes thus might be stronger if physical activity measurements were more accurate.

*Consistency of Findings.* Although the epidemiologic studies of physical activity have varied greatly in methodology, in ways of classifying physical activity, and in populations studied, the findings have been remarkably consistent in supporting a reduction in risk as a function of greater amounts of physical activity, or conversely, an increase in risk as a function of inactivity.

*Temporality.* For most of the health conditions included in this chapter (all-cause mortality, CVD, CHD, hypertension, NIDDM), longitudinal data from cohort studies have been available and have confirmed a temporal sequence in which physical activity patterns are determined prior to development of disease. For obesity and mental health, fewer longitudinal studies have been conducted, and findings have been more equivocal. Perhaps the strongest evidence for temporality comes from two studies of the effect of changes in activity or fitness level. Men who became more active or more fit had a lower mortality rate during follow-up than men who remained inactive or unfit (Paffenbarger et al. 1993; Blair et al. 1995).

*Biological Gradient.* Studies of all-cause mortality, CVD, CHD, and NIDDM have shown a gradient of greater benefit associated with higher amounts of physical activity. Most studies that included more than two categories of amount of physical activity and were therefore able to evaluate a dose-response relationship found a gradient of decreasing risk of disease with increasing amounts of physical activity (see Tables 4-1 through 4-8).

*Biologic Plausibility.* Evidence that physiologic effects of physical activity have beneficial consequences for CHD, NIDDM, and obesity is abundant (see Chapter 3, as well as the biologic plausibility sections of this chapter). Such evidence includes beneficial effects on physiologic risk factors for disease, such as high blood pressure and blood lipoproteins, as well as beneficial effects on circulatory system functioning, blood-clotting mechanisms, insulin production and glucose handling, and caloric balance.

*Experimental Evidence.* Controlled clinical trials have not been conducted for the outcomes of mortality, CVD, cancer, obesity, or NIDDM. However, randomized clinical trials have determined that physical activity improves these diseases' risk factors, such as blood pressure, lipoprotein profile, insulin sensitivity, and body fat.

The information reviewed in this chapter shows that the inverse association between physical activity and several diseases is moderate in magnitude, consistent across studies that differed substantially in methods and populations, and biologically plausible. A dose-response gradient has been observed in most studies that examined more than two levels of activity. For most of the diseases found to be inversely related to physical activity, the temporal sequence of exposure preceding disease has been demonstrated. Although controlled clinical trials have not been conducted (and are not likely to be conducted) for morbidity and mortality related to the diseases of interest, controlled trials have shown that activity can improve physiologic risk factors for these diseases. From this large body of consistent information, it is reasonable to conclude that physical activity is causally related to the health outcomes reported here.

## Population Burden of Sedentary Living

Given that the relationship between activity and several diseases is likely to be causal, it follows that a large number of Americans unnecessarily become ill or die each year because of an inactive way of life. Published estimates of the number of lives lost in a year because of inactivity have ranged from 200,000 for inactivity alone to 300,000 for inactivity and poor diet combined (Hahn et al. 1990; Powell and Blair 1994; McGinnis and Foege 1993). Such estimates are generally derived by calculating the population attributable risk (PAR), which is based on both the relative mortality rate associated with inactivity and the prevalence of inactivity in the population. Such estimates are inherently uncertain because they do not take into account the reality that some people have more than one risk factor for a disease; for these people, the elimination of a single risk factor (e.g., by becoming physically active) may not reduce mortality risk to the level attainable for people who initially have only that one risk factor. PAR methods thus overestimate the proportion of deaths avoidable by eliminating one modifiable risk factor, in this case physical inactivity. On the other hand, PAR estimates of avoidable mortality do not address other important aspects of the population burden of sedentary living. The benefits of reducing the occurrence of CHD, colon cancer, and diabetes greatly surpass the benefits of reducing premature mortality, yet the reductions in avoidable disease, disability, suffering, and health care costs have not been calculated. Similarly, the health benefits of improved mood, quality of life, and functional capacity have not been quantified. Although the total population burden of physical inactivity in the United States has not been quantified, sedentary living habits clearly constitute a major public health problem.

## Dose

Using the epidemiologic literature to derive recommendations for how much and what kind of physical activity a person should obtain is problematic, in part because the methods for measuring and classifying physical activity in epidemiologic studies are not standardized. Measurement of physical activity generally relies on self-reported information in response to questionnaires, although some studies use occupation to categorize a person's presumed level of physical activity at work. Responses to questions or occupational activity categories are usually transformed, using a variety of methods, into estimates of calories expended per week, minutes of activity per week, categories of total activity, or other types of composite scores.

Numerous studies have used this type of information to estimate total amount of activity, and many have been able to explore dose-response relationships across categories of activity amount. For the most part, these studies demonstrate that amount of benefit is directly related to amount of physical activity (see Tables 4-1 through 4-8), rather than showing a threshold level of activity necessary before health benefits accrue. Such studies are less helpful,

however, in assessing the relationship of health benefits to intensity of physical activity (i.e., how hard one must work during the activity itself) because few studies have separately measured or analyzed levels of intensity while taking into account the other dimensions of activity (e.g., frequency, duration, total caloric expenditure). As described earlier, however, for some health benefits (e.g., blood pressure lowering), clinical trials of exercise intensity suggest similar, if not greater, benefit from moderate- as from vigorous-intensity exercise.

It is often asked how little physical activity a person can obtain and still derive health benefit. Although the dose-response relationship appears not to have a lower threshold, thereby indicating that any activity is better than none, some quantitation of a target "dose" of activity is helpful for many people. It has been shown that total amount of physical activity (a combination of intensity, frequency, and duration) is related to health outcomes in a dose-response fashion, but the absolute difference in amount of physical activity in kilocalories of energy expended between exposure categories has not been estimated routinely. Several studies, however, have estimated average caloric expenditure for the activity categories studied and thus allow quantitation of amount of physical activity associated with improved health outcomes. Paffenbarger and colleagues (1986) found that compared with the least active group in the study, those who expended 71–143 kilocalories of energy per day had a 22 percent reduction in overall mortality, and those who expended 143–214 kilocalories per day had a 27 percent reduction. Leon and colleagues (1987) showed that a difference of about 30 minutes per day of activity (light, moderate, and vigorous activity combined), equivalent to an average difference of about 150 kilocalories of energy expended per day, was associated with a 36 percent lower risk of CHD mortality and a 27 percent lower risk of all-cause death, after the analysis adjusted for other factors that can effect CHD and total mortality. Slattery and colleagues (1989) found that a daily average of 73 more kilocalories of total activity than were expended among the least active group was associated with a 16 percent reduction in CHD mortality and a 14 percent reduction in all-cause mortality. Furthermore, in the majority (62 percent) of that study population, no vigorous activity was reported. In that group, a daily average of 150 kilocalories greater expenditure in light-to-moderate activity was associated with a 27 percent lower CHD mortality and a 19 percent lower total mortality. The effects of light-to-moderate activity on CHD death remained significant after the analysis adjusted for potential confounders. Similarly, in a study of NIDDM (Helmrich et al. 1991) that showed a significant inverse trend between kilocalories expended in activity and development of NIDDM, total activity of 140–215 kilocalories per day was associated with a 21 percent reduction in NIDDM onset. In the group that obtained this level of energy expenditure without any vigorous sports participation, the reduction in NIDDM onset was 13 percent.

Based on these studies, it is reasonable to conclude that activity leading to an increase in daily expenditure of approximately 150 kilocalories/day (equivalent to about 1,000 kilocalories/week) is associated with substantial health benefits and that the activity does not need to be vigorous to achieve benefit. It should be emphasized that this is an estimate based on few studies, and that further research will be required to refine it. For example, it is not clear whether it is the total amount of caloric expenditure or the amount of caloric expenditure per unit of body weight that is important. Nonetheless, this amount of physical activity can be obtained in a variety of ways and can vary from day to day to meet the needs and interests of the individual. An average expenditure of 150 kilocalories/day (or 1,000 kilocalories/week) could be achieved by walking briskly for 30 minutes per day, or by a shorter duration of more vigorous activity (e.g., 15 minutes of running at 10 minutes per mile), or by a longer duration of more vigorous activity less frequently (e.g., running at 10 minutes per mile for about 35 minutes 3 times per week). Other sample activities are provided in Table 4-10.

In addition to the health effects associated with a moderate amount of physical activity, the dose-response relationships show that further increases in activity confer additional health benefits. Thus people who are already meeting the moderate activity recommendation can expect to derive additional benefit by increasing their activity. Since amount of activity is a function of intensity, frequency, and duration, increasing the amount of activity can be accomplished by increasing any, or all, of those dimensions.

There is evidence that increasing physical activity, even after years of inactivity, improves health. Studies of the health effects of increasing physical activity or fitness (Paffenbarger et al. 1993; Blair et al. 1995) have shown a reduced mortality rate in men who become more active or more fit compared with those who remain sedentary. This benefit was apparent even for men who became physically active after the age of 60.

Most importantly, a regular pattern of physical activity must be maintained to sustain the physiologic changes that are assumed responsible for the health benefits (see Chapter 3). Thus it is crucial for each person to select physical activities that are sustainable over the course of his or her life. For some people, a vigorous workout at a health club is the most sustainable choice; for others, activities integrated into daily life (e.g., walking to work, gardening and household chores, walking after dinner) may be a more sustainable option. Periodic reevaluation may be necessary to meet changing needs across the life span.

A related issue of pattern of physical activity (frequency and duration in the course of a day) has recently come under review. Three studies have held constant both total amount of activity and intensity of activity while daily pattern was varied (one long session versus shorter, more frequent sessions). Two studies showed equivalent increases in cardiorespiratory fitness (Jakicic et al. 1995; Ebisu 1985). One study showed gains in cardiorespiratory fitness for both the "short bout" and "long bout" groups, although on one of three measures (maximal oxygen uptake versus treadmill test duration and heart rate at submaximal exercise), the gain in fitness was significantly greater in the long bout group (DeBusk et al. 1990). These observations give rise to the notion that intermittent episodes of activity accumulated in the course of a day may have cardiorespiratory fitness benefits comparable to one longer continuous episode. Whether this assumption holds true for the outcomes of disease occurrence and death remains to be determined. Nevertheless, some previous observational studies have shown lower rates of CHD, CVD, and all-cause mortality among people with an active

**Table 4-10.  Duration of various activities to expend 150 kilocalories for an average 70 kg adult**

| Intensity | Activity | Metabolic equivalents METs* | Approximate duration in minutes[†] |
|---|---|---|---|
| Moderate | Volleyball, noncompetitive | 3.0 | 43 |
| Moderate | Walking, moderate pace (3 mph, 20 min/mile) | 3.5 | 37 |
| Moderate | Walking, brisk pace (4 mph, 15 min/mile) | 4.0 | 32 |
| Moderate | Table tennis | 4.0 | 32 |
| Moderate | Raking leaves | 4.5 | 32 |
| Moderate | Social dancing | 4.5 | 29 |
| Moderate | Lawn mowing (powered push mower) | 4.5 | 29 |
| Hard | Jogging (5 mph, 12 min/mile) | 7.0 | 18 |
| Hard | Field hockey | 8.0 | 16 |
| Very hard | Running (6 mph, 10 min/mile) | 10.0 | 13 |

*Based on average METs in Ainsworth et al. 1993.

[†]Formula: $\dfrac{150 \text{ kcal} \times 60 \text{ min/hour}}{\text{METs (kcal/kg/hr)} \times \text{kg}}$ = minutes

lifestyle that included activities such as walking, stair climbing, household or yard work, and gardening—activities that are often performed intermittently (Leon et al. 1987; Paffenbarger et al. 1986). This information, together with evidence that some people may adhere better to an exercise recommendation that allows for accumulating short episodes of activity as an alternative to one longer episode per day (Jakicic et al. 1995), supports the notion that accumulation of physical activity throughout the day is a reasonable alternative to setting aside an uninterrupted period of time for physical activity each day. Although more research is clearly needed to better define the differential effects of various patterns of activity, experts have agreed that intermittent episodes of activity are more beneficial than remaining sedentary. This consensus is reflected in recent physical activity recommendations from the CDC and the ACSM (Pate et al. 1995) and from the NIH Consensus Development Panel on Physical Activity and Cardiovascular Disease (see Chapter 2, Appendix B).

## Conclusions

The findings reviewed in this chapter form the basis for concluding that moderate amounts of activity can protect against several diseases. A greater degree of protection can be achieved by increasing the amount of activity, which can be accomplished by increasing intensity, frequency, or duration. Nonetheless, modest increases in physical activity are likely to be more achievable and sustainable for sedentary people than are more drastic changes, and it is sedentary people who are at greatest risk for poor health related to inactivity. Thus the public health emphasis should be on encouraging those who are inactive to become moderately active. These conclusions are consistent with the recent CDC-ACSM recommendations for physical activity (Pate et al. 1995) and the NIH Consensus Development Conference Statement on Physical Activity and Cardiovascular Health (see Chapter 2, Appendix B), which emphasize the importance of obtaining physical activity of at least moderate amount on a regular basis. The recommendations also encourage those who are already moderately active to become more active to achieve additional health benefits, by increasing the intensity, duration, or frequency of physical activity. Further study is needed to determine which combinations of these interrelated factors are most important for specific health benefits. Most important, however, is the recognition that physical activity recommendations should be tailored to an individual's needs and preferences. Encouraging sedentary people to become moderately active is likely to reduce the burden of unnecessary suffering and death only if the activity can be sustained on a daily basis for many years.

## Chapter Summary

Despite the variety of methods used to measure and classify physical activity, the imprecision of these measures, and the considerable variation in study designs and analytic sophistication, several findings consistently emerge from the epidemiologic literature on physical activity and health. Physical activity of the type that improves cardiorespiratory endurance reduces the risk of developing or dying from CVD (CHD in particular), hypertension, colon cancer, and NIDDM and improves mental health. Findings are highly suggestive that endurance-type physical activity may reduce the risk of developing obesity, osteoporosis, and depression and may improve psychological well-being and quality of life. There is promising evidence that muscle strengthening (resistance) exercise reduces the risk of falling and fractures among the elderly. Furthermore, there appears to be a dose-response relationship between physical activity and disease prevention: higher levels of activity appear to have the most benefit, but lower levels have demonstrable benefits for some diseases as well. For the U.S. population, in which the majority of people are sedentary or only minimally active, achievable increases in physical activity of a moderate amount, including some resistance exercise to strengthen muscle, are likely to substantially improve the health and quality of life of many people.

## Conclusions

### Overall Mortality

1. Higher levels of regular physical activity are associated with lower mortality rates for both older and younger adults.

2. Even those who are moderately active on a regular basis have lower mortality rates than those who are least active.

### Cardiovascular Diseases

1. Regular physical activity or cardiorespiratory fitness decreases the risk of cardiovascular disease mortality in general and of coronary heart disease (CHD) mortality in particular. Existing data are not conclusive regarding a relationship between physical activity and stroke.

2. The level of decreased risk of CHD attributable to regular physical activity is similar to that of other lifestyle factors, such as keeping free from cigarette smoking.

3. Regular physical activity prevents or delays the development of high blood pressure, and exercise reduces blood pressure in people with hypertension.

### Cancer

1. Regular physical activity is associated with a decreased risk of colon cancer.

2. There is no association between physical activity and rectal cancer. Data are too sparse to draw conclusions regarding a relationship between physical activity and endometrial, ovarian, or testicular cancers.

3. Despite numerous studies on the subject, existing data are inconsistent regarding an association between physical activity and breast or prostate cancers.

### Non–Insulin-Dependent Diabetes Mellitus

1. Regular physical activity lowers the risk of developing non–insulin-dependent diabetes mellitus.

149

### Physical Activity and Health

#### Osteoarthritis

1. Regular physical activity is necessary for maintaining normal muscle strength, joint structure, and joint function. In the range recommended for health, physical activity is not associated with joint damage or development of osteoarthritis and may be beneficial for many people with arthritis.

2. Competitive athletics may be associated with the development of osteoarthritis later in life, but sports-related injuries are the likely cause.

#### Osteoporosis

1. Weight-bearing physical activity is essential for normal skeletal development during childhood and adolescence and for achieving and maintaining peak bone mass in young adults.

2. It is unclear whether resistance- or endurance-type physical activity can reduce the accelerated rate of bone loss in postmenopausal women in the absence of estrogen replacement therapy.

#### Falling

1. There is promising evidence that strength training and other forms of exercise in older adults preserve the ability to maintain independent living status and reduce the risk of falling.

#### Obesity

1. Low levels of activity, resulting in fewer kilocalories used than consumed, contribute to the high prevalence of obesity in the United States.

2. Physical activity may favorably affect body fat distribution.

#### Mental Health

1. Physical activity appears to relieve symptoms of depression and anxiety and improve mood.

2. Regular physical activity may reduce the risk of developing depression, although further research is required on this topic.

#### Health-Related Quality of Life

1. Physical activity appears to improve health-related quality of life by enhancing psychological well-being and by improving physical functioning in persons compromised by poor health.

#### Adverse Effects

1. Most musculoskeletal injuries related to physical activity are believed to be preventable by gradually working up to a desired level of activity and by avoiding excessive amounts of activity.

2. Serious cardiovascular events can occur with physical exertion, but the net effect of regular physical activity is a lower risk of mortality from cardiovascular disease.

### Research Needs

1. Delineate the most important features or combinations of features of physical activity (total amount, intensity, duration, frequency, pattern, or type) that confer specific health benefits.

2. Determine specific health benefits of physical activity for women, racial and ethnic minority groups, and people with disabilities.

3. Examine the protective effects of physical activity in conjunction with other lifestyle characteristics and disease prevention behaviors.

4. Examine the types of physical activity that preserve muscle strength and functional capacity in the elderly.

5. Further study the relationship between physical activity in adolescence and early adulthood and the later development of breast cancer.

6. Clarify the role of physical activity in preventing or reducing bone loss after menopause.

# References

Abbott RD, Rodriguez BL, Burchfiel CM, Curb JD. Physical activity in older middle-aged men and reduced risk of stroke: the Honolulu Heart Program. *American Journal of Epidemiology* 1994;139:881–893.

Abraham S, Collins G, Nordsieck M. Relationship of childhood weight status to morbidity in adults. *Health Services and Mental Health Administration Health Reports* 1971;86:273–284.

Adams JE. Injury to the throwing arm: a study of traumatic changes in the elbow joints of boy baseball players. *California Medicine* 1965;102:127–132.

Albanes D. Caloric intake, body weight, and cancer: a review. *Nutrition and Cancer* 1987;9:199–217.

Albanes D, Blair A, Taylor PR. Physical activity and risk of cancer in the NHANES I population. *American Journal of Public Health* 1989;79:744–750.

Allegrante JP, Kovar PA, MacKenzie CR, Peterson MG, Gutin B. A walking education program for patients with osteoarthritis of the knee: theory and intervention strategies. *Health Education Quarterly* 1993;20:63–81.

Allegrucci M, Whitney SL, Irrgang JJ. Clinical implications of secondary impingement of the shoulder in freestyle swimmers. *Journal of Orthopaedic and Sports Physical Therapy* 1994;20:307–318.

Allen SH. Exercise considerations for postmenopausal women with osteoporosis. *Arthritis Care and Research* 1994;7:205–214.

Aloia JF, Vaswani AN, Yeh JK, Cohn SH. Premenopausal bone mass is related to physical activity. *Archives of Internal Medicine* 1988;148:121–123.

Alpert BS, Wilmore JH. Physical activity and blood pressure in adolescents. *Pediatric Exercise Science* 1994;6:361–380.

American Cancer Society. *Cancer facts and figures,* 1996. Atlanta: American Cancer Society, 1996. Publication No. 5008.96.

American College of Sports Medicine. *Guidelines for exercise testing and prescription.* 4th ed. Philadelphia: Lea and Febiger, 1991.

American College of Sports Medicine. Position stand: physical activity, physical fitness, and hypertension. *Medicine and Science in Sports and Exercise* 1993;25:i–x.

American Diabetes Association. Technical review: exercise and NIDDM. *Diabetes Care* 1990;13:785–789.

Anderson SD, Daviskas E, Smith CM. Exercise-induced asthma: a difference in opinion regarding the stimulus. *Allergy Proceedings* 1989;10:215–226.

Arbman G, Axelson O, Fredriksson M, Nilsson E, Sjödahl R. Do occupational factors influence the risk of colon and rectal cancer in different ways? *Cancer* 1993;72: 2543–2549.

Armstrong N, Simons-Morton B. Physical activity and blood lipids in adolescents. *Pediatric Exercise Science* 1994;6:381–405.

Armstrong SJ, Read RA, Ghosh P, Wilson DM. Moderate exercise exacerbates the osteoarthritic lesions produced in cartilage by meniscectomy: a morphological study. *Osteoarthritis and Cartilage* 1993;1:89–96.

Arokoski J, Kiviranta I, Jurvelin J, Tammi M, Helminen HJ. Long-distance running causes site-dependent decrease of cartilage glycosaminoglycan content in the knee joints of beagle dogs. *Arthritis and Rheumatism* 1993;36:1451–1459.

Arraiz GA, Wigle DT, Mao Y. Risk assessment of physical activity and physical fitness in the Canada Health Survey Mortality Follow-up Study. *Journal of Clinical Epidemiology* 1992;45:419–428.

Arroll B, Beaglehole R. Does physical activity lower blood pressure? A critical review of the clinical trials. *Journal of Clinical Epidemiology* 1992;45:439–447.

Bahrke MS, Morgan WP. Anxiety reduction following exercise and meditation. *Cognitive Therapy and Research* 1978;2:323–333.

Ballard-Barbash R, Schatzkin A, Albanes D, Schiffman MH, Kreger BE, Kannel WB, et al. Physical activity and risk of large bowel cancer in the Framingham study. *Cancer Research* 1990;50:3610–3613.

Ballor DL, Keesey RE. A meta-analysis of the factors affecting exercise-induced changes in body mass, fat mass, and fat-free mass in males and females. *International Journal of Obesity* 1991;15:717–726.

Barnard RJ, Jung T, Inkeles SB. Diet and exercise in the treatment of NIDDM: the need for early emphasis. *Diabetes Care* 1994;17:1469–1472.

Bennett GE. Shoulder and elbow lesions of the professional baseball pitcher. *Journal of the American Medical Association* 1941;117:510–514.

Berlin JA, Colditz GA. A meta-analysis of physical activity in the prevention of coronary heart disease. *American Journal of Epidemiology* 1990;132:612–628.

# Physical Activity and Health

Bernstein L, Henderson BE, Hanisch R, Sullivan-Halley J, Ross RK. Physical exercise and reduced risk of breast cancer in young women. *Journal of the National Cancer Institute* 1994;86:1403–1408.

Björntorp P, Krotkiewski M. Exercise treatment in diabetes mellitus. *Acta Medica Scandinavica* 1985;217:3–7.

Björntorp P, Sjöström L, Sullivan L. The role of physical exercise in the management of obesity. In: Munro JF, editor. *The treatment of obesity.* Baltimore: University Park Press, 1979:123–138.

Blackburn H, Prineas R. Diet and hypertension: anthropology, epidemiology, and public health implications. *Progress in Biochemical Pharmacology* 1983;19:31–79.

Blair SN. Physical activity, fitness, and coronary heart disease. In: Bouchard C, Shephard RJ, Stephens T, editors. *Physical activity, fitness, and health: international proceedings and consensus statement.* Champaign, IL: Human Kinetics, 1994:579–590.

Blair SN, Goodyear NN, Gibbons LW, Cooper KH. Physical fitness and incidence of hypertension in healthy normotensive men and women. *Journal of the American Medical Association* 1984;252:487–490.

Blair SN, Kohl HW, Barlow CE. Physical activity, physical fitness, and all-cause mortality in women: do women need to be active? *Journal of the American College of Nutrition* 1993;12:368–371.

Blair SN, Kohl HW, Goodyear NN. Rates and risks for running and exercise injuries: studies in three populations. *Research Quarterly for Exercise and Sport* 1987;58:221–228.

Blair SN, Kohl HW III, Barlow CE, Paffenbarger RS Jr, Gibbons LW, Macera CA. Changes in physical fitness and all-cause mortality: a prospective study of healthy and unhealthy men. *Journal of the American Medical Association* 1995;273:1093–1098.

Blair SN, Kohl HW III, Paffenbarger RS Jr, Clark DG, Cooper KH, Gibbons LW. Physical fitness and all-cause mortality: a prospective study of healthy men and women. *Journal of the American Medical Association* 1989;262:2395–2401.

Blumenthal JA, Emery CF, Madden DJ, George LK, Coleman RE, Riddle MW, et al. Cardiovascular and behavioral effects of aerobic exercise training in healthy older men and women. *Journal of Gerontology* 1989;44:147–157.

Bouchard C, Després J-P, Tremblay A. Exercise and obesity. *Obesity Research* 1993;1:133–147.

Bradfield RB, Paulos J, Grossman L. Energy expenditure and heart rate of obese high school girls. *American Journal of Clinical Nutrition* 1971;24:1482–1488.

Bray GA. Complications of obesity. *Annals of Internal Medicine* 1985;103(Suppl 6, Pt 2):1052–1062.

Bray GA. The energetics of obesity. *Medicine and Science in Sports and Exercise* 1983;15:32–40.

Brown DR. Exercise, fitness, and mental health. In: Bouchard C, Shephard RJ, Stephens T, Sutton JR, McPherson BD, editors. *Exercise, fitness, and health: a consensus of current knowledge.* Champaign, IL: Human Kinetics, 1990:607–626.

Brown DR, Wang Y. The relationships among exercise training, aerobic capacity, and psychological well-being in the general population. *Medicine, Exercise, Nutrition, and Health* 1992;3:125–142.

Brown DR, Wang Y, Ward A, Ebbeling CB, Fortlage L, Puleo E, et al. Chronic psychological effects of exercise and exercise plus cognitive strategies. *Medicine and Science in Sports and Exercise* 1995;27:765–775.

Brownell KD, Stunkard AJ. Physical activity in the development and control of obesity. In: Stunkard AJ, editor. *Obesity.* Philadelphia: W.B. Saunders, 1980:300–324.

Brownson RC, Chang JC, Davis JR, Smith CA. Physical activity on the job and cancer in Missouri. *American Journal of Public Health* 1991;81:639–642.

Brownson RC, Zahm SH, Chang JC, Blair A. Occupational risk of colon cancer: an analysis by anatomic subsite. *American Journal of Epidemiology* 1989;130:675–687.

Brunner D, Manelis G, Modan M, Levin S. Physical activity at work and the incidence of myocardial infarction, angina pectoris, and death due to ischemic heart disease: an epidemiological study in Israeli collective settlements (kibbutzim). *Journal of Chronic Diseases* 1974;27:217–233.

Bullen BA, Reed RB, Mayer J. Physical activity of obese and nonobese adolescent girls appraised by motion picture sampling. *American Journal of Clinical Nutrition* 1964;14:211–223.

Camacho TC, Roberts RE, Lazarus NB, Kaplan GA, Cohen RD. Physical activity and depression: evidence from the Alameda County Study. *American Journal of Epidemiology* 1991;134:220–231.

Cassel J, Heyden S, Bartel AG, Kaplan BH, Tyroler HA, Cornoni JC, et al. Occupation and physical activity and coronary heart disease. *Archives of Internal Medicine* 1971;128:920–928.

Cavanaugh DJ, Cann CE. Brisk walking does not stop bone loss in postmenopausal women. *Bone* 1988;9:201–204.

Cederholm J, Wibell L. Glucose tolerance and physical activity in a health survey of middle-aged subjects. *Acta Medica Scandinavica* 1985;217:373–378.

Chang-Claude J, Frentzel-Beyme R. Dietary and lifestyle determinants of mortality among German vegetarians. *International Journal of Epidemiology* 1993;22:228–236.

Chave SPW, Morris JN, Moss S, Semmence AM. Vigorous exercise in leisure time and the death rate: a study of male civil servants. *Journal of Epidemiology and Community Health* 1978;32:239–243.

Chen MK, Lowenstein FW. Epidemiology of factors related to self-reported diabetes among adults. *American Journal of Preventive Medicine* 1986;2:14–19.

Chesnut CH III. Bone mass and exercise. *American Journal of Medicine* 1993;95(5A Suppl):34S–36S.

Ching PLYH, Willett WC, Rimm EB, Colditz GA, Gortmaker SL, Stampfer MJ. Activity level and risk of overweight in male health professionals. *American Journal of Public Health* 1996;86:25–30.

Chow RK, Harrison JE, Brown CF, Hajek V. Physical fitness effect on bone mass in postmenopausal women. *Archives of Physical Medicine and Rehabilitation* 1986;67:231–234.

Chow W-H, Dosemeci M, Zheng W, Vetter R, McLaughlin JK, Gao Y-T, et al. Physical activity and occupational risk of colon cancer in Shanghai, China. *International Journal of Epidemiology* 1993;22:23–29.

Cohen GC. Cycling injuries. *Canadian Family Physician* 1993;39:628–632.

Cohen MV. *Coronary collaterals: clinical and experimental observations.* Mount Kisco, NY: Futura Publishing Company, 1985.

Conroy BP, Kraemer WJ, Maresh CM, Fleck SJ, Stone MH, Fry AC, et al. Bone mineral density in elite junior Olympic weightlifters. *Medicine and Science in Sports and Exercise* 1993;25:1103–1109.

Cordain L, Latin RW, Behnke JJ. The effects of an aerobic running program on bowel transit time. *Journal of Sports Medicine and Physical Fitness* 1986;26:101–104.

Cramer SR, Nieman DC, Lee JW. The effects of moderate exercise training on psychological well-being and mood state in women. *Journal of Psychosomatic Research* 1991;35:437–449.

Cruz-Vidal M, Costas R Jr, García-Palmieri MR, Sorlie PD, Hertzmark E. Factors related to diabetes mellitus in Puerto Rican men. *Diabetes* 1979;28:300–307.

Cumming RG, Klineberg RJ. Case-control study of risk factors for hip fractures in the elderly. *American Journal of Epidemiology* 1994;139:493–503.

Cummings SR, Kelsey JL, Nevitt MC, O'Dowd KJ. Epidemiology of osteoporosis and osteoporotic fractures. *Epidemiological Reviews* 1985;7:178–208.

Cummings SR, Nevitt MC, Browner WS, Stone K, Fox KM, Ensrud KE, et al. Risk factors for hip fracture in white women. *New England Journal of Medicine* 1995;332:767–773.

Dalsky GP, Stocke KS, Ehsani AA, Slatopolsky E, Lee WC, Birge SJ. Weight-bearing exercise training and lumbar bone mineral content in postmenopausal women. *Annals of Internal Medicine* 1988;108:824–828.

Dannenberg AL, Keller JB, Wilson PWF, Castelli WP. Leisure-time physical activity in the Framingham Offspring Study: description, seasonal variation, and risk factor correlates. *American Journal of Epidemiology* 1989;129:76–88.

Davies MJ, Thomas AC. Plaque fissuring: the cause of acute myocardial infarction, sudden ischaemic death, and crescendo angina. *British Heart Journal* 1985;53:363–373.

Dawson AK, Leon AS, Taylor HL. Effect of submaximal exercise on vulnerability to fibrillation in the canine ventricle. *Circulation* 1979;60:798–804.

DeBusk RF, Stenestrand U, Sheehan M, Haskell WL. Training effects of long versus short bouts of exercise in healthy subjects. *American Journal of Cardiology* 1990;65:1010–1013.

Després J-P, Tremblay A, Nadeau A, Bouchard C. Physical training and changes in regional adipose tissue distribution. *Acta Medica Scandinavica Supplementum* 1988;723:205–212.

DeVries HA. Tranquilizer effect of exercise: a critical review. *Physician and Sportsmedicine* 1981;9:47–55.

DeVries HA, Adams GM. Electromyographic comparison of single doses of exercise and meprobamate as to effects on muscular relaxation. *American Journal of Physical Medicine* 1972;51:130–141.

DiPietro L. Physical activity, body weight, and adiposity: an epidemiologic perspective. *Exercise and Sport Sciences Reviews* 1995;23:275–303.

# Physical Activity and Health

Dishman RK. Mental health. In: Seefeldt V, editor. *Physical activity and well-being*. Reston, VA: American Alliance for Health, Physical Education, Recreation and Dance, 1986:304–341.

Donahue RP, Abbott RD, Reed DM, Yano K. Physical activity and coronary heart disease in middle-aged and elderly men: the Honolulu Heart Program. *American Journal of Public Health* 1988;78:683–685.

Donaldson CL, Hulley SB, Vogel JM, Hattner RS, Bayers JH, McMillan DE. Effect of prolonged bed rest on bone mineral. *Metabolism: Clinical and Experimental* 1970;19:1071–1084.

Dorgan JF, Brown C, Barrett M, Splansky GL, Kreger BE, D'Agostino RB, et al. Physical activity and risk of breast cancer in the Framingham Heart Study. *American Journal of Epidemiology* 1994;139:662–669.

Dosemeci M, Hayes RB, Vetter R, Hoover RN, Tucker M, Engin K, et al. Occupational physical activity, socioeconomic status, and risks of 15 cancer sites in Turkey. *Cancer Causes and Control* 1993;4:313–321.

Dowse GK, Zimmet PZ, Gareeboo H, Alberti KGMM, Tuomilehto J, Finch CF, et al. Abdominal obesity and physical inactivity as risk factors for NIDDM and impaired glucose tolerance in Indian, Creole, and Chinese Mauritians. *Diabetes Care* 1991;14:271–282.

Doyne EJ, Ossip-Klein DJ, Bowman ED, Osborn KM, McDougall-Wilson IB, Neimeyer RA. Running versus weight lifting in the treatment of depression. *Journal of Consulting and Clinical Psychology* 1987;55:748–754.

Drinkwater BL. Exercise in the prevention of osteoporosis. *Osteoporosis International* 1993;1:S169–S171.

Drinkwater BL, Nilson K, Chesnut CH III, Bremner WJ, Shainholtz S, Southworth MB. Bone mineral content of amenorrheic and eumenorrheic athletes. *New England Journal of Medicine* 1984;311:277–281.

Duncan JJ, Gordon NF, Scott CB. Women walking for health and fitness: how much is enough? *Journal of the American Medical Association* 1991;266:3295–3299.

Dunn JE, Rudberg MA, Furner SE, Cassel CK. Mortality, disability, and falls in older persons: the role of underlying disease and disability. *American Journal of Public Health* 1992;82:395–400.

Durstine JL, Haskell WL. Effects of exercise training on plasma lipids and lipoproteins. *Exercise and Sport Sciences Reviews* 1994;22:477–521.

Dustman RE, Emmerson R, Shearer D. Physical activity, age, and cognitive-neuropsychological function. *Journal of Aging and Physical Activity* 1994;2:143–181.

Dyer RG. Traditional treatment of obesity: does it work? *Baillieres Clinical Endocrinology and Metabolism* 1994;8:661–688.

Ebisu T. Splitting the distance of endurance running: on cardiovascular endurance and blood lipids. *Japanese Journal of Physical Education* 1985;30:37–43.

Ekelund LG, Haskell WL, Johnson JL, Whaley FS, Criqui MH, Sheps DS. Physical fitness as a predictor of cardiovascular mortality in asymptomatic North American men: the Lipid Research Clinics Mortality Follow-up Study. *New England Journal of Medicine* 1988;319:1379–1384.

England AC III, Fraser DW, Hightower AW, Tirinnanzi R, Greenberg DJ, Powell KE, et al. Preventing severe heat injury in runners: suggestions from the 1979 Peachtree Road Race experience. *Annals of Internal Medicine* 1982;97:196–201.

Epstein LH, Wing RR. Aerobic exercise and weight. *Addictive Behaviors* 1980;5:371–388.

Erikssen J. Physical fitness and coronary heart disease morbidity and mortality: a prospective study in apparently healthy, middle-aged men. *Acta Medica Scandinavica Supplementum* 1986;711:189–192.

Eriksson K-F, Lindgärde F. Prevention of type 2 (non-insulin-dependent) diabetes mellitus by diet and physical exercise. *Diabetologia* 1991;34:891–898.

Ettinger WH Jr, Afable RF. Physical disability from knee osteoarthritis: the role of exercise as an intervention. *Medicine and Science in Sports and Exercise* 1994;26:1435–1440.

Ewart CK. Psychological effects of resistive weight training: implications for cardiac patients. *Medicine and Science in Sports and Exercise* 1989;21:683–688.

Ewbank PP, Darga LL, Lucas CP. Physical activity as a predictor of weight maintenance in previously obese subjects. *Obesity Research* 1995;3:257–263.

Fagard R, Bielen E, Hespel P, Lijnen P, Staessen J, Vanhees L, et al. Physical exercise in hypertension. In: Laragh JH, Brenner BM, editors. *Hypertension: pathophysiology, diagnosis, and management*. Vol. 2. New York: Raven Press, 1990:1985–1998.

Falk E. Unstable angina with fatal outcome: dynamic coronary thrombosis leading to infarction and/or sudden death: autopsy evidence of recurrent mural thrombosis with peripheral embolization culminating in total vascular occlusion. *Circulation* 1985;71:699–708.

Farmer ME, Harris T, Madans JH, Wallace RB, Cornoni-Huntley J, White LR. Anthropometric indicators and hip fracture: the NHANES I Epidemiologic Follow-up Study. *Journal of the American Geriatrics Society* 1989;37:9–16.

Farmer ME, Locke BZ, Moscicki EK, Dannenberg AL, Larson DB, Radloff LS. Physical activity and depressive symptoms: the NHANES I Epidemiologic Follow-up Study. *American Journal of Epidemiology* 1988;128:1340–1351.

Fechner-Bates S, Coyne JC, Schwenk TL. The relationship of self-reported distress to depressive disorders and other psychopathology. *Journal of Consulting and Clinical Psychology* 1994;62:550–559.

Federation of American Societies for Experimental Biology, Life Sciences Research Office. *Third report on nutrition monitoring in the United States.* Vol. 1. Washington, DC: Interagency Board for Nutrition Monitoring and Related Research, 1995:211–219.

Feskens EJ, Loeber JG, Kromhout D. Diet and physical activity as determinants of hyperinsulinemia: the Zutphen Elderly Study. *American Journal of Epidemiology* 1994;140:350–360.

Fiatarone MA, O'Neill EF, Ryan ND, Clements KM, Solares GR, Nelson ME, et al. Exercise training and nutritional supplementation for physical frailty in very elderly people. *New England Journal of Medicine* 1994;330:1769–1775.

Fisch A, Pichard E, Prazuck T, Leblanc H, Sidibe Y, Brücker G. Prevalence and risk factors of diabetes mellitus in the rural region of Mali (West Africa): a practical approach. *Diabetologia* 1987;30:859–862.

Fisher NM, Gresham GE, Abrams M, Hicks J, Horrigan D, Pendergast DR. Quantitative effects of physical therapy on muscular and functional performance in subjects with osteoarthritis of the knees. *Archives of Physical Medicine and Rehabilitation* 1993;74:840–847.

Fisher NM, Kame VD Jr, Rouse L, Pendergast DR. Quantitative evaluation of a home exercise program on muscle and functional capacity of patients with osteoarthritis. *American Journal of Physical Medicine and Rehabilitation* 1994;73:413–420.

Fisher NM, Pendergast DR. Effects of a muscle exercise program on exercise capacity in subjects with osteoarthritis. *Archives of Physical Medicine and Rehabilitation* 1994;75:792–797.

Fisher NM, Pendergast DR, Gresham GE, Calkins E. Muscle rehabilitation: its effect on muscular and functional performance of patients with knee osteoarthritis. *Archives of Physical Medicine and Rehabilitation* 1991;72:367–374.

Folsom AR, Caspersen CJ, Taylor HL, Jacobs DR Jr, Luepker RV, Gomez-Marin O, et al. Leisure-time physical activity and its relationship to coronary risk factors in a population-based sample: the Minnesota Heart Survey. *American Journal of Epidemiology* 1985;121:570–579.

Folsom AR, Prineas RJ, Kaye SA, Munger RG. Incidence of hypertension and stroke in relation to body fat distribution and other risk factors in older women. *Stroke* 1990;21:701–706.

Fraser G, Pearce N. Occupational physical activity and risk of cancer of the colon and rectum in New Zealand males. *Cancer Causes and Control* 1993;4:45–50.

Fredriksson M, Bengtsson NO, Hardell L, Axelson O. Colon cancer, physical activity, and occupational exposures: a case-control study. *Cancer* 1989;63:1838–1842.

French SA, Jeffery RW, Forster JL, McGovern PG, Kelder SH, Baxter JE. Predictors of weight change over two years among a population of working adults: the Healthy Worker Project. *International Journal of Obesity* 1994;18:145–154.

Friedenreich CM, Rohan TE. Physical activity and risk of breast cancer. *European Journal of Cancer Prevention* 1995;4:145–151.

Frisch RE, Wyshak G, Albright NL, Albright TE, Schiff I, Jones KP, et al. Lower prevalence of breast cancer and cancers of the reproductive system among former college athletes compared to nonathletes. *British Journal of Cancer* 1985;52:885–891.

Frisch RE, Wyshak G, Albright NL, Albright TE, Schiff I, Witschi J, et al. Lower lifetime occurrence of breast cancer and cancers of the reproductive system among former college athletes. *American Journal of Clinical Nutrition* 1987;45:328–335.

Frisch RE, Wyshak G, Albright TE, Albright NL, Schiff I. Lower prevalence of diabetes in female former college athletes compared with nonathletes. *Diabetes* 1986;35:1101–1105.

Frizzell RT, Lang GH, Lowance DC, Lathan SR. Hyponatremia and ultra-marathon running. *Journal of the American Medical Association* 1986;255:772–774.

Garabrant DH, Peters JM, Mack TM, Bernstein L. Job activity and colon cancer risk. *American Journal of Epidemiology* 1984;119:1005–1014.

Garcia-Palmieri MR, Costas R Jr, Cruz-Vidal M, Sorlie PD, Havlik RJ. Increased physical activity: a protective factor against heart attacks in Puerto Rico. *American Journal of Cardiology* 1982;50:749–755.

Garfinkel L, Stellman SD. Mortality by relative weight and exercise. *Cancer* 1988;62:1844–1850.

Garn SM, Leonard WR, Hawthorne VM. Three limitations of the body mass index. *American Journal of Clinical Nutrition* 1986;44:996–997.

Gerhardsson M, Steineck G, Hagman U, Rieger Å, Norell SE. Physical activity and colon cancer: a case-referent study in Stockholm. *International Journal of Cancer* 1990;46:985–989.

Gerhardsson M, Floderus B, Norell SE. Physical activity and colon cancer risk. *International Journal of Epidemiology* 1988;17:743–746.

Gerhardsson M, Norell SE, Kiviranta H, Pederson NL, Ahlbom A. Sedentary jobs and colon cancer. *American Journal of Epidemiology* 1986;123:775–780.

Getz GS. The involvement of lipoproteins in atherogenesis: evolving concepts. *Annals of the New York Academy of Sciences* 1990;598:17–28.

Gibbons LW, Blair SN, Cooper KH, Smith M. Association between coronary heart disease risk factors and physical fitness in healthy adult women. *Circulation* 1983;67:977–983.

Gilligan C, Checovich MM, Smith EL. Osteoporosis. In: Skinner JS, editor. *Exercise testing and exercise prescription for special cases: theoretical basis and clinical application.* 2nd ed. Philadelphia: Lea and Febiger, 1993: 127–137.

Gillum RF. Trends in acute myocardial infarction and coronary heart disease death in the United States. *Journal of the American College of Cardiology* 1994;23: 1273–1277.

Giovannucci E, Ascherio A, Rimm EB, Colditz GA, Stampfer M, Willett WC. Physical activity, obesity, and risk for colon cancer and adenoma in men. *Annals of Internal Medicine* 1995;122:327–334.

Goldberg AP. Aerobic and resistive exercise modify risk factors for coronary heart disease. *Medicine and Science in Sports and Exercise* 1989;21:669–674.

Gordon NF, Scott CB. The role of exercise in the primary and secondary prevention of coronary artery disease. *Clinics in Sports Medicine* 1991;10:87–103.

Grimston SK, Willows ND, Hanley DA. Mechanical loading regime and its relationship to bone mineral density in children. *Medicine and Science in Sports and Exercise* 1993;25:1203–1210.

Grodzinsky AJ. Age-related changes in cartilage: physical properties and cellular response to loading. In: Buckwalter JA, Goldberg VM, Woo SLY, editors. *Musculoskeletal soft-tissue aging: impact on mobility.* Rosemont, IL: American Academy of Orthopedic Surgeons, 1993:137–149.

Gudat U, Berger M, Lefèbvre PJ. Physical activity, fitness, and non-insulin-dependent (type II) diabetes mellitus. In: Bouchard C, Shephard RJ, Stephens T, editors. *Physical activity, fitness, and health: international proceedings and consensus statement.* Champaign, IL: Human Kinetics, 1994:669–683.

Hagberg JM, Montain SJ, Martin WH III, Ehsani AA. Effect of exercise training in 60- to 69-year-old persons with essential hypertension. *American Journal of Cardiology* 1989;64:348–353.

Hahn RA, Teutsch SM, Rothenberg RB, Marks JS. Excess deaths from nine chronic diseases in the United States, 1986. *Journal of the American Medical Association* 1990;264:2654–2659.

Hall AC, Urban JPG, Gehl KA. The effects of hydrostatic pressure on matrix synthesis in articular cartilage. *Journal of Orthopaedic Research* 1991;9:1–10.

Hambrecht R, Niebauer J, Marburger C, Grunze M, Kälberer B, Hauer K, et al. Various intensities of leisure-time physical activity in patients with coronary artery disease: effects on cardiorespiratory fitness and progression of coronary atherosclerotic lesions. *Journal of the American College of Cardiology* 1993;22:468–477.

Hara H, Kawase T, Yamakido M, Nishimoto Y. Comparative observation of micro- and macroangiopathies in Japanese diabetics in Japan and U.S.A. In: Abe H, Hoshi M, editors. *Diabetic microangiopathy.* Basel: Karger, 1983.

Harmsen P, Rosengren A, Tsipogianni A, Wilhelmsen L. Risk factors for stroke in middle-aged men in Göteborg, Sweden. *Stroke* 1990;21:223–229.

Harris MI. Classification, diagnostic criteria, and screening for diabetes. In: Harris MI, Cowie CC, Stern MP, Boyko EJ, Reiber GE, Bennett PH, editors. *Diabetes in America*. Bethesda, MD: National Institutes of Health, National Institute of Diabetes and Digestive and Kidney Diseases, 1995:15–36. NIH Publication No. 95-1468.

Harris MI. Epidemiological correlates of NIDDM in Hispanics, whites, and blacks in the U.S. population. *Diabetes Care* 1991;14(Suppl 3):639–648.

Harris MI, Hadden WC, Knowler WC, Bennett PH. Prevalence of diabetes and impaired glucose tolerance and plasma glucose levels in U.S. population aged 20–74 yr. *Diabetes* 1987;36:523–534.

Harrison GG. Height-weight Tables. *Annals of Internal Medicine* 1985;103(Suppl 6, Pt 2):989–994.

Haskell WL. Physical activity in the prevention and management of coronary heart disease. *Physical Activity and Fitness Research* 1995;Series 2:1–7.

Haskell WL, Alderman EL, Fair JM, Maron DJ, Mackey SF, Superko HR, et al. Effects of intensive multiple risk factor reduction on coronary atherosclerosis and clinical cardiac events in men and women with coronary artery disease: the Stanford Coronary Risk Intervention Project (SCRIP). *Circulation* 1994;89:975–990.

Hein HO, Suadicani P, Gyntelberg F. Physical fitness or physical activity as a predictor of ischaemic heart disease: a 17-year follow-up in the Copenhagen Male Study. *Journal of Internal Medicine* 1992;232:471–479.

Heinonen A, Oja P, Kannus P, Sievanen H, Haapasalo H, Manttari A, Vuori I. Bone mineral density in female athletes representing sports with different loading characteristics of the skeleton. *Bone* 1995;17:197–203.

Helmrich SP, Ragland DR, Leung RW, Paffenbarger RS Jr. Physical activity and reduced occurrence of non-insulin-dependent diabetes mellitus. *New England Journal of Medicine* 1991;325:147–152.

Herman B, Schmitz PIM, Leyten ACM, Van Luijk JH, Frenken CWGM, Op de Coul AAW, et al. Multivariate logistic analysis of risk factors for stroke in Tilburg, The Netherlands. *American Journal of Epidemiology* 1983;118:514–525.

Hill AB. The environment and disease: association or causation? *Proceedings of the Royal Society of Medicine* 1965;58:295–300.

Hill JO, Drougas HJ, Peters JC. Physical activity, fitness, and moderate obesity. In: Bouchard C, Shephard RJ, Stephens T, editors. *Physical activity, fitness, and health: international proceedings and consensus statement*. Champaign, IL: Human Kinetics, 1994:684–695.

Hoeberigs JH. Factors related to the incidence of running injuries: a review. *Sports Medicine* 1992;13:408–422.

Holbrook TL, Barrett-Connor E, Wingard DL. The association of lifetime weight and weight control patterns with diabetes among men and women in an adult community. *International Journal of Obesity* 1989;13:723–729.

Hollenbeck CB, Haskell W, Rosenthal M, Reaven GM. Effect of habitual physical activity on regulation of insulin-stimulated glucose disposal in older males. *Journal of the American Geriatrics Society* 1984;33:273–277.

Holloszy JO, Schultz J, Kusnierkiewicz J, Hagberg JM, Ehsani AA. Effects of exercise on glucose tolerance and insulin resistance: brief review and some preliminary results. *Acta Medica Scandinavica Supplementum* 1986;711:55–65.

Holman H, Mazonson P, Lorig K. Health education for self-management has significant early and sustained benefits in chronic arthritis. *Transactions of the Association of American Physicians* 1989;102:204–208.

Horton ES. Exercise and decreased risk of NIDDM. *New England Journal of Medicine* 1991;325:196–198.

Howell DW. Musculoskeletal profile and incidence of musculoskeletal injuries in lightweight women rowers. *American Journal of Sports Medicine* 1984;12:278–282.

Hubert HB, Feinleib M, McNamara PM, Castelli WP. Obesity as an independent risk factor for cardiovascular disease: a 26-year follow-up of participants in the Framingham Heart Study. *Circulation* 1983;67:968–977.

Hughes JR, Casal DC, Leon AS. Psychological effects of exercise: a randomized cross-over trial. *Journal of Psychosomatic Research* 1986;30:355–360.

Jacobson PC, Beaver W, Grubb SA, Taft TN, Talmage RV. Bone density in women: college athletes and older athletic women. *Journal of Orthopaedic Research* 1984;2:328–332.

Jaglal SB, Kreiger N, Darlington G. Past and recent physical activity and risk of hip fracture. *American Journal of Epidemiology* 1993;138:107–118.

157

Jakicic JM, Wing RR, Butler BA, Robertson RJ. Prescribing exercise in multiple short bouts versus one continuous bout: effects on adherence, cardiorespiratory fitness, and weight loss in overweight women. *International Journal of Obesity* 1995;19:893–901.

Jarebinski M, Adanja B, Vlajinac H. Case-control study of relationship of some biosocial correlates to rectal cancer patients in Belgrade, Yugoslavia. *Neoplasma* 1989;36: 369–374.

Jarrett RJ, Shipley MJ, Hunt R. Physical activity, glucose tolerance, and diabetes mellitus: the Whitehall Study. *Diabetic Medicine* 1986;3:549–551.

Johansson S, Rosengren A, Tsipogianni A, Ulvenstam G, Wiklund I, Wilhelmsen L. Physical inactivity as a risk factor for primary and secondary coronary events in Göteborg, Sweden. *European Heart Journal* 1988;9 (Suppl L):8–19.

Johnson JE, Sim FH, Scott SG. Musculoskeletal injuries in competitive swimmers. *Mayo Clinic Proceedings* 1987; 62:289–304.

Johnson ML, Burke BS, Mayer J. Relative importance of inactivity and overeating in the energy balance of obese high school girls. *American Journal of Clinical Nutrition* 1956;4:37–44.

Johnston FE. Health implications of childhood obesity. *Annals of Internal Medicine* 1985;103 (Suppl 6, Pt 2): 1068–1072.

Jones BH, Cowan DN, Knapik JJ. Exercise, training, and injuries. *Sports Medicine* 1994;18:202–214.

Jorgensen CR, Gobel FL, Taylor HL, Wang Y. Myocardial blood flow and oxygen consumption during exercise. *Annals of the New York Academy of Sciences* 1977;301: 213–223.

Kahn HA. The relationship of reported coronary heart disease mortality to physical activity of work. *American Journal of Public Health* 1963;53:1058–1067.

Kamien M. A rational management of tennis elbow. *Sports Medicine* 1990;9:173–191.

Kannel WB, Belanger A, D'Agostino R, Israel I. Physical activity and physical demand on the job and risk of cardiovascular disease and death: the Framingham study. *American Heart Journal* 1986;112:820–825.

Kannel WB, Sorlie P. Some health benefits of physical activity: the Framingham study. *Archives of Internal Medicine* 1979;139:857–861.

Kaplan GA, Seeman TE, Cohen RD, Knudsen LP, Guralnik J. Mortality among the elderly in the Alameda County Study: behavioral and demographic risk factors. *American Journal of Public Health* 1987;77:307–312.

Kaplan RM, Bush JW. Health-related quality of life measurement for evaluation research and policy analysis. *Health Psychology* 1982;1:61–80.

Kato I, Tominaga S, Ikari A. A case-control study of male colorectal cancer in Aichi Prefecture, Japan: with special reference to occupational activity level, drinking habits, and family history. *Japanese Journal of Cancer Research* 1990;81:115–121.

Kawate R, Yamakido M, Nishimoto Y, Bennett PH, Hamman RF, Knowler WC. Diabetes mellitus and its vascular complications in Japanese migrants on the island of Hawaii. *Diabetes Care* 1979;2:161–170.

Kaye SA, Folsom AR, Prineas RJ, Potter JD, Gapstur SM. The association of body fat distribution with lifestyle and reproductive factors in a population study of premenopausal women. *International Journal of Obesity* 1990;14:583–591.

Kaye SA, Folsom AR, Sprafka JM, Prineas RJ, Wallace RB. Increased incidence of diabetes mellitus in relation to abdominal adiposity in older women. *Journal of Clinical Epidemiology* 1991;44:329–334.

Kayman S, Bruvold W, Stern JS. Maintenance and relapse after weight loss in women: behavioral aspects. *American Journal of Clinical Nutrition* 1990;52:800–807.

Kelley G, McClellan P. Antihypertensive effects of aerobic exercise: a brief meta-analytic review of randomized controlled trials. *American Journal of Hypertension* 1994;7:115–119.

Kessler RC, McGonagle KA, Zhao S, Nelson CB, Hughes M, Eshleman S, et al. Lifetime and 12-month prevalence of DSM-III-R psychiatric disorders in the United States: results from the National Comorbidity Survey. *Archives of General Psychiatry* 1994;51:8–19.

Kiely DK, Wolf PA, Cupples LA, Beiser AS, Kannel WB. Physical activity and stroke risk: the Framingham study. *American Journal of Epidemiology* 1994;140:608–620.

King AC, Taylor CB, Haskell WL. Effects of differing intensities and formats of 12 months of exercise training on psychological outcomes in older adults. *Health Psychology* 1993;12:292–300.

King AC, Taylor CB, Haskell WL, DeBusk RF. Influence of regular aerobic exercise on psychological health: a randomized, controlled trial of healthy middle-aged adults. *Health Psychology* 1989;8:305–324.

King H, Kriska AM. Prevention of type II diabetes by physical training: epidemiology considerations and study methods. *Diabetes Care* 1992;15:1794–1799.

King H, Taylor R, Zimmet P, Pargeter K, Raper LR, Berike T, et al. Non-insulin-dependent diabetes mellitus (NIDDM) in a newly independent Pacific nation: The Republic of Kiribati. *Diabetes Care* 1984;7:409–415.

King H, Zimmet P, Raper LR, Balkau B. Risk factors for diabetes in three Pacific populations. *American Journal of Epidemiology* 1984;119:396–409.

Kirchner EM, Lewis RD, O'Connor PJ. Effect of past gymnastics participation on adult bone mass. *Journal of Applied Physiology* 1996;80:225–232.

Klein MH, Greist JH, Gurman AS, Neimeyer RA, Lesser DP, Bushnell NJ, et al. A comparative outcome study of group psychotherapy vs exercise treatments for depression. *International Journal of Mental Health* 1985;13: 148–177.

Klesges RC, Klesges LM, Eck LH, Shelton ML. A longitudinal analysis of accelerated weight gain in preschool children. *Pediatrics* 1995;95:126–130.

Klesges RC, Klesges LM, Haddock CK, Eck LH. A longitudinal analysis of the impact of dietary intake and physical activity on weight change in adults. *American Journal of Clinical Nutrition* 1992;55:818–822.

Kohl HW III, Powell KE, Gordon NF, Blair SN, Paffenbarger RS Jr. Physical activity, physical fitness, and sudden cardiac death. *Epidemiologic Reviews* 1992;14:37–58.

Kohrt WM, Snead DB, Slatopolsky E, Birge SJ Jr. Additive effects of weight-bearing exercise and estrogen on bone mineral density in older women. *Journal of Bone and Mineral Research* 1995;10:1303–1311.

Koivisto VA, Soman V, Conrad P, Hendler R, Nadel E, Felig P. Insulin binding to monocytes in trained athletes: changes in the resting state and after exercise. *Journal of Clinical Investigation* 1979;64:1011–1015.

Koivisto VA, Yki-Järvinen H, DeFronzo RA. Physical training and insulin sensitivity. *Diabetes/Metabolism Reviews* 1986;1:445–481.

Kokkinos PF, Hurley BF, Vaccaro P, Patterson JC, Gardner LB, Ostrove SM, et al. Effects of low- and high-repetition resistive training on lipoprotein-lipid profiles. *Medicine and Science in Sports and Exercise* 1988;20:50–54.

Kono S, Shinchi K, Ikeda N, Yanai F, Imanishi K. Physical activity, dietary habits, and adenomatous polyps of the sigmoid colon: a study of self-defense officials in Japan. *Journal of Clinical Epidemiology* 1991;44:1255–1261.

Koplan JP. Cardiovascular deaths while running. *Journal of the American Medical Association* 1979;242:2578–2579.

Koplan JP, Powell KE, Sikes RK, Shirley RW, Campbell CC. An epidemiologic study of the benefits and risks of running. *Journal of the American Medical Association* 1982;248:3118–3121.

Krall LP, Beaser RS. *Joslin diabetes manual*. 12th ed. Philadelphia: Lea and Febiger, 1989.

Kramsch DM, Aspen AJ, Abramowitz BM, Kreimendahl T, Hood WB Jr. Reduction of coronary atherosclerosis by moderate conditioning exercise in monkeys on an atherogenic diet. *New England Journal of Medicine* 1981;305:1483–1489.

Kraus JF, Conroy C. Mortality and morbidity from injuries in sports and recreation. *Annual Review of Public Health* 1984;5:163–192.

Kriska AM, Bennett PH. An epidemiological perspective of the relationship between physical activity and NIDDM: from activity assessment to intervention. *Diabetes/Metabolism Reviews* 1992;8:355–372.

Kriska AM, Blair SN, Pereira MA. The potential role of physical activity in the prevention of noninsulin-dependent diabetes mellitus: the epidemiological evidence. *Exercise and Sport Sciences Reviews* 1994; 22:121–143.

Kriska AM, Gregg EW, Utter AC, Knowler WC, Narayan V, Bennett PH. Association of physical activity and plasma insulin levels in a population at high risk for NIDDM. *Medicine and Science in Sports and Exercise* 1993;26(5 Suppl):S121.

Kriska AM, LaPorte RE, Pettitt DJ, Charles MA, Nelson RG, Kuller LH, et al. The association of physical activity with obesity, fat distribution, and glucose intolerance in Pima Indians. *Diabetologia* 1993;36:863–869.

Krølner B, Toft B, Pors Nielsen S, Tøndevold E. Physical exercise as prophylaxis against involutional vertebral bone loss: a controlled trial. *Clinical Science* 1983; 64:541–546.

Krotkiewski M. Can body fat patterning be changed? *Acta Medica Scandinavica Supplementum* 1988;723:213–223.

Krotkiewski M. Physical training in the prophylaxis and treatment of obesity, hypertension, and diabetes. *Scandinavian Journal of Rehabilitation Medicine Supplement* 1983;9:55–70.

# Physical Activity and Health

Krummel D, Etherton TD, Peterson S, Kris-Etherton PM. Effects of exercise on plasma lipids and lipoproteins of women. *Proceedings of the Society for Experimental Biology and Medicine* 1993;204:123–137.

Ku LC, Shapiro LR, Crawford PB, Huenemann RL. Body composition and physical activity in 8-year-old children. *American Journal of Clinical Nutrition* 1981; 34:2770–2775.

Kuczmarski RJ. Prevalence of overweight and weight gain in the United States. *American Journal of Clinical Nutrition* 1992;55:495S–502S.

Kuczmarski RJ, Flegal KM, Campbell SM, Johnson CL. Increasing prevalence of overweight among US adults: the National Health and Nutrition Examination Surveys, 1960 to 1991. *Journal of the American Medical Association* 1994;272:205–211.

Kuipers H. Exercise-induced muscle damage. *International Journal of Sports Medicine* 1994;15:132–135.

Kujala UM, Kaprio J, Sarna S. Osteoarthritis of weight-bearing joints of lower limbs in former elite male athletes. *British Medical Journal* 1994;308:231–234.

Kujala UM, Kettunen J, Paananen H, Aalto T, Battié MC, Impivaara O, et al. Knee osteoarthritis in former runners, soccer players, weight lifters, and shooters. *Arthritis and Rheumatism* 1995;38:539–546.

Kune GA, Kune S, Watson LF. Body weight and physical activity as predictors of colorectal cancer risk. *Nutrition and Cancer* 1990;13:9–17.

LaCroix AZ, Leveille SG, Hecht JA, Grothaus LC, Wagner EH. Does walking decrease the risk of cardiovascular disease hospitalizations and death in older adults? *Journal of the American Geriatrics Society* 1996;44:113–120.

LaFontaine TP, DiLorenzo TM, Frensch PA, Stucky-Ropp RC, Bargman EP, McDonald DG. Aerobic exercise and mood: a brief review, 1985–1990. *Sports Medicine* 1992;13:160–170.

Lai J-S, Lan C, Wong M-K, Teng S-H. Two-year trends in cardiorespiratory function among older Tai Chi Chuan practitioners and sedentary subjects. *Journal of the American Geriatrics Society* 1995;43:1222–1227.

Lammi M. *Influences of in vivo and in vitro loading on the proteoglycan syntheses of articular cartilage chondrocytes.* Kuopio, Finland: Kuopio University, 1993.

Lampman RM, Schteingart DE. Effects of exercise training on glucose control, lipid metabolism, and insulin sensitivity in hypertriglyceridemia and non-insulin-dependent diabetes mellitus. *Medicine and Science in Sports and Exercise* 1991;23:703–712.

Landers DM, Petruzzello SJ. Physical activity, fitness, and anxiety. In: Bouchard C, Shephard RJ, Stephens T, editors. *Physical activity, fitness, and health: international proceedings and consensus statement.* Champaign, IL: Human Kinetics, 1994:868–882.

Lane NE. Exercise: a cause of osteoarthritis. *Journal of Rheumatology* 1995;22 (Suppl 43):3–6.

Lane NE, Bloch DA, Jones HH, Marshall WH, Wood PD, Fries JF. Long-distance running, bone density, and osteoarthritis. *Journal of the American Medical Association* 1986;255:1147–1151.

Lane NE, Michel B, Bjorkengren A, Oehlert J, Shi H, Bloch DA, et al. The risk of osteoarthritis with running and aging: a 5-year longitudinal study. *Journal of Rheumatology* 1993;20:461–468.

Lanyon LE. Functional strain in bone tissue as an objective, and controlling stimulus for adaptive bone remodelling. *Journal of Biomechanics* 1987;20:1083–1093.

Lanyon LE. Osteocytes, strain detection, bone modeling and remodeling. *Calcified Tissue International* 1993;53 (1 Suppl):S102–S107.

Lanyon LE. Using functional loading to influence bone mass and architecture: objectives, mechanisms, and relationship with estrogen of the mechanically adaptive process in bone. *Bone* 1996;18(1 Suppl):37S–43S.

Lapidus L, Bengtsson C. Socioeconomic factors and physical activity in relation to cardiovascular disease and death: a 12-year follow-up of participants in a population study of women in Gothenburg, Sweden. *British Heart Journal* 1986;55:295–301.

LaPorte RE, Cauley JA, Kinsey CM, Corbett W, Robertson R, Black-Sandler R, et al. The epidemiology of physical activity in children, college students, middle-aged men, menopausal females, and monkeys. *Journal of Chronic Diseases* 1982;35:787–795.

Laughlin MH. Effects of exercise training on coronary circulation: introduction. *Medicine and Science in Sports and Exercise* 1994;26:1226–1229.

Le Marchand L, Kolonel LN, Yoshizawa CN. Lifetime occupational physical activity and prostate cancer risk. *American Journal of Epidemiology* 1991;133:103–111.

Lee I-M. Physical activity, fitness, and cancer. In: Bouchard C, Shephard RJ, Stephens T, editors. *Physical activity, fitness, and health: international proceedings and consensus statement.* Champaign, IL: Human Kinetics, 1994:814–831.

Lee I-M, Manson JE, Hennekens CH, Paffenbarger RS Jr. Body weight and mortality: a 27-year follow-up of middle-aged men. *Journal of the American Medical Association* 1993;270:2823–2828.

Lee I-M, Paffenbarger RS Jr, Hsieh C-C. Physical activity and risk of developing colorectal cancer among college alumni. *Journal of the National Cancer Institute* 1991;83:1324–1329.

Lee I-M, Paffenbarger RS Jr, Hsieh C-C. Physical activity and risk of prostatic cancer among college alumni. *American Journal of Epidemiology* 1992;135:169–179.

Lee J, Lauer RM, Clarke WR. Lipoproteins in the progeny of young men with coronary artery disease: children with increased risk. *Pediatrics* 1986;78:330–337.

Leibel RL, Rosenbaum M, Hirsch J. Changes in energy expenditure resulting from altered body weight. *New England Journal of Medicine* 1995;332:621–628.

Lennon D, Nagle F, Stratman F, Shrago E, Dennis S. Diet and exercise training effects on resting metabolic rate. *International Journal of Obesity* 1985;9:39–47.

Lennox SS, Bedell JR, Stone AA. The effect of exercise on normal mood. *Journal of Psychosomatic Research* 1990;34:629–636.

Leon AS. Effects of exercise conditioning on physiologic precursors of coronary heart disease. *Journal of Cardiopulmonary Rehabilitation* 1991a;11:46–57.

Leon AS. Patients with diabetes mellitus. In: Franklin BA, Gordon S, Timmis GC, editors. *Exercise in modern medicine.* Baltimore: Williams and Wilkins, 1989:118–145.

Leon AS. Physical activity and risk of ischemic heart disease: an update, 1990. In: Oja P, Telama R, editors. *Sport for all.* New York: Elsevier, 1991b:251–64.

Leon AS. Recent advances in the management of hypertension. *Journal of Cardiopulmonary Rehabilitation* 1991c;11:182–191.

Leon AS. The role of exercise in the prevention and management of diabetes mellitus and blood lipid disorders. In: Shephard RJ, Miller HS Jr, editors. *Exercise and the heart in health and disease.* New York: Marcel Dekker, 1992:299–368.

Leon AS, Bloor CM. Effects of exercise and its cessation on the heart and its blood supply. *Journal of Applied Physiology* 1968;24:485–490.

Leon AS, Bloor CM. The effect of complete and partial deconditioning on exercise-induced cardiovascular changes in the rat. *Advances in Cardiology* 1976;18:81–92.

Leon AS, Connett J. Physical activity and 10.5 year mortality in the Multiple Risk Factor Intervention Trial (MRFIT). *International Journal of Epidemiology* 1991;20:690–697.

Leon AS, Connett J, Jacobs DR Jr, Rauramaa R. Leisure-time physical activity levels and risk of coronary heart disease and death: the Multiple Risk Factor Intervention Trial. *Journal of the American Medical Association* 1987;258:2388–2395.

Levi F, La Vecchia C, Negri E, Franceschi S. Selected physical activities and the risk of endometrial cancer. *British Journal of Cancer* 1993;67:846–851.

Levitt NS, Katzenellenbogen JM, Bradshaw D, Hoffman MN, Bonnici F. The prevalence and identification of risk factors for NIDDM in urban Africans in Cape Town, South Africa. *Diabetes Care* 1993;16:601–607.

Lie H, Mundal R, Erikssen J. Coronary risk factors and incidence of coronary death in relation to physical fitness: seven-year follow-up study of middle-aged and elderly men. *European Heart Journal* 1985;6:147–157.

Lillioja S, Bogardus C. Obesity and insulin resistance: lessons learned from the Pima Indians. *Diabetes/Metabolism Reviews* 1988;4:517–540.

Lindberg H, Roos H, Gårdsell P. Prevalence of coxarthrosis in former soccer players: 286 players compared with matched controls. *Acta Orthopaedica Scandinavica* 1993;64:165–167.

Lindgärde F, Malmquist J, Balke B. Physical fitness, insulin secretion, and glucose tolerance in healthy males and mild type-2 diabetes. *Acta Diabetologica Latina* 1983;20:33–40.

Lindgärde F, Saltin B. Daily physical activity, work capacity, and glucose tolerance in lean and obese normoglycaemic middle-aged men. *Diabetologia* 1981;20:134–138.

Lindsted KD, Tonstad S, Kuzma JW. Self-report of physical activity and patterns of mortality in Seventh-day Adventist men. *Journal of Clinical Epidemiology* 1991;44:355–364.

Little J, Logan RFA, Hawtin PG, Hardcastle JD, Turner ID. Colorectal adenomas and energy intake, body size, and physical activity: a case-control study of subjects participating in the Nottingham faecal occult blood screening programme. *British Journal of Cancer* 1993;67:172–176.

Longnecker MP, De Verdier MG, Frumkin H, Carpenter C. A case-control study of physical activity in relation to risk of cancer of the right colon and rectum in men. *International Journal of Epidemiology* 1995;24:42–50.

Lynge E, Thygesen L. Use of surveillance systems for occupational cancer: data from the Danish National system. *International Journal of Epidemiology* 1988;17:493–500.

Macera CA. Lower extremity injuries in runners: advances in prediction. *Sports Medicine* 1992;13:50–57.

Macera CA, Pate RR, Powell KE, Jackson KL, Kendrick JS, Craven TE. Predicting lower extremity injuries among habitual runners. *Archives of Inernal Medicine* 1989;149:2565–2568.

Mahoney LT, Lauer RM, Lee J, Clarke WR. Factors affecting tracking of coronary heart disease risk factors in children: the Muscatine Study. *Annals of the New York Academy of Sciences* 1991;623:120–132.

Manson JE, Nathan DM, Krolewski AS, Stampfer MJ, Willett WC, Hennekens CH. A prospective study of exercise and incidence of diabetes among U.S. male physicians. *Journal of the American Medical Association* 1992;268:63–67.

Manson JE, Rimm EB, Stampfer MJ, Colditz GA, Willett WC, Krolewski AS, et al. Physical activity and incidence of non-insulin-dependent diabetes mellitus in women. *Lancet* 1991;338:774778.

Manson JE, Willett WC, Stampfer MJ, Colditz GA, Hunter DJ, Hankinson SE, et al. Body weight and mortality among women. *New England Journal of Medicine* 1995;333:677–685.

Marceau M, Kouame N, Lacourciere Y, Cleroux J. Effects of different training intensities on 24 hour blood pressure in hypertensive subjects. *Circulation* 1993; 88:2803–2811.

Marcus PM, Newcomb PA, Storer BE. Early adulthood physical activity and colon cancer risk among Wisconsin women. *Cancer Epidemiology, Biomarkers and Prevention* 1994;3:641–644.

Marcus R, Cann C, Madvig P, Minkoff J, Goddard M, Bayer M, et al. Menstrual function and bone mass in elite women distance runners: endocrine and metabolic features. *Annals of Internal Medicine* 1985;102:158–163.

Markowitz S, Morabia A, Garibaldi K, Wynder E. Effect of occupational and recreational activity on the risk of colorectal cancer among males: a case-control study. *International Journal of Epidemiology* 1992;21:1057–1062.

Marti B. Benefits and risks of running among women: an epidemiologic study. *International Journal of Sports Medicine* 1988;9:92–98.

Marti B, Minder CE. Physische berufsaktivität und kolonkarzinommortalität bei Schweizer männern 1979–1982 [Physical occupational activity and colonic carcinoma mortality in Swiss men, 1979–1982]. *Sozial- und Präventivmedizin* 1989;34:30–37.

Marti B, Vader JP, Minder CE, Abelin T. On the epidemiology of running injuries: the 1984 Bern Grand-Prix study. *American Journal of Sports Medicine* 1988;16: 285–294.

Martinsen EW, Medhus A, Sandvik L. Effects of aerobic exercise on depression: a controlled study. *British Medical Journal* 1985;291:109–110.

Martinsen EW, Stephens T. Exercise and mental health in clinical and free-living populations. In: Dishman RK, editor. *Advances in exercise adherence.* Champaign, IL: Human Kinetics, 1994:55–72.

Matsusaki M, Ikeda M, Tashiro E, Koga M, Miura S, Ideishi M, et al. Influence of workload on the antihypertensive effect of exercise. *Clinical and Experimental Pharmacology and Physiology* 1992;19:471–479.

McAuley E. Physical activity and psychosocial outcomes. In: Bouchard C, Shephard RJ, Stephens T, editors. *Physical activity, fitness, and health: international proceedings and consensus statement.* Champaign, IL: Human Kinetics, 1994:551–568.

McAuley E, Rudolph D. Physical activity, aging, and psychological well-being. *Journal of Aging and Physical Activity* 1995;3:67–96.

McDonald DG, Hodgdon JA. *The psychological effects of aerobic fitness training: research and theory.* New York: Springer-Verlag, 1991.

McGinnis JM, Foege WH. Actual causes of death in the United States. *Journal of the American Medical Association* 1993;270:2207–2212.

McKeigue PM, Pierpoint T, Ferrie JE, Marmot MG. Relationship of glucose intolerance and hyperinsulinaemia to body fat pattern in south Asians and Europeans. *Diabetologia* 1992;35:785–791.

Mellion MB. Common cycling injuries: management and prevention. *Sports Medicine* 1991;11:52–70.

Menotti A, Keys A, Blackburn H, Aravanis C, Dontas A, Fidanza F, et al. Twenty-year stroke mortality and prediction in twelve cohorts of the Seven Countries Study. *International Journal of Epidemiology* 1990;19: 309–315.

Menotti A, Seccareccia F. Physical activity at work and job responsibility as risk factors for fatal coronary heart disease and other causes of death. *Journal of Epidemiology and Community Health* 1985;39:325–329.

Metropolitan Life Insurance Company. New weight standards for men and women. *Statistical Bulletin of the Metropolitan Life Insurance Company* 1959;40:1–4.

Meyer HE, Tverdal A, Falch JA. Risk factors for hip fracture in middle-aged Norwegian women and men. *American Journal of Epidemiology* 1993;137:1203–1211.

Michel BA, Bloch DA, Fries JF. Weight-bearing exercise, overexercise, and lumbar bone density over age 50 years. *Archives of Internal Medicine* 1989;149:2325–2329.

Mink PJ, Folsom AR, Sellers TA, Kushi LH. Physical activity, waist-to-hip ratio, and other risk factors for ovarian cancer: a follow-up study of older women. *Epidemiology* 1996;7:38–45.

Minor MA. Physical activity and management of arthritis. *Annals of Behavioral Medicine* 1991;13:117–124.

Minor MA, Brown JD. Exercise maintenance of persons with arthritis after participation in a class experience. *Health Education Quarterly* 1993;20:83–95.

Minor MA, Hewett JE, Webel RR, Anderson SK, Kay DR. Efficacy of physical conditioning exercise in patients with rheumatoid arthritis and osteoarthritis. *Arthritis and Rheumatism* 1989;32:1396–1405.

Minor MA, Hewett JE, Webel RR, Dreisinger TE, Kay DR. Exercise tolerance and disease-related measures in patients with rheumatoid arthritis and osteoarthritis. *Journal of Rheumatology* 1988;15:905–911.

Mittendorf R, Longnecker MP, Newcomb PA, Dietz AT, Greenberg ER, Bogdan GF, et al. Strenuous physical activity in young adulthood and risk of breast cancer (United States). *Cancer Causes and Control* 1995;6:347–353.

Mittleman MA, Maclure M, Tofler GH, Sherwood JB, Goldberg RJ, Muller JE. Triggering of acute myocardial infarction by heavy physical exertion: protection against triggering by regular exertion. *New England Journal of Medicine* 1993;329:1677–1683.

Montoye HJ, Block WD, Metzner H, Keller JB. Habitual physical activity and glucose tolerance: males age 16–64 in a total community. *Diabetes* 1977;26:172–176.

Moore M. Endorphins and exercise: a puzzling relationship. *Physician and Sportsmedicine* 1982;10:111–114.

Moore LL, Nguyen US, Rothman KJ, Cupples LA, Ellison RC. Preschool physical activity level and change in body fatness in young children: the Framingham Children's Study. *American Journal of Epidemiology* 1995;142:982–988.

Morgan WP. Anxiety reduction following acute physical activity. *Psychiatric Annals* 1979a;9:36–45.

Morgan WP. Negative addiction in runners. *Physician and Sportsmedicine* 1979b;7:57–70.

Morgan WP. Physical activity, fitness, and depression. In: Bouchard C, Shephard RJ, Stephens T, editors. *Physical activity, fitness, and health: international proceedings and consensus statement.* Champaign, IL: Human Kinetics, 1994:851–867.

Morgan WP. Psychological benefits of physical activity. In: Nagle FJ, Montoye HJ, editors. *Exercise in health and disease.* Springfield, IL: Charles C. Thomas, 1981:299–314.

Morgan WP, Brown DR, Raglin JS, O'Connor PJ, Ellickson KA. Psychological monitoring of overtraining and staleness. *British Journal of Sports Medicine* 1987;21:107–114.

Morgan WP, Goldston SE, editors. *Exercise and mental health.* Washington, DC: Hemisphere Publishing, 1987.

Morgan WP, Horstman DH, Cymerman A, Stokes J. Use of exercise as a relaxation technique. *Primary Cardiology* 1980;6:48–57.

Morgan WP, Roberts JA, Brand FR, Feinerman AD. Psychological effect of chronic physical activity. *Medicine and Science in Sports* 1970;2:213–217.

Morris JN, Chave SPW, Adam C, Sirey C, Epstein L, Sheehan DJ. Vigorous exercise in leisure-time and the incidence of coronary heart disease. *Lancet* 1973;1:333–339.

Morris JN, Clayton DG, Everitt MG, Semmence AM, Burgess EH. Exercise in leisure time: coronary attack and death rates. *British Heart Journal* 1990;63:325–334.

Morris JN, Crawford MD. Coronary heart disease and physical activity of work: evidence of a national necropsy survey. *British Medical Journal* 1958;2:1485–1496.

Morris JN, Everitt MG, Pollard R, Chave SPW, Semmence AM. Vigorous exercise in leisure time: protection against coronary heart disease. *Lancet* 1980;2:1207–1210.

Morris JN, Heady JA, Raffle PAB, Roberts CG, Parks JW. Coronary heart disease and physical activity of work. *Lancet* 1953;2:1111–1120.

## Physical Activity and Health

Morris JN, Kagan A, Pattison DC, Gardner MJ, Raffle PAB. Incidence and prediction of ischemic heart disease in London busmen. *Lancet* 1966;2:553–559.

Moses J, Steptoe A, Mathews A, Edwards S. The effects of exercise training on mental well-being in the normal population: a controlled trial. *Journal of Psychosomatic Research* 1989;33:47–61.

Must A, Jacques PF, Dallal GE, Bajema CJ, Dietz WH. Long-term morbidity and mortality of overweight adolescents: a follow-up of the Harvard Growth Study of 1922 to 1935. *New England Journal of Medicine* 1992;327:1350–1355.

Nagulesparan M, Savage PJ, Bennion LJ, Unger RH, Bennett PH. Diminished effect of caloric restriction on control of hyperglycemia with increasing known duration of type II diabetes mellitus. *Journal of Clinical Endocrinology and Metabolism* 1981;53:560–568.

National Advisory Mental Health Council. Health care reform for Americans with severe mental illnesses: report of the National Advisory Mental Health Council. *American Journal of Psychiatry* 1993;150:1447–1465.

National Center for Health Statistics. *Vital Statistics of the United States, 1990, Vol. 2, Mortality, Part A.* Hyattsville, MD: U.S. Department of Health and Human Services, Public Health Service, Centers for Disease Control and Prevention, National Center for Health Statistics, 1994. DHHS Publication No. (PHS) 95-1102.

National Center for Health Statistics, Gardner P, Hudson BL. *Advance report of final mortality statistics, 1993.* Hyattsville, MD: U.S. Department of Health and Human Services, Public Health Service, Centers for Disease Control and Prevention, National Center for Health Statistics, 1996. (Monthly vital statistics report; Vol. 44, No. 4, Suppl).

National Institutes of Health. Consensus Conference: Osteoporosis. *Journal of the American Medical Association* 1984;252:799–802.

National Institutes of Health. Health implications of obesity: National Institutes of Health Consensus Development Conference Statement. *Annals of Internal Medicine* 1985;103(Suppl 6, Pt 2):1073–1077.

National Institutes of Health. *The Fifth Report of the Joint National Committee on Detection, Evaluation, and Treatment of High Blood Pressure.* Bethesda, MD: National Institutes of Health, National Heart, Lung, and Blood Institute, 1992:1–48. NIH Publication No. 93-1088.

Nelson ME, Fisher EC, Dilmanian FA, Dallal GE, Evans WJ. A one-year walking program and increased dietary calcium in postmenopausal women: effects on bone. *American Journal of Clinical Nutrition* 1991;53:1304–1311.

Newsholme EA, Parry-Billings M. Effects of exercise on the immune system. In: Bouchard C, Shephard RJ, Stephens T, editors. *Physical activity, fitness, and health: international proceedings and consensus statement.* Champaign, IL: Human Kinetics, 1994:451–455.

Nichols DL, Sanborn CF, Bonnick SL, Ben-Ezra V, Gench B, DiMarco NM. The effects of gymnastics training on bone mineral density. *Medicine and Science in Sports and Exercise* 1994;26:1220–1225.

Nieto FJ, Szklo M, Comstock GW. Childhood weight and growth rate as predictors of adult mortality. *American Journal of Epidemiology* 1992;136:201–213.

North TC, McCullagh P, Tran ZV. Effect of exercise on depression. *Exercise and Sport Sciences Reviews* 1990;18:379–415.

Obarzanek E, Schreiber GB, Crawford PB, Goldman SR, Barrier PM, Frederick MM, et al. Energy intake and physical activity in relation to indexes of body fat: the National Heart, Lung, and Blood Institute Growth and Health Study. *American Journal of Clinical Nutrition* 1994;60:15–22.

O'Connor GT, Buring JE, Yusuf S, Goldhaber SZ, Olmstead EM, Paffenbarger RS Jr, et al. An overview of randomized trials of rehabilitation with exercise after myocardial infarction. *Circulation* 1989;80:234–244.

Oliveria SA, Kohl HW III, Trichopoulos D, Blair SN. The association between cardiorespiratory fitness and prostate cancer. *Medicine and Science in Sports and Exercise* 1996;28:97–104.

Ornish D, Brown SE, Scherwitz LW, Billings JH, Armstrong WT, Ports TA, et al. Can lifestyle changes reverse coronary heart disease? The Lifestyle Heart Trial. *Lancet* 1990;336:129–133.

Oscai LB. The role of exercise in weight control. *Exercise and Sport Sciences Reviews* 1973;1:103–123.

Overholser KA, Laughlin MH, Bhatte MJ. Exercise training-induced increase in coronary transport capacity. *Medicine and Science in Sports and Exercise* 1994;26:1239–1244.

Paffenbarger RS Jr. Contributions of epidemiology to exercise science and cardiovascular health. *Medicine and Science in Sports and Exercise* 1988;20:426–438.

Paffenbarger RS Jr. Factors predisposing to fatal stroke in longshoremen. *Preventive Medicine* 1972;1:522–527.

Paffenbarger RS Jr, Hale WE. Work activity and coronary heart mortality. *New England Journal of Medicine* 1975;292:545–550.

Paffenbarger RS Jr, Hale WE, Brand RJ, Hyde RT. Work-energy level, personal characteristics, and fatal heart attack: a birth-cohort effect. *American Journal of Epidemiology* 1977;105:200–213.

Paffenbarger RS Jr, Hyde RT, Wing AL. Physical activity and incidence of cancer in diverse populations: a preliminary report. *American Journal of Clinical Nutrition* 1987;45:312–317.

Paffenbarger RS Jr, Hyde RT, Wing AL, Hsieh C-C. Physical activity, all-cause mortality, and longevity of college alumni. *New England Journal of Medicine* 1986;314:605–613.

Paffenbarger RS Jr, Hyde RT, Wing AL, Lee I-M, Jung DL, Kampert JB. The association of changes in physical activity level and other lifestyle characteristics with mortality among men. *New England Journal of Medicine* 1993;328:538–545.

Paffenbarger RS Jr, Hyde RT, Wing AL, Lee I-M, Kampert JB. Some interrelations of physical activity, physiological fitness, health, and longevity. In: Bouchard C, Shephard RJ, Stephens T, editors. *Physical activity, fitness, and health: international proceedings and consensus statement.* Champaign, IL: Human Kinetics, 1994:119–133.

Paffenbarger RS Jr, Hyde RT, Wing AL, Steinmetz CH. A natural history of athleticism and cardiovascular health. *Journal of the American Medical Association* 1984; 252:491–495.

Paffenbarger RS Jr, Jung DL, Leung RW, Hyde RT. Physical activity and hypertension: an epidemiological view. *Annals of Medicine* 1991;23:319–327.

Paffenbarger RS Jr, Lee I-M, Leung R. Physical activity and personal characteristics associated with depression and suicide in American college men. *Acta Psychiatrica Scandinavica Supplementum* 1994;377:16–22.

Paffenbarger RS Jr, Thorne MC, Wing AL. Chronic disease in former college students: characteristics in youth predisposing to hypertension in later years. *American Journal of Epidemiology* 1968;88:25–32.

Paffenbarger RS Jr, Williams JL. Chronic disease in former college students: early precursors of fatal stroke. *American Journal of Public Health* 1967;57:1290–1299.

Paffenbarger RS Jr, Wing AL, Hyde RT. Physical activity as an index of heart attack risk in college alumni. *American Journal of Epidemiology* 1978;108:161–175.

Paffenbarger RS Jr, Wing AL, Hyde RT, Jung DL. Physical activity and incidence of hypertension in college alumni. *American Journal of Epidemiology* 1983;117:245–257.

Pan X, Li G, Hu Y. [Effect of dietary and/or exercise intervention on incidence of diabetes in 530 subjects with impaired glucose tolerance from 1986–1992]. *Chinese Journal of Internal Medicine* 1995;34:108–112.

Panush RS, Hanson CS, Caldwell JR, Longley S, Stork J, Thoburn R. Is running associated with osteoarthritis? An eight-year follow-up study. *Journal of Clinical Rheumatology* 1995;1:35–39.

Panush RS, Lane NE. Exercise and the musculoskeletal system. *Bailliere's Clinical Rheumatology* 1994;8:79–102.

Panush RS, Schmidt C, Caldwell JR, Edwards NL, Longley S, Yonker R, et al. Is running associated with degenerative joint disease? *Journal of the American Medical Association* 1986;255:1152–1154.

Pate RR, Pratt M, Blair SN, Haskell WL, Macera CA, Bouchard C, et al. Physical activity and public health: a recommendation from the Centers for Disease Control and Prevention and the American College of Sports Medicine. *Journal of the American Medical Association* 1995;273:402–407.

Pekkanen J, Marti B, Nissinen A, Tuomilehto J, Punsar S, Karvonen MJ. Reduction of premature mortality by high physical activity: a 20-year follow-up of middle-aged Finnish men. *Lancet* 1987;1:1473–1477.

Peters RK, Cady LD Jr, Bischoff DP, Bernstein L, Pike MC. Physical fitness and subsequent myocardial infarction in healthy workers. *Journal of the American Medical Association* 1983;249:3052–3056.

Peters RK, Garabrant DH, Yu MC, Mack TM. A case-control study of occupational and dietary factors in colorectal cancer in young men by subsite. *Cancer Research* 1989;49:5459–5468.

Pfeiffer RP, Kronisch RL. Off-road cycling injuries: an overview. *Sports Medicine* 1995;19:311–325.

Pi-Sunyer FX. Exercise in the treatment of obesity. In: *Obesity and weight control: the health professional's guide to understanding and treatment.* Rockville, MD: Aspen Publishers, 1988:241–255.

165

# Physical Activity and Health

Pitsillides AA, Rawlinson SCF, Suswillo RFL, Bourrin S, Zaman G, Lanyon LE. Mechanical strain-induced NO production by bone cells: a possible role in adaptive bone (re)modeling. *FASEB Journal* 1995;9:1614–1622.

Plante TG, Rodin J. Physical fitness and enhanced psychological health. *Current Psychology: Research and Reviews* 1990;9:3–24.

Pocock NA, Eisman JA, Yeates MG, Sambrook PN, Eberl S. Physical fitness is a major determinant of femoral neck and lumbar spine bone mineral density. *Journal of Clinical Investigation* 1986;78:618–621.

Polednak AP. College athletes, body size, and cancer mortality. *Cancer* 1976;38:382–387.

Polivy J. Physical activity, fitness, and compulsive behaviors. In: Bouchard C, Shephard RJ, Stephens T, editors. *Physical activity, fitness, and health: international proceedings and consensus statement.* Champaign, IL: Human Kinetics, 1994:883–897.

Pollock ML, Carroll JF, Graves JE, Leggett SH, Braith RW, Limacher M, et al. Injuries and adherence to walk/jog and resistance training programs in the elderly. *Medicine and Science in Sports and Exercise* 1991;23:1194–1200.

Pollock ML, Gettman LR, Milesis CA, Bah MD, Durstine L, Johnson RB. Effects of frequency and duration of training on attrition and incidence of injury. *Medicine and Science in Sports* 1977;9:31–36.

Pomrehn PR, Wallace RB, Burmeister LF. Ischemic heart disease mortality in Iowa farmers: the influence of lifestyle. *Journal of the American Medical Association* 1982;248:1073–1076.

Powell KE, Blair SN. The public health burdens of sedentary living habits: theoretical but realistic estimates. *Medicine and Science in Sports and Exercise* 1994;26:851–856.

Powell KE, Thompson PD, Caspersen CJ, Kendrick JS. Physical activity and the incidence of coronary heart disease. *Annual Review of Public Health* 1987;8:253–287.

Prince RL, Smith M, Dick IM, Price RI, Webb PG, Henderson NK, et al. Prevention of postmenopausal osteoporosis: a comparative study of exercise, calcium supplementation, and hormone-replacement therapy. *New England Journal of Medicine* 1991:325:1189–1195.

Province MA, Hadley EC, Hornbrook MC, Lipsitz LA, Miller JP, Mulrow CD, et al. The effects of exercise on falls in elderly patients: a preplanned meta-analysis of the FICSIT trials. *Journal of the American Medical Association* 1995;273:1341–1347.

Pruitt LA, Jackson RD, Bartels RL, Lehnhard HJ. Weight-training effects on bone mineral density in early postmenopausal women. *Journal of Bone and Mineral Research* 1992;7:179–185.

Puett DW, Griffin MR. Published trials of nonmedicinal and noninvasive therapies for hip and knee osteoarthritis. *Annals of Internal Medicine* 1994;121:133–140.

Pukkala E, Poskiparta M, Apter D, Vihko V. Life-long physical activity and cancer risk among Finnish female teachers. *European Journal of Cancer Prevention* 1993;2:369–376.

Raglin JS. Exercise and mental health: beneficial and detrimental effects. *Sports Medicine* 1990;9:323–329.

Raglin JS, Morgan WP. Influence of exercise and quiet rest on state anxiety and blood pressure. *Medicine and Science in Sports and Exercise* 1987;19:456–463.

Rall KL, McElroy GL, Keats TE. A study of long-term effects of football injury to the knee. *Missouri Medicine* 1964;61:435–438.

Ramaiya KL, Swai ABM, McLarty DG, Alberti KGMM. Impaired glucose tolerance and diabetes mellitus in Hindu Indian immigrants in Dar es Salaam. *Diabetic Medicine* 1991;8:738–744.

Rankin JW. Diet, exercise, and osteoporosis. *American College of Sports Medicine News*, 1993;3:1–4.

Ransford CP. A role for amines in the antidepressant effect of exercise: a review. *Medicine and Science in Sports and Exercise* 1982;14:1–10.

Rauramaa R, Rankinen T, Tuomainen P, Väisänen S, Mercuri M. Inverse relationship between cardiorespiratory fitness and carotid atherosclerosis. *Atherosclerosis* 1995;112:213–221.

Ravussin E, Bennett PH, Valencia ME, Schulz LO, Esparza J. Effects of a traditional lifestyle on obesity in Pima Indians. *Diabetes Care* 1994;17:1067–1074.

Recker RR, Davies KM, Hinders SM, Heaney RP, Stegman MR, Kimmel DB. Bone gain in young adult women. *Journal of the American Medical Association* 1992;268:2403–2408.

Regensteiner JG, Shetterly SM, Mayer EJ, Eckel RH, Haskell WL, Baxter J, et al. Relationship between habitual physical activity and insulin area among individuals with impaired glucose tolerance: the San Luis Valley Diabetes Study. *Diabetes Care* 1995;18:490–497.

Regier DA, Narrow WE, Rae DS, Manderscheid RW, Locke BZ, Goodwin FK. The de facto U.S. mental and addictive disorders service system: epidemiologic catchment area prospective 1-year prevalence rates of disorders and services. Archives of General Psychiatry 1993;50:85–94.

Rejeski WJ, Brawley LR, Schumaker SA. Physical activity and health-related quality of life. Exercise and Sport Sciences Reviews 1996;24:71–108.

Rejeski WJ, Gauvin L, Hobson ML, Norris JL. Effects of baseline responses, in-task feelings, and duration of activity on exercise-induced feeling states in women. Health Psychology 1995;14:350–359.

Richie DH, Kelso SF, Bellucci PA. Aerobic dance injuries: a retrospective study of instructors and participants. Physician and Sportsmedicine 1985;13:130–140.

Richter EA, Ruderman NB, Schneider SH. Diabetes and exercise. American Journal of Medicine 1981;70:201–209.

Robinson TL, Snow-Harter C, Taaffe DR, Gillis D, Shaw J, Marcus R. Gymnasts exhibit higher bone mass than runners despite similar prevalence of amenorrhea and oligomenorrhea. Journal of Bone and Mineral Research 1995;10:26–35.

Rodriguez BL, Curb JD, Burchfiel CM, Abbott RD, Petrovitch H, Masaki K, et al. Physical activity and 23-year incidence of coronary heart disease morbidity and mortality among middle-aged men: the Honolulu Heart Program. Circulation 1994;89:2540–2544.

Rolf C. Overuse injuries of the lower extremity in runners. Scandinavian Journal of Medicine and Science in Sports 1995;5:181–190.

Rönnemaa T, Mattila K, Lehtonen A, Kallio V. A controlled randomized study on the effect of long-term physical exercise on the metabolic control in type 2 diabetic patients. Acta Medica Scandinavica 1986; 220:219–224.

Roos H, Lindberg H, Gardsell P, Lohmander LS, Wingstrand H. The prevalence of gonarthrosis and its relation to meniscectomy in former soccer players. American Journal of Sports Medicine 1994;22:219–222.

Rosenman RH, Bawol RD, Oscherwitz M. A 4-year prospective study of the relationship of different habitual vocational physical activity to risk and incidence of ischemic heart disease in volunteer male federal employees. Annals of the New York Academy of Sciences 1977;301:627–641.

Ross CE, Hayes D. Exercise and psychologic well-being in the community. American Journal of Epidemiology 1988;127:762–771.

Roth DL. Acute emotional and psychophysiological effects of aerobic exercise. Psychophysiology 1989;26:593–602.

Rubin K, Schirduan V, Gendreau P, Sarfarazi M, Mendola R, Dalsky G. Predictors of axial and peripheral bone mineral density in healthy children and adolescents, with special attention to the role of puberty. Journal of Pediatrics 1993;123:863–870.

Sallis JF, Patterson TL, McKenzie TL, Nader PR. Family variables and physical activity in preschool children. Journal of Developmental and Behavioral Pediatrics 1988; 9:57–61.

Salonen JT, Puska P, Tuomilehto J. Physical activity and risk of myocardial infarction, cerebral stroke, and death: a longitudinal study in Eastern Finland. American Journal of Epidemiology 1982;115:526–537.

Salonen JT, Slater JS, Tuomilehto J, Rauramaa R. Leisure time and occupational physical activity: risk of death from ischemic heart disease. American Journal of Epidemiology 1988;127:87–94.

Saltin B, Lindgärde F, Houston M, Horlin R, Nygaard E, Gad P. Physical training and glucose tolerance in middle-aged men with chemical diabetes. Diabetes 1979;28:30–32.

Sandler RB, Cauley JA, Sashin D, Scialabba MA, Kriska AM. The effect of grip strength on radial bone in postmenopausal women. Journal of Orthopaedic Research 1989;7:440–444.

Sandler RS, Pritchard ML, Bangdiwala SI. Physical activity and the risk of colorectal adenomas. Epidemiology 1995;6:602–606.

Sandvik L, Erikssen J, Thaulow E, Erikssen G, Mundal R, Rodahl K. Physical fitness as a predictor of mortality among healthy, middle-aged Norwegian men. New England Journal of Medicine 1993;328:533–537.

Scheuer J. Effects of physical training on myocardial vascularity and perfusion. Circulation 1982;66:491–495.

Schneider SH, Amorosa LF, Khachadurian AK, Ruderman NB. Studies on the mechanism of improved glucose control during regular exercise in type 2 (non-insulin-dependent) diabetes. Diabetologia 1984;26:355–360.

# Physical Activity and Health

Schranz A, Tuomilehto J, Marti B, Jarrett RJ, Grabauskas V, Vassallo A. Low physical activity and worsening of glucose tolerance: results from a 2-year follow-up of a population sample in Malta. *Diabetes Research and Clinical Practice* 1991;11:127–136.

Schuler G, Hambrecht R, Schlierf G, Niebauer J, Hauer K, Neumann J, et al. Regular physical exercise and low fat diet: effects on progression of coronary artery disease. *Circulation* 1992;86:1–11.

Seccareccia F, Menotti A. Physical activity, physical fitness, and mortality in a sample of middle-aged men followed up 25 years. *Journal of Sports Medicine and Physical Fitness* 1992; 32:206–213.

Seidell JC, Cigolini M, Deslypere J-P, Charzewska J, Ellsinger B-M, Cruz A. Body fat distribution in relation to physical activity and smoking habits in 38-year-old European men. *American Journal of Epidemiology* 1991;133:257–265.

Severson RK, Nomura AMY, Grove JS, Stemmermann GN. A prospective analysis of physical activity and cancer. *American Journal of Epidemiology* 1989;130:522–529.

Shangold MM. Exercise and the adult female: hormonal and endocrine effects. *Exercise and Sport Sciences Reviews* 1984;12:53–79.

Shaper AG, Wannamethee G. Physical activity and ischaemic heart disease in middle-aged British men. *British Heart Journal* 1991;66:384–394.

Shaper AG, Wannamethee G, Walker M. Physical activity, hypertension, and risk of heart attack in men without evidence of ischaemic heart disease. *Journal of Human Hypertension* 1994;8:3–10.

Shear CL, Freedman DS, Burke GL, Harsha DW, Webber LS, Berenson GS. Secular trends of obesity in early life: the Bogalusa Heart Study. *American Journal of Public Health* 1988;78:75–77.

Shephard RJ. Exercise in the prevention and treatment of cancer: an update. *Sports Medicine* 1993;15:258–280.

Shephard RJ, Verde TJ, Thomas SG, Shek P. Physical activity and the immune system. *Canadian Journal of Sport Sciences* 1991;16:163–185.

Sherman SE, D'Agostino RB, Cobb JL, Kannel WB. Physical activity and mortality in women in the Framingham Heart Study. *American Heart Journal* 1994;128:879–884.

Shimegi S, Yanagita M, Okano H, Yamada M, Fukui H, Fukumura Y, et al. Physical exercise increases bone mineral density in postmenopausal women. *Endocrine Journal* 1994;41:49–56.

Shu XO, Hatch MC, Zheng W, Gao YT, Brinton LA. Physical activity and risk of endometrial cancer. *Epidemiology* 1993;4:342–349.

Shumaker SA, Anderson RT, Czajkowski SM. Psychological tests and scales. In: Spilker B, editor. *Quality of life assessments in clinical trials*. New York: Raven Press, 1990:95–113.

Sime WE. Discussion: exercise, fitness, and mental health. In: Bouchard C, Shephard RJ, Stephens T, Sutton JR, McPherson BD, editors. *Exercise, fitness, and health: a consensus of current knowledge*. Champaign, IL: Human Kinetics, 1990:627–633.

Simons AD, McGowan CR, Epstein LH, Kupfer DJ, Robertson RJ. Exercise as a treatment for depression: an update. *Clinical Psychology Review* 1985;5;553–568.

Simons CW, Birkimer JC. An exploration of factors predicting the effects of aerobic conditioning on mood state. *Journal of Psychosomatic Research* 1988;32:63–75.

Sinaki M, McPhee MC, Hodgson SF, Merritt JM, Offord KP. Relationship between bone mineral density of spine and strength of back extensors in healthy postmenopausal women. *Mayo Clinic Proceedings* 1986;61:116–122.

Sinaki M, Offord KP. Physical activity in postmenopausal women: effect on back muscle strength and bone mineral density of the spine. *Archives of Physical Medicine and Rehabilitation* 1988;69:277–280.

Sinert R, Kohl L, Rainone T, Scalea T. Exercise-induced rhabdomyolysis. *Annals of Emergency Medicine* 1994;23:1301–1306.

Siscovick DS, Weiss NS, Fletcher RH, Lasky T. The incidence of primary cardiac arrest during vigorous exercise. *New England Journal of Medicine* 1984; 311:874–877.

Slattery ML, Jacobs DR Jr. Physical fitness and cardiovascular disease mortality: the U.S. Railroad Study. *American Journal of Epidemiology* 1988;127:571–580.

Slattery ML, Jacobs DR Jr, Nichaman MZ. Leisure-time physical activity and coronary heart disease death: the U.S. Railroad Study. *Circulation* 1989;79:304–311.

Slattery ML, McDonald A, Bild DE, Caan BJ, Hilner JE, Jacobs DR Jr, et al. Associations of body fat and its distribution with dietary intake, physical activity, alcohol, and smoking in blacks and whites. *American Journal of Clinical Nutrition* 1992;55:943–950.

Slattery ML, Schumacher MC, Smith KR, West DW, Abd-Elghany N. Physical activity, diet, and risk of colon cancer in Utah. *American Journal of Epidemiology* 1988;128:989–999.

Smith TW, Leon AS. *Coronary heart disease: a behavioral perspective*. Champaign, IL: Research Press, 1992:9–20.

Sobolski J, Kornitzer M, DeBacker G, Dramaix M, Abramowicz M, Degre S, et al. Protection against ischemic heart disease in the Belgian Physical Fitness Study: physical fitness rather than physical activity? *American Journal of Epidemiology* 1987;125:601–610.

Stamler R, Stamler J, Gosch FC, Civinelli J, Fishman J, McKeever P, et al. Primary prevention of hypertension by nutritional-hygienic means: final report of a randomized, controlled trial. *Journal of the American Medical Association* 1989;262:1801–1807.

Stary HC. Evolution and progression of atherosclerotic lesions in coronary arteries of children and young adults. *Arteriosclerosis* 1989;9(Suppl 1):119–132.

Stefanick ML. Exercise and weight control. *Exercise and Sport Sciences Reviews* 1993;21:363–396.

Stefanick ML, Wood PD. Physical activity, lipid and lipoprotein metabolism, and lipid transport. In: Bouchard C, Shephard RJ, Stephens T, editors. *Physical activity, fitness, and health: international proceedings and consensus statement*. Champaign, IL: Human Kinetics, 1994:417–431.

Stefanik PA, Heald FP, Mayer J. Caloric intake in relation to energy output of obese and nonobese adolescent boys. *American Journal of Clinical Nutrition* 1959;7:55–62.

Stender M, Hense HW, Döring A, Keil U. Physical activity at work and cardiovascular disease risk: results from the MONICA Augsburg Study. *International Journal of Epidemiology* 1993;22:644–650.

Stephens T. Physical activity and mental health in the United States and Canada: evidence from four population surveys. *Preventive Medicine* 1988;17:35–47.

Stephens T, Craig CL. *The well-being of Canadians: highlights of the 1988 Campbell's Survey*. Ottawa: Canadian Fitness and Lifestyle Research Institute, 1990.

Steptoe A, Edwards S, Moses J, Mathews A. The effects of exercise training on mood and perceived coping ability in anxious adults from the general population. *Journal of Psychosomatic Research* 1989;33:537–547.

Sternfeld B, Williams CS, Quesenberry CP, Satariano WA, Sidney S. Lifetime physical activity and incidence of breast cancer. *Medicine and Science in Sports and Exercise* 1993;25(5 Suppl):S147.

Stewart AL, Hays RD, Wells KB, Rogers WH, Spritzer KL, Greenfield S. Long-term functioning and well-being outcomes associated with physical activity and exercise in patients with chronic conditions in the Medical Outcomes Study. *Journal of Clinical Epidemiology* 1994; 47:719–730.

Stewart AL, King AC, Haskell WL. Endurance exercise and health-related quality of life in 50–65-year-old adults. *Gerontologist* 1993:33:782–9.

Strazzullo P, Cappuccio FP, Trevisan M, De Leo A, Krogh V, Giorgione N, et al. Leisure-time physical activity and blood pressure in schoolchildren. *American Journal of Epidemiology* 1988;127:726–733.

Sturgeon SR, Brinton LA, Berman ML, Mortel R, Twiggs LB, Barrett RJ, et al. Past and present physical activity and endometrial cancer risk. *British Journal of Cancer* 1993;68:584–589.

Superko HR. Exercise training, serum lipids, and lipoprotein particles: is there a change threshold? *Medicine and Science in Sports and Exercise* 1991;23:677–685.

Surgenor S, Uphold RE. Acute hyponatremia in ultra-endurance athletes. *American Journal of Emergency Medicine* 1994;12:441–444.

Taioli E, Barone J, Wynder EL. A case-control study on breast cancer and body mass: the American Health Foundation, Division of Epidemiology. *European Journal of Cancer* 1995;31A:723–728.

Tall AR. Plasma high density lipoproteins: metabolism and relationship to atherogenesis. *Journal of Clinical Investigation* 1990;86:379–384.

Talmage RV, Stinnett SS, Landwehr JT, Vincent LM, McCartney WH. Age-related loss of bone mineral density in non-athletic and athletic women. *Bone and Mineral* 1986;1:115–125.

Tang LY, Raab-Cullen DM, Yee JA, Jee WSS, Kimmel DB. Prostaglandin E$_2$ increases skeletal response. *Journal of Bone and Mineral Research* 1995;10:S246.

Task Force on Blood Pressure Control in Children. Report of the Second Task Force on Blood Pressure Control in Children—1987. *Pediatrics* 1987;79:1–25.

Taylor CB, Sallis JF, Needle R. The relation of physical activity and exercise to mental health. *Public Health Reports* 1985;100:195–202.

Taylor HL, Klepetar E, Keys A, Parlin W, Blackburn H, Puchner T. Death rates among physically active and sedentary employees of the railroad industry. *American Journal of Public Health* 1962;52:1697–1707.

Taylor R, Ram P, Zimmet P, Raper LR, Ringrose H. Physical activity and prevalence of diabetes in Melanesian and Indian men in Fiji. *Diabetologia* 1984;27:578–582.

Taylor RJ, Bennett PH, LeGonidec G, Lacoste J, Combe D, Joffres M, et al. The prevalence of diabetes mellitus in a traditional-living Polynesian population: the Wallis Island survey. *American Journal of Public Health* 1983;6:334–340.

Tell GS, Vellar OD. Physical fitness, physical activity, and cardiovascular disease risk factors in adolescents: the Oslo Youth Study. *Preventive Medicine* 1988;17:12–24.

Thomas JR, Landers DM, Salazar W, Etnier J. Exercise and cognitive function. In: Bouchard C, Shephard RJ, Stephens T, editors. *Physical activity, fitness, and health: international proceedings and consensus statement.* Champaign, IL: Human Kinetics, 1994:521–529.

Thompson JK, Jarvie GJ, Lahey BB, Cureton KJ. Exercise and obesity: etiology, physiology, and intervention. *Psychological Bulletin* 1982;91:55–79.

Thompson PD, Funk EJ, Carleton RA, Sturner WQ. Incidence of death during jogging in Rhode Island from 1975 through 1980. *Journal of the American Medical Association* 1982;247:2535–2538.

Thompson PD, Mitchell JH. Exercise and sudden cardiac death: protection or provocation? *New England Journal of Medicine* 1984;311:914–915.

Thor P, Konturek JW, Konturek SJ, Anderson JH. Role of prostaglandins in control of intestinal motility. *American Journal of Physiology* 1985;248:G353–G359.

Thune I, Lund E. Physical activity and the risk of prostate and testicular cancer: a cohort study of 53,000 Norwegian men. *Cancer Causes and Control* 1994;5:549–556.

Tinetti ME, Baker DI, McAvay G, Claus EB, Garrett P, Gottschalk M, et al. A multifactorial intervention to reduce the risk of falling among elderly people living in the community. *New England Journal of Medicine* 1994;331:821–827.

Tinetti ME, Speechley M, Ginter SF. Risk factors for falls among elderly persons living in the community. *New England Journal of Medicine* 1988;319:1701–1707.

Tipton CM. Exercise and resting blood pressure. In: Eckert HM, Montoye HJ, editors. *Exercise and health.* Champaign, IL: Human Kinetics, 1984:32–41.

Tomanek RJ. Exercise-induced coronary angiogenesis: a review. *Medicine and Science in Sports and Exercise* 1994;26:1245–1251.

Tremblay A, Després J-P, Leblanc C, Craig CL, Ferris B, Stephens T, et al. Effect of intensity of physical activity on body fatness and fat distribution. *American Journal of Clinical Nutrition* 1990;51:153–157.

Troiano RP, Flegal KM, Kuczmarski RJ, Campbell SM, Johnson CL. Overweight prevalence and trends for children and adolescents: the National Health and Nutrition Examination Surveys, 1963 to 1991. *Archives of Pediatrics and Adolescent Medicine* 1995; 149:1085–1091.

Troisi RJ, Heinold JW, Vokonas PS, Weiss ST. Cigarette smoking, dietary intake, and physical activity: effects on body fat distribution—the Normative Aging Study. *American Journal of Clinical Nutrition* 1991;53:1104–1111.

Trovati M, Carta Q, Cavalot F, Vitali S, Banaudi C, Lucchina PG, et al. Influence of physical training on blood glucose control, glucose tolerance, insulin secretion, and insulin action in noninsulin-dependent-diabetes patients. *Diabetes Care* 1984;7:416–420.

Tsopanakis AD, Sgouraki EP, Pavlou KN, Nadel ER, Bussolari SR. Lipids and lipoprotein profiles in a 4-hour endurance test on a recumbent cycloergometer. *American Journal of Clinical Nutrition* 1989;49:980–984.

Turner CH, Owan I, Takano Y, Madali S, Murrell GA. Nitric oxide plays a role in bone mechanotrasduction. *Journal of Bone and Mineral Research* 1995;10:S235.

Turner CH, Takano Y, Owan I. Aging changes mechanical loading thresholds for bone formation in rats. *Journal of Bone and Mineral Research* 1995;10:240.

Tutton PJM, Barkla DH. Influence of prostaglandin analogues on epithelial cell proliferation and xenograft growth. *British Journal of Cancer* 1980;41:47–51.

Underwood FB, Laughlin MH, Sturek M. Altered control of calcium in coronary smooth muscle cells by exercise training. *Medicine and Science in Sports and Exercise* 1994;26:1230–1238.

United Kingdom Testicular Cancer Study Group. Aetiology of testicular cancer: association with congenital abnormalities, age at puberty, infertility, and exercise. *British Medical Journal* 1994;308:1393–1399.

U.S. Department of Health and Human Services. *Health, United States, 1994.* Hyattsville, MD: U.S. Department of Health and Human Services, Public Health Service, Centers for Disease Control and Prevention, National Center for Health Statistics, 1995. DHHS Publication No. (PHS)95-1232.

Uusitupa M, Siitonen O, Pyörälä K, Aro A, Hersio K, Penttilä I, Voutilainen E. The relationship of cardio-vascular risk factors to the prevalence of coronary heart disease in newly diagnosed type 2 (non-insulin-dependent) diabetes. *Diabetologia* 1985;28:653–659.

Van Mechelen W. Running injuries: a review of the epidemiological literature. *Sports Medicine* 1992; 14:320–335.

Vena JE, Graham S, Zielezny M, Brasure J, Swanson MK. Occupational exercise and risk of cancer. *American Journal of Clinical Nutrition* 1987;45:318–327.

Vena JE, Graham S, Zielezny M, Swanson MK, Barnes RE, Nolan J. Lifetime occupational exercise and colon cancer. *American Journal of Epidemiology* 1985;122:357–365.

Vetter R, Dosemeci M, Blair A, Wacholder S, Unsal M, Engin K, et al. Occupational physical activity and colon cancer risk in Turkey. *European Journal of Epidemiology* 1992;8:845–850.

Vincelette P, Laurin CA, Lévesque HP. The footballer's ankle and foot. *Canadian Medical Association Journal* 1972;107:872–877.

Vineis P, Ciccone G, Magnino A. Asbestos exposure, physical activity, and colon cancer: a case control study. *Tumori* 1993;79:301–303.

Vlajinac H, Jarebinski M, Adanja B. Relationship of some biosocial factors to colon cancer in Belgrade (Yugoslavia). *Neoplasma* 1987;34:503–507.

Voorrips LE, Meijers JHH, Sol P, Seidell JC, van Staveren WA. History of body weight and physical activity of elderly women differing in current physical activity. *International Journal of Obesity* 1992;16:199–205.

Wahrenberg H, Bolinder J, Arner P. Adrenergic regulation of lipolysis in human fat cells during exercise. *European Journal of Clinical Investigation* 1991;21: 534–541.

Wallberg-Henriksson H. Exercise and diabetes mellitus. *Exercise and Sport Sciences Reviews* 1992;20:339–368.

Walter SD, Hart LE, McIntosh JM, Sutton JR. The Ontario cohort study of running-related injuries. *Archives of Internal Medicine* 1989;149:2561–2564.

Wang JT, Ho LT, Tang KT, Wang LM, Chen Y-DI, Reaven GM. Effect of habitual physical activity on age-related glucose intolerance. *Journal of the American Geriatrics Society* 1989; 37:203–209.

Wannamethee G, Shaper AG. Physical activity and stroke in British middle-aged men. *British Medical Journal* 1992;304:597–601.

Webber LS, Srinivasan SR, Wattigney WA, Berenson GS. Tracking of serum lipids and lipoproteins from childhood to adulthood: the Bogalusa Heart Study. *American Journal of Epidemiology* 1991;133:884–899.

West DW, Slattery ML, Robison LM, French TK, Mahoney AW. Adult dietary intake and prostate cancer risk in Utah: a case-control study with special emphasis on aggressive tumors. *Cancer Causes and Control* 1991;2:85–94.

West KM. *Epidemiology of diabetes and its vascular lesions.* New York: Elsevier, 1978.

Weyerer S. Physical inactivity and depression in the community: evidence from the Upper Bavarian Field Study. *International Journal of Sports Medicine* 1992;13:492–496.

Whittemore AS, Wu-Williams AH, Lee M, Shu Z, Gallagher RP, Deng-ao J, et al. Diet, physical activity, and colorectal cancer among Chinese in North America and China. *Journal of the National Cancer Institute* 1990;82:915–926.

Wilfley D, Kunce J. Differential physical and psychological effects of exercise. *Journal of Counseling Psychology* 1986;33:337–342.

Willett WC, Manson JE, Stampfer MJ, Colditz GA, Rosner B, Speizer FE, et al. Weight, weight change, and coronary heart disease in women: risk within the 'normal' weight range. *Journal of the American Medical Association* 1995;273:461–465.

Willett WC, Stampfer MJ, Colditz GA, Rosner BA, Speizer FE. Relation of meat, fat, and fiber intake to the risk of colon cancer in a prospective study among women. *New England Journal of Medicine* 1990;323:1664–1672.

Williamson DF, Madans J, Anda RF, Kleinman JC, Kahn HS, Byers T. Recreational physical activity and ten-year weight change in a US national cohort. *International Journal of Obesity* 1993;17:279–286.

Willich SN, Lewis M, Löwel H, Arntz H-R, Schubert F, Schröder R. Physical exertion as a trigger of acute myocardial infarction. *New England Journal of Medicine* 1993;329:1684–1690.

Wilmore JH. Body composition in sport and exercise: directions for future research. *Medicine and Science in Sports and Exercise* 1983;15:21–31.

Wing RR, Matthews KA, Kuller LH, Meilahn EN, Plantinga P. Waist-to-hip ratio in middle-aged women: associations with behavioral and psychosocial factors and with changes in cardiovascular risk factors. *Arteriosclerosis and Thrombosis* 1991;11:1250–1257.

Wolf AM, Gortmaker SL, Cheung L, Gray HM, Herzog DB, Colditz GA. Activity, inactivity, and obesity: racial, ethnic, and age differences among schoolgirls. *American Journal of Public Health* 1993;83: 1625–1627.

Wolf SL, Barnhart HX, Kutner NG, McNeely E, Coogler C, Xu T, et al. Reducing frailty and falls in older persons: an investigation of Tai Chi and computerized balance training. *Journal of the American Geriatrics Society* 1996;44:489–497.

Wolfson L, Whipple R, Derby C, Judge J, King M, Amerman P, et al. Balance and strength training in older adults: intervention gains and Tai Chi maintenance. *Journal of the American Geriatrics Society* 1996;44:498–506.

Woo R, Garrow JS, Pi-Sunyer FX. Effect of exercise on spontaneous calorie intake in obesity. *American Journal of Clinical Nutrition* 1982a;36:470–477.

Woo R, Garrow JS, Pi-Sunyer FX. Voluntary food intake during prolonged exercise in obese women. *American Journal of Clinical Nutrition* 1982b;36:478–484.

World Health Organization. Constitution of the World Health Organization. *Chronicle of the World Health Organization* 1947;1:29–43.

Wu AH, Paganini-Hill A, Ross RK, Henderson BE. Alcohol, physical activity, and other risk factors for colorectal cancer: a prospective study. *British Journal of Cancer* 1987;55:687–694.

Yano K, Reed DM, McGee DL. Ten-year incidence of coronary heart disease in the Honolulu Heart Program: relationship to biologic and lifestyle characteristics. *American Journal of Epidemiology* 1984;119: 653–666.

Yanowitz FG. Atherosclerosis: processes vs origins. In:Yanowitz F, editor. *Coronary heart disease prevention*. New York: Marcel Dekker, 1992:17–31.

Yu H, Harris RE, Wynder EL. Case-control study of prostate cancer and socioeconomic factors. *Prostate* 1988;13:317–325.

Zheng W, Shu XO, McLaughlin JK, Chow WH, Gao YT, Blot WJ. Occupational physical activity and the incidence of cancer of the breast, corpus uteri, and ovary in Shanghai. *Cancer* 1993;71:3620–3624.

Zimmet P, Faaiuso S, Ainuu J, Whitehouse S, Milne B, DeBoer W. The prevalence of diabetes in the rural and urban Polynesian population of Western Samoa. *Diabetes* 1981;30:45–51.

Zimmet PZ. Kelly West Lecture 1991 challenges in diabetes epidemiology—from West to the rest. *Diabetes Care* 1992;15:232–252.

## Contents

## Introduction

This chapter documents patterns and trends of reported leisure-time physical activity of adults and adolescents in the United States and compares the findings to the goals set by *Healthy People 2000* (U.S. Department of Health and Human Services [USDHHS] 1990; see Chapter 2, Appendix A, for the 1995 revised *Healthy People 2000* objectives for physical activity and fitness). The information presented here is based on cross-sectional data from national- and state-based surveillance systems, sponsored by the Centers for Disease Control and Prevention (CDC), that track health behaviors including leisure-time physical activity. Although self-reported survey information about physical activity is likely to contain errors of overreporting, there is no other feasible way to estimate physical activity patterns of a population. Moreover, there is no widely accepted "gold standard" methodology for measuring physical activity (see Chapter 2).

Occupational and most domestic physical activities are not presented because such information is not available. Most national goals address leisure-time rather than occupational physical activity because people have more personal control over how they spend their leisure time and because most people do not have jobs that require regular physical exertion. Nonetheless, measuring only leisure-time physical activity leads to an underestimate of total physical activity, especially for those people with physically demanding jobs.

Five surveys provided data on physical activity for this review: 1) the National Health Interview Survey (NHIS), which included questions on physical activity among adults in 1985, 1990, and 1991; 2) the Behavioral Risk Factor Surveillance System (BRFSS), a state-based survey of adults that was conducted monthly by state health departments, in collaboration with the CDC, and included questions on physical activity from 1986 through 1992 and in 1994; 3) the Third National Health and Nutrition Examination Survey (NHANES III) of U.S. adults from 1988 through 1994 (data from Phase I, 1988–1991, were available for presentation in this report); 4) the 1992 household-based NHIS Youth Risk Behavior Survey (NHIS-YRBS) of 12- through 21-year-olds; and 5) the national school-based Youth Risk Behavior Survey (YRBS), which was conducted in 1991, 1993, and 1995 among students in grades 9–12. The methodologies of these surveys are summarized in Table 5-1 and are described in detail in Appendices A and B of this chapter.

When adult data from the NHIS, BRFSS, and NHANES III are presented for comparison, they are shown from the most nearly contemporaneous survey years. Otherwise, the most recent data are presented. For determining trends, BRFSS data are restricted to those states that collected physical activity information each year.

Responses to questions included in the surveys were compiled (see Appendix B) into categories approximately corresponding to the *Healthy People 2000* physical activity objectives. These objectives are based on the health-related physical activity dimensions of caloric expenditure, aerobic intensity, flexibility, and muscle strength (Caspersen 1994). Thus the "regular, sustained physical activity" category used here pertains to total caloric expenditure and includes a summation of activities of any intensity, whereas the "regular, vigorous" category pertains to aerobic intensity and therefore includes only activities of vigorous intensity. Because some activities (e.g., vigorous activity of 30 minutes duration) fall into both of these categories, the categories are not mutually exclusive. Adding together the proportion of people in each category thus yields an

# Physical Activity and Health

**Table 5-1.** Sources of national and state-based data on physical activity*

| Survey title | Abbreviated title | Sponsor | Mode of survey administration | Years | Population, age | Response rate | Sample size | Physical activity measure† |
|---|---|---|---|---|---|---|---|---|
| **Adults** | | | | | | | | |
| National Health Interview Survey | NHIS | National Center for Health Statistics (NCHS), Centers for Disease Control and Prevention (CDC) | Household interview | 1985, 1990, 1991 | US, 18+ years | 83–88% | 36,399 in 1985, 41,104 in 1990, 43,732 in 1991 | F/I/T/D over past 2 weeks |
| Behavioral Risk Factor Surveillance System | BRFSS | National Center for Chronic Disease Prevention and Health Promotion (NCCDPHP), CDC | Telephone interview | 1986–1991 | 25 states‡ and D.C., 18+ years | 62–71% | Approx. 35,000–50,000 | F/I/T/D over past month |
| | | | | 1992 | 48 states and D.C. 18+ years | 71% | 96,343 | |
| | | | | 1994 | 49 states and D.C. 18+ years | 70% | 106,030 | |
| Third National Health and Nutrition Examination Survey | NHANES III | NCHS, CDC | Household interview | 1988–91 (Phase I) | US, 18+ years | 82% | 9,901 | F/T over past month |
| **Youths** | | | | | | | | |
| Youth Risk Behavior Survey | YRBS | NCCDPHP, CDC | Self-administered in school | 1991, 1993, 1995 | US, 9th–12th grades (approximately 15–18 years) | 70–78% of selected schools; 86–90% of students | 12,272 in 1991, 16,296 in 1993, 10,904 in 1995 | F/I/T/D over past week |
| National Health Interview Survey-Youth Risk Behavior Survey | NHIS-YRBS | NCHS, CDC | Household administration via audiotape and self-completed answer sheets | 1992 | US, 12–21 years | 74% | 10,645 | F/I/T over past week |

*Available at the time this report was compiled.
†F = frequency; I = intensity; T = type; D = duration.
‡Alabama, Arizona, California, Florida, Georgia, Hawaii, Idaho, Illinois, Indiana, Kentucky, Massachusetts, Minnesota, Missouri, Montana, New Mexico, New York, North Carolina, North Dakota, Ohio, Rhode Island, South Carolina, Tennessee, Utah, West Virginia, and Wisconsin.

overestimate of the proportion of people who are regularly physically active. More clear-cut is the category of inactivity, which is considered to be the most detrimental to health and is thus important to monitor as an indicator of need for intervention. Measures of stretching and strength training are also derived, when possible, from the survey responses.

The various surveys differ in the means by which they are conducted, in the wording of questions, in the time of year, in population sampling frames, in response rates, and in definitions of physical activity—all of which may cause differences in the resulting physical activity estimates. However, even with these differences, the data from the several data collection systems reveal a number of consistencies in patterns and trends in self-reported leisure-time physical activity.

## Physical Activity among Adults in the United States

### Recent Patterns of Leisure-Time Physical Activity

#### Physical Inactivity during Leisure Time

Physical inactivity during leisure time is one of the easiest measures to define in population surveys. Inactivity was conceptualized in the NHIS, BRFSS, and NHANES III as no reported leisure-time physical activity in the previous 2 to 4 weeks. Healthy People 2000 objective 1.5 states that the proportion of leisure-time physical inactivity among people aged 6 years and older should be no more than 15 percent by the year 2000 (USDHHS 1990).

The proportion of U.S. adults aged 18 years and older who were classified as physically inactive during leisure time varied somewhat among the three recent surveys (Table 5-2). In the 1991 NHIS, 24.3 percent reported no activity in the previous 2 weeks. In the 1992 BRFSS, 28.7 percent of adults reported no activity during the previous month. In the 1988–1991 NHANES III, in which for operational reasons participants tended to be surveyed in the North in the summer and the South in the winter, the prevalence of inactivity during the previous month was somewhat lower—21.7 percent.

Thus, despite minor differences, the surveys are consistent in finding that about one-fourth of U.S.

adults do not engage in any leisure-time physical activity, a proportion far from the 15 percent target of Healthy People 2000 objective 1.5. Also evident across the surveys is that more women than men are physically inactive (Figure 5-1). The ratio of physical inactivity prevalence for women relative to that for men ranged from 1.2 to 1.7 across the three surveys. Findings for racial and ethnic groups, unadjusted for socioeconomic differences, were generally in accord across the surveys (Table 5-2): whites had a lower prevalence of leisure-time inactivity than blacks, Hispanics, and persons categorized as "other."

Among the sex-specific racial and ethnic groups, white men were the least likely to be inactive (< 26 percent). White women had a prevalence of inactivity (23.1–29.0 percent) similar to that among black men and lower than that among Hispanic men. At least one-third of black women and Hispanic women reported no physical activity in their leisure time.

In all three surveys, the prevalence of physical inactivity was higher in older groups (Figure 5-1). Fewer than one in four adults aged 18–29 years engaged in no physical activity, whereas about one in three men and one in two women over 74 years of age were inactive (Table 5-2). For the most part, the prevalence of physical inactivity was greater among persons with lower levels of education and income. For example, there was twofold to threefold more inactivity from lowest to highest income categories: only 10.9 to 17.8 percent of participants with an annual family income of $50,000 or more reported no leisure-time physical activities, whereas 30.3 to 41.5 percent of those with an income less than $10,000 reported this.

The prevalence of inactivity among adults tended to be lower in the north central and western states than in the northeastern and southern states (Table 5-2). Participants surveyed in the winter months reported being physically inactive substantially more often than did those surveyed during the summer months (Figure 5-2). In the 1994 BRFSS, state-specific prevalences of physical inactivity from 49 states and the District of Columbia ranged from 17.2 to 48.6 (Table 5-3).

### Regular, Sustained Physical Activity during Leisure Time

Healthy People 2000 objective 1.3 proposes that at least 30 percent of people aged 6 years and older should engage regularly, preferably daily, in light to

# Physical Activity and Health

Table 5-2.  Percentage of adults aged 18+ years reporting no participation in leisure-time physical activity, by various demographic characteristics, National Health Interview Survey (NHIS), Third National Health and Nutrition Examination Survey (NHANES III), and Behavioral Risk Factor Surveillance System (BRFSS), United States

| Demographic group | 1991 NHIS* | 1988–1991 NHANES III* | 1992 BRFSS*† |
|---|---|---|---|
| Overall | 24.3  (23.2, 25.3)† | 21.7 (19.0, 24.5) | 28.7 (28.3, 29.1) |
| **Sex** | | | |
| Males | 21.4  (20.2, 22.6) | 15.8 (12.4, 19.2) | 26.5 (25.9, 27.1) |
| Females | 26.9  (25.8, 28.0) | 27.1 (23.0, 31.3) | 30.7 (30.1, 31.3) |
| **Race/Ethnicity** | | | |
| White, non-Hispanic | 22.5  (21.4, 23.7) | 18.2 (15.6, 20.8) | 26.8 (26.4, 27.2) |
| Males | 20.3  (19.0, 21.6) | 12.9  (9.6, 16.1) | 25.3 (24.7, 25.9) |
| Females | 24.6  (23.4, 25.8) | 23.1 (19.0, 27.1) | 28.2 (27.6, 28.8) |
| Black, non-Hispanic | 28.4  (26.4, 30.4) | 30.4 (25.6, 35.3) | 38.5 (36.9, 40.1) |
| Males | 22.5  (20.0, 25.0) | 20.6 (14.5, 26.8) | 33.1 (30.9, 35.3) |
| Females | 33.2  (30.8, 35.6) | 38.1 (30.9, 45.2) | 42.7 (40.7, 44.7) |
| Hispanic§ | 33.6  (31.0, 36.3) | 36.0 (32.5, 39.5) | 34.8 (32.8, 36.8) |
| Males | 29.6  (26.0, 33.2) | 29.1 (24.3, 33.9) | 30.2 (27.3, 33.1) |
| Females | 37.4  (34.1, 40.8) | 43.8 (38.5, 49.1) | 39.0 (36.5, 41.5) |
| Other | 26.7  (23.4, 30.0) | | 31.4 (28.9, 33.9) |
| Males | 22.8  (18.2, 27.3) | ‖ | 27.6 (24.1, 31.1) |
| Females | 30.8  (27.0, 34.7) | | 35.8 (32.3, 39.3) |
| **Age (years)** | | | |
| **Males** | | | |
| 18–29 | 17.6  (15.8, 19.4) | 12.5  (9.0, 16.0) | 18.9 (17.7, 20.1) |
| 30–44 | 21.1  (19.8, 22.5) | 14.5 (10.9, 18.1) | 25.0 (24.0, 26.0) |
| 45–64 | 23.9  (22.1, 25.7) | 16.9 (13.0, 20.8) | 32.0 (30.8, 33.2) |
| 65–74 | 23.0  (20.4, 25.6) | 17.5 (12.2, 22.8) | 33.2 (31.2, 35.2) |
| 75+ | 27.1  (23.8, 30.4) | 34.5 (28.0, 41.1) | 38.2 (35.3, 41.1) |
| **Females** | | | |
| 18–29 | 25.0  (23.4, 26.6) | 17.4 (13.4, 21.4) | 25.4 (24.2, 26.6) |
| 30–44 | 25.2  (23.8, 26.6) | 24.9 (20.6, 29.3) | 26.9 (25.9, 27.9) |
| 45–64 | 27.4  (25.9, 28.9) | 29.4 (24.6, 34.2) | 32.1 (30.9, 33.3) |
| 65–74 | 27.8  (25.7, 29.9) | 32.5 (25.9, 39.2) | 36.6 (34.8, 38.4) |
| 75+ | 37.9  (35.3, 40.6) | 54.3 (47.9, 60.6) | 50.5 (48.5, 52.5) |
| **Education** | | | |
| < 12 yrs | 37.1  (35.3, 38.9) | 34.5 (31.2, 37.8) | 46.5 (45.3, 47.7) |
| 12 yrs | 25.9  (24.7, 27.1) | 20.8 (17.4, 24.3) | 32.8 (32.1, 33.6) |
| Some college (13–15 yrs) | 19.0  (17.8, 20.2) | 15.7 (11.4, 19.9) | 22.6 (21.9, 23.4) |
| College (16+ yrs) | 14.2  (13.1, 15.3) | 11.1  (6.9, 15.4) | 17.8 (17.0, 18.5) |
| **Income¶** | | | |
| < $10,000 | 30.3  (28.4, 32.2) | 34.5 (30.3, 38.7) | 41.5 (40.1, 42.9) |
| $10,000–19,999 | 30.2  (28.5, 32.0) | 28.5 (24.5, 32.6) | 34.6 (33.6, 35.6) |
| $20,000–34,999 | 24.3  (22.9, 25.7) | 18.7 (14.8, 22.6) | 26.9 (26.1, 27.7) |
| $35,000–49,999 | 19.5  (18.1, 20.9) | 15.9 (10.9, 20.9) | 23.0 (22.0, 24.0) |
| $50,000+ | 14.4  (13.2, 15.6) | 10.9  (6.7, 15.1) | 17.7 (16.9, 18.5) |
| **Geographic region** | | | |
| Northeast | 25.9  (24.5, 27.3) | 21.6  (8.5, 34.6) | 29.5 (28.5, 30.5) |
| North Central | 20.8  (18.7, 22.9) | 16.7  (7.6, 25.8) | 28.6 (27.8, 29.4) |
| South | 27.0  (25.2, 28.8) | 24.8 (18.4, 31.1) | 32.4 (31.6, 33.2) |
| West | 22.5  (19.5, 25.5) | 22.6 (14.8, 30.5) | 22.0 (21.0, 23.0) |

Sources: Centers for Disease Control and Prevention, National Center for Health Statistics, NHIS, public use data tapes, 1991; Centers for Disease Control and Prevention, National Center for Health Statistics, NHANES, public use data tapes, 1988–1991; Centers for Disease Control and Prevention, National Center for Chronic Disease Prevention and Health Promotion, BRFSS, 1992.

*NHIS asked about the prior 2 weeks; BRFSS asked about the prior month. †Based on data from 48 states and the District of Columbia.
‡95% confidence intervals. §Hispanic reflects Mexican-Americans in NHANES III. ‖Estimates unreliable.
¶Annual income per family (NHIS) or household (BRFSS).

Figure 5-1. Percentage of adults aged 18+ years reporting no participation in leisure-time physical activity by sex and age

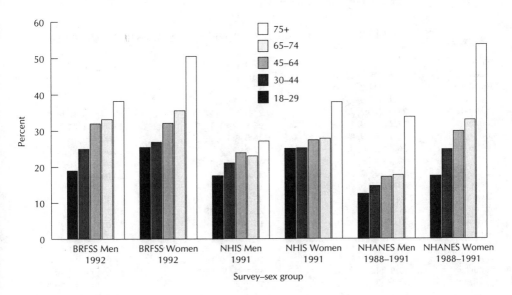

Figure 5-2. Percentage of adults aged 18+ years reporting no participation in leisure-time physical activity by month

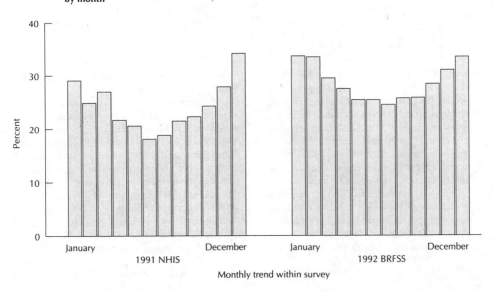

Table 5-3.  Percentage of adults aged 18+ years reporting participation in no activity; regular, sustained activity; and regular, vigorous activity, by state,* Behavioral Risk Factor Surveillance System (BRFSS), 1994, United States

| | No activity | Regular, sustained activity | Regular, vigorous activity |
|---|---|---|---|
| **Overall** | **29.4**  (29.0, 29.8)[†] | **19.7**  (19.3, 20.1) | **14.0** (13.6, 14.4) |
| Alabama | **45.9**  (43.2, 48.6) | **17.1**  (14.9, 19.3) | **11.2**  (9.4, 13.0) |
| Alaska | **22.8**  (19.9, 25.7) | **28.3**  (24.8, 31.8) | **15.1** (12.4, 17.8) |
| Arizona | **23.7**  (21.2, 26.2) | **17.8**  (15.4, 20.2) | **17.9** (15.4, 20.4) |
| Arkansas | **35.1**  (32.6, 37.6) | **17.2**  (15.0, 19.4) | **10.7**  (9.1, 12.3) |
| California | **21.8**  (20.2, 23.4) | **21.9**  (20.3, 23.5) | **15.7** (14.5, 16.9) |
| Colorado | **17.2**  (15.0, 19.4) | **26.5**  (24.1, 28.9) | **15.9** (14.1, 17.7) |
| Connecticut | **22.1**  (19.9, 24.3) | **26.9**  (24.5, 29.3) | **16.9** (14.9, 18.9) |
| Delaware | **36.4**  (34.0, 38.8) | **17.7**  (15.7, 19.7) | **14.1** (12.5, 15.7) |
| D.C. | **48.6**  (45.3, 51.9) | **11.6**  (9.4, 13.8) | **8.7**  (6.9, 10.5) |
| Florida | **28.0**  (26.2, 29.8) | **23.8**  (22.2, 25.4) | **20.0** (18.6, 21.4) |
| Georgia | **33.0**  (30.6, 35.4) | **18.0**  (16.0, 20.0) | **13.5** (11.9, 15.1) |
| Hawaii | **20.8**  (18.6, 23.0) | **25.5**  (23.3, 27.7) | **18.3** (16.3, 20.3) |
| Idaho | **21.9**  (19.7, 24.1) | **26.3**  (23.8, 28.8) | **15.7** (13.7, 17.7) |
| Illinois | **33.5**  (31.1, 35.9) | **15.7**  (13.9, 17.5) | **14.6** (12.8, 16.4) |
| Indiana | **29.7**  (27.7, 31.7) | **18.8**  (17.0, 20.6) | **13.0** (11.4, 14.6) |
| Iowa | **33.2**  (31.2, 35.2) | **15.9**  (14.3, 17.5) | **13.3** (11.9, 14.7) |
| Kansas | **34.5**  (31.8, 37.2) | **16.8**  (14.6, 19.0) | **13.9** (11.9, 15.9) |
| Kentucky | **45.9**  (43.5, 48.3) | **13.2**  (11.6, 14.8) | **11.3**  (9.9, 12.7) |
| Louisiana | **33.5**  (30.8, 36.2) | **16.8**  (14.8, 18.8) | **11.3**  (9.5, 13.1) |
| Maine | **40.7**  (37.8, 43.6) | **13.0**  (11.0, 15.0) | **11.3**  (9.5, 13.1) |
| Maryland | **30.5**  (28.9, 32.1) | **17.6**  (16.2, 19.0) | **14.5** (13.3, 15.7) |
| Massachusetts | **24.0**  (21.6, 26.4) | **23.2**  (21.0, 25.4) | **17.4** (15.4, 19.4) |
| Michigan | **23.1**  (21.1, 25.1) | **21.8**  (19.8, 23.8) | **14.5** (12.9, 16.1) |
| Minnesota | **21.8**  (20.4, 23.2) | **20.1**  (18.7, 21.5) | **15.4** (14.2, 16.6) |
| Mississippi | **38.5**  (35.6, 41.4) | **14.0**  (12.0, 16.0) | **9.8**  (8.2, 11.4) |

moderate physical activity requiring sustained, rhythmic muscular movements for at least 30 minutes per day (USDHHS 1990). Regular, sustained activity derived from the NHIS and the BRFSS was defined as any type or intensity of activity that occurs 5 times or more per week and 30 minutes or more per occasion (see Appendix B ). This definition approximates the activity goal of the *Healthy People 2000* objective but includes vigorous activity of at least 30 minutes duration as well. Comparable information was unavailable in the NHANES III. The percentage of U.S. adults meeting this definition of regular, sustained activity during leisure time was about 22 percent in the two surveys (23.5 in the NHIS and 20.1 in the BRFSS; see

Table 5-4)—8 percentage points lower than the *Healthy People 2000* target.

The prevalence of regular, sustained activity was somewhat higher among men than women; male:female ratios were 1.1:1.3. The two surveys found no consistent association between racial/ethnic groups and participation in regular, sustained activity. The prevalence of regular, sustained activity tended to be higher among 18- through 29-year-olds than among other age groups, and it was lowest ($\leq 15$ percent) among women aged 75 years and older. Education and income levels were associated positively with regular, sustained activity. For example, adults with a college education had an approximately 50 percent higher prevalence of regular, sustained activity than those with fewer than 12 years of

**Table 5-3.** *Continued*

| | No activity | Regular, sustained activity | Regular, vigorous activity |
|---|---|---|---|
| Missouri | **32.0** (29.3, 34.7) | **18.0** (15.8, 20.2) | **10.8** (9.0, 12.6) |
| Montana | **21.0** (18.6, 23.4) | **21.8** (19.3, 24.3) | **15.0** (12.6, 17.4) |
| Nebraska | **24.3** (22.1, 26.5) | **16.7** (14.7, 18.7) | **14.7** (12.9, 16.5) |
| Nevada | **21.7** (19.5, 23.9) | **25.3** (22.9, 27.7) | **14.1** (12.3, 15.9) |
| New Hampshire | **25.8** (23.3, 28.3) | **21.2** (19.0, 23.4) | **17.0** (14.8, 19.2) |
| New Jersey | **30.9** (28.2, 33.6) | **20.7** (18.3, 23.1) | **11.6** (9.8, 13.4) |
| New Mexico | **19.8** (17.3, 22.3) | **25.5** (22.6, 28.4) | **18.4** (16.0, 20.8) |
| New York | **37.1** (34.7, 39.5) | **14.8** (13.2, 16.4) | **10.6** (9.2, 12.0) |
| North Carolina | **42.8** (40.3, 45.3) | **12.7** (11.1, 14.3) | **9.3** (7.9, 10.7) |
| North Dakota | **32.0** (29.6, 34.4) | **20.2** (18.0, 22.4) | **13.9** (12.1, 15.7) |
| Ohio | **38.0** (35.1, 40.9) | **15.9** (13.7, 18.1) | **12.4** (10.4, 14.4) |
| Oklahoma | **30.4** (28.0, 32.8) | **23.0** (20.8, 25.2) | **11.1** (9.5, 12.7) |
| Oregon | **20.8** (19.2, 22.4) | **27.3** (25.3, 29.3) | **18.7** (17.1, 20.3) |
| Pennsylvania | **26.5** (24.9, 28.1) | **21.2** (19.6, 22.8) | **14.5** (13.3, 15.7) |
| South Carolina | **31.4** (29.2, 33.6) | **15.1** (13.3, 16.9) | **11.9** (10.3, 13.5) |
| South Dakota | **30.8** (28.4, 33.2) | **19.4** (17.4, 21.4) | **11.9** (10.3, 13.5) |
| Tennessee | **39.7** (37.7, 41.7) | **15.0** (13.6, 16.4) | **12.7** (11.3, 14.1) |
| Texas | **27.8** (25.1, 30.5) | **20.7** (18.2, 23.2) | **13.0** (11.0, 15.0) |
| Utah | **21.0** (18.8, 23.2) | **21.6** (19.4, 23.8) | **14.3** (12.5, 16.1) |
| Vermont | **23.3** (21.5, 25.1) | **25.7** (23.7, 27.7) | **18.4** (16.6, 20.2) |
| Virginia | **23.0** (20.6, 25.4) | **24.6** (22.2, 27.0) | **14.6** (12.8, 16.4) |
| Washington | **18.2** (16.8, 19.6) | **25.7** (24.1, 27.3) | **16.8** (15.4, 18.2) |
| West Virginia | **45.3** (43.1, 47.5) | **14.3** (12.7, 15.9) | **9.8** (8.4, 11.2) |
| Wisconsin | **25.9** (23.2, 28.6) | **22.7** (20.2, 25.2) | **12.7** (10.7, 14.7) |
| Wyoming | **20.9** (18.4, 23.4) | **27.9** (24.8, 31.0) | **16.3** (13.9, 18.7) |

Source: Centers for Disease Control and Prevention, National Center for Chronic Disease Prevention and Health Promotion, BRFSS, 1994.

*Includes 49 states and the District of Columbia. Data for Rhode Island were unavailable.
†95% confidence intervals.

education. Among the regions of the United States, the West tended to have the highest prevalence of adults participating in regular, sustained activity (Table 5-4). Regular, sustained activity, which comprises many outdoor activities, was most prevalent in the summer. In the 1994 BRFSS, state-specific prevalences of regular, sustained activity ranged from 11.6 to 28.3 (Table 5-3).

### Regular, Vigorous Physical Activity during Leisure Time

People who exercise both regularly and vigorously would be expected to improve cardiovascular fitness the most. The NHIS and the BRFSS defined regular, vigorous physical activity as rhythmic contraction of large muscle groups, performed at 50 percent or more of estimated age- and sex-specific maximum cardiorespiratory capacity, 3 times per week or more for at least 20 minutes per occasion (see Appendix B). The prevalence of regular, vigorous leisure-time activity reported by U.S. adults was about 15 percent (16.4 percent in the 1991 NHIS and 14.2 percent in the 1992 BRFSS; see Table 5-5). This prevalence is lower than the goal stated in *Healthy People 2000* objective 1.4, which is to have at least 20 percent of people aged 18 years and older engage in vigorous physical activity at 50 percent or more of individual cardiorespiratory capacity 3 days or more per week for 20 minutes or more per occasion (USDHHS 1990).

181

# Physical Activity and Health

**Table 5-4.** Percentage of adults aged 18+ years reporting participation in regular, sustained physical activity (5+ times per week for 30+ minutes per occasion), by various demographic characteristics, National Health Interview Survey (NHIS) and Behavioral Risk Factor Surveillance System (BRFSS), United States

| Demographic group | 1991 NHIS* | 1992 BRFSS*[†] |
|---|---|---|
| Overall | 23.5 (22.9, 24.1)[‡] | 20.1 (19.7, 20.5) |
| **Sex** | | |
| Males | 26.6 (25.7, 27.5) | 21.5 (20.9, 22.1) |
| Females | 20.7 (19.9, 21.5) | 18.9 (18.4, 19.3) |
| **Race/Ethnicity** | | |
| White, non-Hispanic | 24.0 (23.2, 24.7) | 20.8 (20.4, 21.2) |
| Males | 26.7 (25.7, 27.6) | 21.9 (21.3, 22.5) |
| Females | 21.5 (20.6, 22.4) | 19.8 (19.2, 20.4) |
| Black, non-Hispanic | 22.9 (21.4, 24.4) | 15.2 (14.0, 16.4) |
| Males | 28.9 (26.6, 31.3) | 18.5 (16.5, 20.5) |
| Females | 18.0 (16.2, 19.8) | 12.6 (11.4, 13.8) |
| Hispanic | 20.0 (18.1, 21.9) | 20.1 (18.5, 21.7) |
| Males | 23.7 (20.6, 26.7) | 21.4 (18.9, 23.9) |
| Females | 16.5 (14.3, 18.7) | 18.9 (16.7, 21.1) |
| Other | 23.4 (20.5, 26.2) | 17.3 (15.1, 19.5) |
| Males | 25.5 (21.0, 30.0) | 19.7 (16.6, 22.8) |
| Females | 21.1 (17.7, 24.6) | 14.5 (12.0, 17.0) |
| **Age (years)** | | |
| **Males** | | |
| 18–29 | 32.0 (30.2, 33.7) | 26.8 (25.4, 28.2) |
| 30–44 | 24.1 (22.8, 25.3) | 17.4 (16.6, 18.2) |
| 45–64 | 24.2 (22.8, 25.6) | 18.9 (17.7, 20.1) |
| 65–74 | 29.2 (27.0, 31.4) | 26.8 (24.8, 28.8) |
| 75+ | 24.6 (21.8, 27.4) | 23.2 (20.5, 25.9) |
| **Females** | | |
| 18–29 | 23.2 (21.6, 24.8) | 19.9 (18.7, 21.1) |
| 30–44 | 20.4 (19.4, 21.4) | 18.5 (17.7, 19.3) |
| 45–64 | 20.6 (19.4, 21.8) | 19.4 (18.4, 20.4) |
| 65–74 | 21.3 (19.5, 23.0) | 19.0 (17.6, 20.4) |
| 75+ | 13.8 (12.2, 15.4) | 15.0 (13.4, 16.6) |
| **Education** | | |
| < 12 yrs | 18.1 (17.0, 19.2) | 15.6 (14.6, 16.6) |
| 12 yrs | 21.9 (21.0, 22.7) | 17.8 (17.2, 18.4) |
| Some college (13–15 yrs) | 26.8 (25.7, 28.0) | 22.7 (21.9, 23.5) |
| College (16+ yrs) | 28.5 (27.3, 29.6) | 23.5 (22.7, 24.3) |
| **Income[§]** | | |
| < $10,000 | 23.6 (21.8, 25.5) | 17.6 (16.6, 18.6) |
| $10,000–19,999 | 20.4 (19.3, 21.4) | 18.7 (17.9, 19.5) |
| $20,000–34,999 | 23.2 (22.2, 24.2) | 20.3 (19.5, 21.1) |
| $35,000–49,999 | 23.9 (22.7, 25.1) | 20.9 (19.9, 21.9) |
| $50,000+ | 28.0 (26.8, 29.2) | 23.5 (22.5, 24.5) |
| **Geographic region** | | |
| Northeast | 23.9 (22.8, 25.0) | 20.2 (19.2, 21.2) |
| North Central | 24.2 (22.7, 25.6) | 18.2 (17.4, 19.0) |
| South | 21.1 (19.9, 22.2) | 19.0 (18.4, 19.6) |
| West | 26.1 (24.6, 27.5) | 24.0 (23.0, 25.0) |

Sources: Centers for Disease Control and Prevention, National Center for Health Statistics, NHIS, public use data tapes, 1991; Centers for Disease Control and Prevention, National Center for Chronic Disease Prevention and Health Promotion, BRFSS, 1992.

*Based on data from 48 states and the District of Columbia.

[†]NHIS asked about the prior 2 weeks; BRFSS asked about the prior month.

[‡]95% confidence intervals.

[§]Annual income per family (NHIS) or household (BRFSS).

Table 5-5. Percentage of adults aged 18+ years participating in regular, vigorous physical activity (3+ times per week for 20+ minutes per occasion at 50+ percent of estimated age- and sex-specific maximum cardiorespiratory capacity), by various demographic characteristics, National Health Interview Survey (NHIS) and Behavioral Risk Factor Surveillance System (BRFSS), United States

| Demographic group | 1991 NHIS* | 1992 BRFSS*† |
|---|---|---|
| Overall | 16.4 (15.9, 16.9)‡ | 14.4 (14.0, 14.8) |
| **Sex** | | |
| Males | 18.1 (17.4, 18.8) | 12.9 (12.5, 13.3) |
| Females | 14.9 (14.3, 15.5) | 15.8 (15.4, 16.2) |
| **Race/Ethnicity** | | |
| White, non-Hispanic | 17.2 (16.6, 17.7) | 15.3 (14.9, 15.7) |
| Males | 18.6 (17.9, 19.3) | 13.3 (12.7, 13.9) |
| Females | 15.9 (15.2, 16.6) | 17.1 (16.5, 17.7) |
| Black, non-Hispanic | 12.9 (11.7, 14.0) | 9.4 (8.6, 10.2) |
| Males | 16.0 (13.9, 18.0) | 9.5 (8.1, 10.9) |
| Females | 10.4 (9.0, 11.7) | 9.4 (8.4, 10.4) |
| Hispanic | 13.6 (11.9, 15.2) | 11.9 (10.5, 13.3) |
| Males | 15.6 (12.9, 18.3) | 12.4 (10.2, 14.6) |
| Females | 11.7 (9.9, 13.4) | 11.4 (9.8, 13.0) |
| Other | 16.8 (14.5, 19.1) | 11.8 (10.0, 13.6) |
| Males | 18.8 (15.2, 22.3) | 11.5 (9.0, 14.0) |
| Females | 14.8 (11.9, 17.8) | 12.2 (10.0, 14.4) |
| **Age (years)** | | |
| Males | | |
| 18–29 | 19.7 (18.3, 21.1) | 8.0 (7.2, 8.8) |
| 30–44 | 13.7 (12.8, 14.6) | 11.1 (10.3, 11.9) |
| 45–64 | 14.9 (13.7, 16.1) | 16.3 (15.3, 17.3) |
| 65–74 | 27.3 (25.2, 29.5) | 20.6 (18.8, 22.4) |
| 75+ | 38.3 (35.2, 41.5) | 20.6 (18.1, 23.1) |
| Females | | |
| 18–29 | 16.0 (14.7, 17.3) | 11.4 (10.6, 12.2) |
| 30–44 | 13.3 (12.4, 14.1) | 18.0 (17.2, 18.8) |
| 45–64 | 12.1 (11.1, 13.0) | 17.7 (16.7, 18.7) |
| 65–74 | 18.5 (16.9, 20.1) | 16.5 (15.1, 17.9) |
| 75+ | 22.6 (20.5, 24.7) | 12.8 (11.4, 14.2) |
| **Education** | | |
| < 12 yrs | 11.9 (11.1, 12.8) | 8.2 (7.4, 9.0) |
| 12 yrs | 13.6 (13.0, 14.3) | 11.5 (10.9, 12.1) |
| Some college (13–15 yrs) | 18.9 (17.9, 19.9) | 14.9 (14.3, 15.5) |
| College (16+ yrs) | 23.5 (22.4, 24.6) | 21.9 (21.1, 22.7) |
| **Income§** | | |
| < $10,000 | 15.5 (14.1, 17.0) | 9.0 (8.2, 9.8) |
| $10,000–19,999 | 14.4 (13.5, 15.4) | 10.8 (10.2, 11.4) |
| $20,000–34,999 | 15.5 (14.6, 16.4) | 14.2 (13.6, 14.8) |
| $35,000–49,999 | 16.0 (14.9, 17.0) | 16.3 (15.5, 17.1) |
| $50,000+ | 21.5 (20.4, 22.6) | 20.5 (19.5, 21.5) |
| **Geographic region** | | |
| Northeast | 16.1 (15.2, 16.9) | 13.8 (13.0, 14.6) |
| North Central | 16.5 (15.5, 17.5) | 13.7 (13.1, 14.3) |
| South | 14.7 (13.9, 15.5) | 13.8 (13.2, 14.4) |
| West | 19.2 (17.9, 20.5) | 16.8 (16.0, 17.6) |

Sources: Centers for Disease Control and Prevention, National Center for Health Statistics, NHIS, 1991; Centers for Disease Control and Prevention, National Center for Chronic Disease Prevention and Health Promotion, BRFSS, 1992.

*NHIS asked about the prior 2 weeks; BRFSS asked about the prior month.
†Based on data from 48 states and the District of Columbia.
‡95% confidence intervals.
§Annual income per family (NHIS) or household (BRFSS).

183

The proportion performing regular, vigorous activity was 3 percentage points higher among men than women in the NHIS, but it was 3 percentage points higher among women than men in the BRFSS. This difference between sexes in the surveys may be related to the BRFSS's use of a correction procedure (based on speeds of activities like walking, jogging, and swimming) to create intensity coding (Appendix B; Caspersen and Powell [unpublished technical monograph] 1986; Caspersen and Merritt 1995). Regular, vigorous activity tended to be more prevalent among whites than among blacks and Hispanics (Table 5-5). These racial and ethnic patterns were somewhat more striking among women than among men.

The relationship between regular, vigorous physical activity and age varied somewhat between the two surveys. In the NHIS, the prevalence of regular, vigorous activity was higher for men and women aged 18–29 years than for those aged 30–64 years, but it was highest among men and women aged 65 years and older. Among men participating in the BRFSS, regular, vigorous activity increased with age from those 18–29 years old to those ≥ 65 years old. Among women participating in the BRFSS, the prevalence of regular, vigorous activity was higher for those aged 30–74 years than for those aged 18–29 years and ≥ 75 years.

The finding of generally lower prevalences of regular, vigorous activity among younger than older adults (Table 5-5) may seem unexpected. It is explained partly by both the greater leisure time of older adults and the use of an age-related relative intensity classification (Caspersen, Pollard, Pratt 1987; Stephens and Caspersen 1994; Caspersen and Merritt 1995). Because cardiorespiratory capacity declines with age, activities that would be moderately intense for young adults, such as walking, become more vigorous for older people. If the two surveys had instead used an absolute intensity classification, the estimated prevalence of people engaging in regular, vigorous physical activity would have fallen dramatically with age. (This age-related drop in activities of high absolute intensity is shown in Table 5-6 and described in the next section.) Likewise, the male:female ratio of vigorous activity prevalence in Table 5-5 would rise if an absolute intensity classification were used, because women have a lower average cardiorespiratory capacity than men.

In both surveys, the proportion of adults reporting regular, vigorous activity was higher in each successive educational category (Table 5-5). Adults who had college degrees reported regular, vigorous activity approximately two to three times more often than those who had not completed high school. In the NHIS, a similar positive association was seen between income and regular, vigorous physical activity. In the BRFSS, the prevalence of regular, vigorous physical activity was highest at the highest income level. The prevalence of regular, vigorous physical activity was not consistently related to employment status or marital status in the two surveys. It was higher in the West than in other regions of the United States and in warmer than in colder months. In the 1994 BRFSS, state-specific prevalences of regular, vigorous activity ranged from 6.7 to 16.9 (Table 5-3).

### Participation in Specific Physical Activities

NHIS participants reported specific activities in the previous 2 weeks (Table 5-6). By far, walking was the most commonly reported leisure-time physical activity, followed by gardening or yard work, stretching exercises, bicycling, strengthening exercises, stair climbing, jogging or running, aerobics or aerobic dancing, and swimming. Because these percentages are based on all participants in the year-round NHIS, they underestimate the overall prevalence of participation in seasonal activities, such as skiing.

Substantial differences exist between the sexes for many activities. Gardening or yard work, strengthening exercises, jogging or running, and vigorous or contact sports were more commonly reported by men than women. Women reported walking and aerobics or aerobic dancing more often than men and reported participation in stretching exercises, bicycling, stair climbing, and swimming about as often as men. Participation in most activities, especially weight lifting and vigorous or contact sports, declined substantially with age (Table 5-6). The prevalence of walking, gardening or yard work, and golf tended to remain stable or increase with age. Among adults aged 65 years and older, walking (> 40 percent prevalence) and gardening or yard work (> 20 percent prevalence) were by far the most popular activities.

**Table 5-6.** Percentage of adults aged 18+ years reporting participation in selected common physical activities in the prior 2 weeks, by sex and age, National Health Interview Survey (NHIS), United States, 1991

| Activity category | Males | | | | | | Females | | | | | | All ages and sexes |
|---|---|---|---|---|---|---|---|---|---|---|---|---|---|
| | 18–29 | 30–44 | 45–64 | 65–74 | 75+ | All | 18–29 | 30–44 | 45–64 | 65–74 | 75+ | All | |
| Walking for exercise | 32.8 | 37.6 | 43.3 | 50.1 | 47.1 | 39.4 | 47.4 | 49.1 | 49.4 | 50.1 | 40.5 | 48.3 | 44.1 |
| Gardening or yard work | 22.2 | 36.0 | 39.8 | 42.6 | 38.4 | 34.2 | 15.4 | 28.6 | 29.6 | 28.2 | 21.5 | 25.1 | 29.4 |
| Stretching exercises | 32.1 | 27.2 | 20.0 | 15.5 | 15.7 | 25.0 | 32.5 | 27.7 | 21.4 | 21.9 | 17.9 | 26.0 | 25.5 |
| Weight lifting or other exercise to increase muscle strength | 33.6 | 21.2 | 12.2 | 6.4 | 4.7 | 20.0 | 14.5 | 10.6 | 5.1 | 2.8 | 1.1 | 8.8 | 14.1 |
| Jogging or running | 22.6 | 14.1 | 7.7 | 1.4 | 0.5 | 12.8 | 11.6 | 6.5 | 2.5 | 0.8 | 0.4 | 5.7 | 9.1 |
| Aerobics or aerobic dance | 3.4 | 3.3 | 2.1 | 1.6 | 1.0 | 2.8 | 19.3 | 12.3 | 6.6 | 4.2 | 1.6 | 11.1 | 7.1 |
| Riding a bicycle or exercise bike | 18.7 | 18.5 | 14.0 | 10.8 | 8.4 | 16.2 | 17.4 | 16.9 | 12.6 | 11.4 | 6.0 | 14.6 | 15.4 |
| Stair climbing | 10.5 | 11.4 | 9.6 | 6.0 | 4.0 | 9.9 | 14.6 | 12.8 | 10.3 | 7.3 | 5.6 | 11.6 | 10.8 |
| Swimming for exercise | 10.1 | 7.6 | 5.3 | 3.1 | 1.4 | 6.9 | 8.0 | 7.5 | 4.6 | 4.2 | 1.5 | 6.2 | 6.5 |
| Tennis | 5.7 | 3.3 | 2.9 | 1.1 | 0.4 | 3.5 | 3.1 | 2.4 | 1.3 | 0.6 | 0.1 | 2.0 | 2.7 |
| Bowling | 7.0 | 5.2 | 3.0 | 2.8 | 1.6 | 4.7 | 4.8 | 4.2 | 2.8 | 2.5 | 1.1 | 3.6 | 4.1 |
| Golf | 7.9 | 8.6 | 7.9 | 9.7 | 4.9 | 8.2 | 1.4 | 1.7 | 2.2 | 3.3 | 0.7 | 1.8 | 4.9 |
| Baseball or softball | 11.0 | 6.9 | 1.8 | 0.4 | — | 5.8 | 3.2 | 1.7 | 0.3 | 0.2 | — | 1.4 | 3.5 |
| Handball, racquet-ball, or squash | 5.2 | 2.8 | 1.5 | 0.3 | — | 2.7 | 1.0 | 0.4 | 0.4 | 0.1 | — | 0.5 | 1.6 |
| Skiing | 1.5 | 1.0 | 0.4 | 0.1 | — | 0.9 | 0.9 | 0.6 | 0.3 | 0.0 | — | 0.5 | 0.7 |
| Cross country skiing | 0.1 | 0.5 | 0.5 | 0.2 | 0.4 | 0.4 | 0.3 | 0.4 | 0.6 | 0.2 | 0.2 | 0.4 | 0.4 |
| Water skiing | 1.5 | 0.7 | 0.3 | — | — | 0.7 | 0.7 | 0.5 | 0.1 | 0.0 | — | 0.4 | 0.5 |
| Basketball | 24.2 | 10.5 | 2.4 | 0.1 | 0.1 | 10.5 | 3.1 | 1.7 | 0.4 | — | 0.2 | 1.5 | 5.8 |
| Volleyball | 6.8 | 3.0 | 1.1 | 0.2 | 0.2 | 3.1 | 4.4 | 1.9 | 0.5 | 0.0 | 0.1 | 1.8 | 2.5 |
| Soccer | 3.3 | 1.4 | 0.3 | 0.1 | — | 1.4 | 0.9 | 0.4 | 0.1 | — | — | 0.4 | 0.9 |
| Football | 7.6 | 1.8 | 0.4 | 0.2 | — | 2.7 | 0.7 | 0.4 | 0.0 | — | — | 0.3 | 1.5 |
| Other sports | 8.6 | 7.9 | 6.0 | 6.2 | 5.2 | 7.3 | 4.5 | 4.5 | 3.6 | 4.3 | 2.8 | 4.1 | 5.7 |

Note: 0.0 = quantity less than 0.05 but greater than zero; — = quantity is equal to zero.
Source: Centers for Disease Control and Prevention, National Center for Health Statistics, NHIS, 1991.

185

*Healthy People 2000* objective 1.6 recommends that at least 40 percent of people aged 6 years and older should regularly perform physical activities that enhance and maintain muscular strength, muscular endurance, and flexibility (USDHHS 1990). National surveys have not quantified all these activities but have inquired about specific sentinel activities, such as weight lifting and stretching. In the 1991 NHIS, 14.1 percent of adults reported "weight lifting and other exercises to increase muscle strength" in the previous 2 weeks (Table 5-7). Participation in strengthening activities was more than twice as prevalent among men than women. Black men tended to have the highest participation (26.2 percent) and black women the lowest (6.9 percent). Participation was much higher among younger than older adults, among the more affluent than the less affluent, and in the West than in other regions of the United States.

Of special concern, given the promising evidence that strengthening exercises provide substantial benefit to the elderly (see Chapter 4), is the low prevalence of strengthening activities among those aged 65 or older ($\leq$ 6.4 percent in men and $\leq$ 2.8 percent in women; see Table 5-7).

Adult participation in stretching activity over the previous 2 weeks was 25.5 percent in the NHIS (Table 5-7). Stretching participation declined with age and tended to be associated positively with levels of education and income and to be lower in the South than in other regions of the United States.

## Leisure-Time Physical Activity among Adults with Disabilities

Although little information is available on physical activity patterns among people with disabilities, one recent analysis was based on the special NHIS Health Promotion and Disease Prevention Supplement from 1991. Heath and colleagues (1995) compared physical activity patterns among people with disabilities (i.e., activity limitations due to a chronic health problem or impairment) to those among people without disabilities. People with disabilities were less likely to report engaging in regular moderate physical activity (27.2 percent) than were people without disabilities (37.4 percent). People with disabilities were also less likely to report engaging in regular vigorous physical activity (9.6 percent vs. 14.2 percent). Correspondingly, people with disabilities were more likely to report being inactive (32 percent vs. 27 percent).

## Trends in Leisure-Time Physical Activity

Until the 20th century, people performed most physical activity as part of their occupations or in subsistence activities. In Western populations, occupation-related physical demands have declined, and the availability of leisure time has grown. It is generally believed that over the past 30 years, as both the popularity of sports and public awareness of the role of physical activity in maintaining health have increased, physical activity performed during leisure time has increased (Stephens 1987; Jacobs et al. 1991). Stephens concluded that the increase was greater among women than men and among older than younger adults and that the rate of increase probably was more pronounced in the 1970s than between 1980 and 1985 (Stephens 1987). However, no systematic data were collected on physical activity among U.S. adults until the 1980s.

Even now, few national data are available on consistently measured trends in physical activity. The NHIS has data from 1985, 1990, and 1991, and the BRFSS has consistent data from the same 25 states and the District of Columbia for each year between 1986 and 1992 and for 1994. According to the NHIS, participation in leisure-time physical activity among adults changed very little between the mid-1980s and the early 1990s (Table 5-8 and Figure 5-3). Similarly, in the BRFSS (Table 5-8 and Figure 5-4), little improvement was evident from 1986 through 1994.

# Physical Activity among Adolescents and Young Adults in the United States

The most recent U.S. data on the prevalence of physical activity among young people are from the 1992 household-based NHIS-YRBS, which sampled all young people aged 12–21 years, and the 1995 school-based YRBS, which included students in grades 9–12. Variations in estimates between the NHIS-YRBS and the YRBS may be due not only to the distinct populations represented in each survey but also to the time of year each survey was conducted, the mode of administration, the specific wording of

Table 5-7. Percentage of adults aged 18+ years reporting participation in any strengthening activities* or stretching exercises in the prior 2 weeks, by various demographic characteristics, National Health Interview Survey (NHIS), United States, 1991

| Demographic group | Strengthening activities | Stretching exercises |
|---|---|---|
| Overall | 14.1 (13.6, 14.6)† | 25.5 (24.7, 26.4) |
| **Sex** | | |
| Males | 20.0 (19.2, 20.7) | 25.0 (24.0, 26.1) |
| Females | 8.8 (8.3, 9.2) | 26.0 (25.1, 27.0) |
| **Race/Ethnicity** | | |
| White, non-Hispanic | 13.7 (13.2, 14.2) | 25.9 (24.9, 26.8) |
| Males | 18.8 (18.0, 19.6) | 24.9 (23.8, 26.0) |
| Females | 9.0 (8.5, 9.6) | 26.7 (25.7, 27.8) |
| Black, non-Hispanic | 15.5 (14.2, 16.9) | 24.2 (22.5, 26.0) |
| Males | 26.2 (23.7, 28.7) | 24.7 (22.1, 27.3) |
| Females | 6.9 (5.8, 8.0) | 23.9 (21.7, 26.0) |
| Hispanic | 15.8 (13.9, 17.6) | 22.4 (19.9, 24.9) |
| Males | 23.4 (20.3, 26.5) | 23.6 (20.4, 26.7) |
| Females | 8.6 (7.0, 10.3) | 21.3 (18.3, 24.3) |
| Other | 14.9 (12.3, 17.5) | 30.0 (26.2, 33.8) |
| Males | 20.3 (16.0, 24.7) | 31.4 (26.0, 36.8) |
| Females | 9.2 (6.6, 11.7) | 28.5 (24.3, 32.7) |
| **Age (years)** | | |
| **Males** | | |
| 18–29 | 33.6 (31.7, 35.5) | 32.1 (30.1, 34.2) |
| 30–44 | 21.2 (20.1, 22.3) | 27.2 (25.8, 28.6) |
| 45–64 | 12.2 (11.1, 13.4) | 20.0 (18.6, 21.5) |
| 65–74 | 6.4 (5.1, 7.7) | 15.5 (13.4, 17.6) |
| 75+ | 4.7 (3.1, 6.3) | 15.7 (13.2, 18.3) |
| **Females** | | |
| 18–29 | 14.5 (13.3, 15.6) | 32.5 (30.7, 34.2) |
| 30–44 | 10.6 (9.9, 11.4) | 27.7 (26.3, 29.0) |
| 45–64 | 5.1 (4.5, 5.8) | 21.4 (20.1, 22.8) |
| 65–74 | 2.8 (2.0, 3.7) | 21.9 (20.0, 23.8) |
| 75+ | 1.1 (0.7, 1.6) | 17.9 (16.0, 19.9) |
| **Education** | | |
| < 12 yrs | 7.4 (6.6, 8.1) | 14.7 (13.5, 15.8) |
| 12 yrs | 12.3 (11.7, 13.0) | 22.6 (21.7, 23.6) |
| Some college (13–15 yrs) | 18.3 (17.3, 19.2) | 31.3 (29.9, 32.7) |
| College (16+ yrs) | 19.6 (18.6, 20.6) | 35.4 (34.0, 36.9) |
| **Income‡** | | |
| < $10,000 | 12.9 (11.4, 14.4) | 23.4 (21.7, 25.1) |
| $10,000–$19,999 | 10.7 (9.8, 11.6) | 21.0 (19.7, 22.3) |
| $20,000–$34,999 | 14.3 (13.4, 15.1) | 25.6 (24.4, 26.9) |
| $35,000–$49,999 | 15.3 (14.3, 16.3) | 28.9 (27.4, 30.4) |
| $50,000+ | 19.1 (18.1, 20.2) | 33.5 (32.1, 34.9) |
| **Geographic region** | | |
| Northeast | 13.8 (12.9, 14.8) | 24.9 (23.6, 26.2) |
| North Central | 14.5 (13.6, 15.3) | 28.5 (26.5, 30.6) |
| South | 12.4 (11.6, 13.3) | 20.8 (19.2, 22.4) |
| West | 16.5 (15.4, 17.7) | 29.9 (28.1, 31.7) |

Source: Centers for Disease Control and Prevention, National Center for Health Statistics, NHIS, 1991.

*Strengthening activities include weight lifting and other exercises to increase muscle strength.
†95% confidence intervals.
‡Annual income per family.

187

**Table 5-8.** Trends in the percentage of adults aged 18+ years reporting participation in no activity; regular, sustained activity; and regular, vigorous activity, by sex, National Health Interview Survey (NHIS) and Behavioral Risk Factor Surveillance System (BRFSS), United States, from 1985-1994

| | 1985, 1990, 1991 NHIS | | | 1986-1994 BRFSS* | | |
|---|---|---|---|---|---|---|
| | Males | Females | Total | Males | Females | Total |
| **No activity** | | | | | | |
| 1985 | 19.9 (18.8, 20.9)† | 26.3 (25.3, 27.3) | 23.2 (22.3, 24.1) | | | |
| 1986 | | | | 31.2 (30.0, 32.4) | 34.3 (33.3, 35.3) | 32.8 (32.0, 33.6) |
| 1987 | | | | 29.6 (28.4, 30.8) | 33.9 (32.9, 34.9) | 31.8 (31.0, 32.6) |
| 1988 | | | | 27.5 (26.5, 28.5) | 31.5 (30.5, 32.5) | 29.6 (28.8, 30.4) |
| 1989 | | | | 28.8 (27.8, 29.8) | 33.6 (32.6, 34.6) | 31.3 (30.5, 32.1) |
| 1990 | 24.9 (23.9, 25.9) | 32.4 (31.4, 33.4) | 28.3 (28.0, 29.7) | 28.6 (27.6, 29.6) | 32.3 (31.3, 33.3) | 30.5 (29.7, 31.3) |
| 1991 | 21.4 (20.2, 22.6) | 26.9 (25.8, 28.0) | 24.3 (23.2, 25.3) | 29.0 (28.0, 30.0) | 32.8 (32.0, 33.6) | 31.0 (30.4, 31.6) |
| 1992 | | | | 26.7 (25.9, 27.5) | 31.4 (30.6, 32.2) | 29.2 (28.6, 29.8) |
| 1993 | | | | | | |
| 1994 | | | | 28.7 (27.9, 29.5) | 33.0 (32.2, 33.8) | 30.9 (30.3, 31.5) |
| **Regular, sustained activity** | | | | | | |
| 1985 | 27.5 (26.6, 28.4) | 22.5 (21.7, 23.3) | 24.9 (24.2, 25.5) | | | |
| 1986 | | | | | | |
| 1987 | | | | 19.5 (18.5, 20.5) | 18.1 (17.3, 18.9) | 18.8 (18.2, 19.4) |
| 1988 | | | | 20.0 (18.8, 21.2) | 17.6 (16.8, 18.4) | 18.8 (18.2, 19.4) |
| 1989 | | | | 20.5 (19.5, 21.5) | 19.6 (18.8, 20.4) | 20.0 (19.4, 20.6) |
| 1990 | 29.0 (28.1, 29.9) | 22.7 (22.0, 23.4) | 25.7 (25.1, 26.3) | 20.0 (19.0, 21.0) | 18.0 (17.2, 18.8) | 19.0 (18.4, 19.6) |
| 1991 | 26.6 (25.7, 27.5) | 20.7 (19.9, 21.5) | 23.5 (22.9, 24.1) | 20.5 (19.5, 21.5) | 18.5 (17.7, 19.3) | 19.4 (18.8, 20.0) |
| 1992 | | | | 19.5 (18.7, 20.3) | 18.3 (17.5, 19.1) | 18.9 (18.3, 19.5) |
| 1993 | | | | 21.0 (20.2, 21.8) | 18.4 (17.8, 19.0) | 19.7 (19.1, 20.3) |
| 1994 | | | | 19.3 (18.5, 20.1) | 18.1 (17.5, 18.7) | 18.7 (18.1, 19.3) |
| **Regular, vigorous activity** | | | | | | |
| 1985 | 17.2 (16.1, 18.3) | 15.1 (14.3, 15.8) | 16.1 (15.3, 16.8) | | | |
| 1986 | | | | 11.2 (10.4, 12.0) | 10.3 (9.7, 10.9) | 10.7 (10.1, 11.3) |
| 1987 | | | | 10.7 (9.9, 11.5) | 10.6 (10.0, 11.2) | 10.7 (10.1, 11.3) |
| 1988 | | | | 11.1 (10.3, 11.9) | 12.3 (11.5, 13.1) | 11.7 (11.1, 12.3) |
| 1989 | | | | 11.3 (10.5, 12.1) | 11.9 (11.3, 12.5) | 11.6 (11.2, 12.0) |
| 1990 | 18.9 (18.1, 19.7) | 15.9 (15.3, 16.4) | 17.3 (16.8, 17.8) | 11.0 (10.2, 11.8) | 12.9 (12.3, 13.5) | 12.0 (11.6, 12.4) |
| 1991 | 18.1 (17.4, 18.8) | 14.9 (14.3, 15.5) | 16.4 (15.9, 16.9) | 11.2 (10.6, 11.8) | 12.6 (12.0, 13.2) | 11.9 (11.5, 12.3) |
| 1992 | | | | 11.8 (11.2, 12.4) | 12.2 (11.6, 12.8) | 12.0 (11.6, 12.4) |
| 1993 | | | | | | |
| 1994 | | | | 11.4 (10.8, 12.0) | 11.4 (10.8, 12.0) | 11.4 (11.0, 11.8) |

Sources: Centers for Disease Control and Prevention, National Center for Health Statistics, NHIS, 1985, 1990, 1991; Centers for Disease Control and Prevention, National Center for Chronic Disease Prevention and Health Promotion, BRFSS, 1986-1992 and 1994.

*25 states and the District of Columbia
†95% confidence intervals.

questions, and the age of respondents. Trends over time can be monitored only with the YRBS, which was conducted in 1991 and 1993 as well as in 1995. An assessment of the test-retest reliability of the YRBS indicated that the four physical activity items included in the study had a kappa value (an indicator of reliability) in the "substantial" (i.e., 61–80) or "almost perfect" (i.e., 81–100) range (Brener et al. 1995).

## Physical Inactivity

*Healthy People 2000* objective 1.5 calls for reducing to no more than 15 percent the proportion of people aged 6 years and older who are inactive (USDHHS 1990). For this report, inactivity was defined as performing no vigorous activity (exercise or sports participation that made the respondent "sweat or breathe hard" for at least 20 minutes) and performing

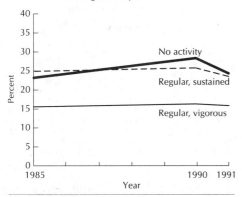

**Figure 5-3. Trends in leisure-time physical activity of adults aged 18+ years, NHIS**

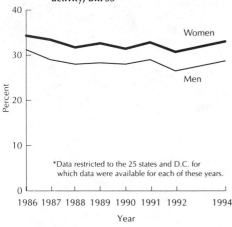

**Figure 5-4. Trends in the percentage of adults aged 18+ years participating in no leisure-time activity, BRFSS\***

*Data restricted to the 25 states and D.C. for which data were available for each of these years.

no light to moderate activity (walking or bicycling for at least 30 minutes) during any of the 7 days preceding the survey. Among 12- through 21-year-olds surveyed in the 1992 NHIS-YRBS, the prevalence of inactivity in the previous week was 13.7 percent and was higher among females than males (15.3 percent vs. 12.1 percent) (Table 5-9). Overall, there was no difference among racial and ethnic groups, but black females had a higher prevalence

than white females (20.2 percent vs. 13.7 percent). For both males and females, inactivity increased with age.

Similarly, in the 1995 school-based YRBS, the prevalence of inactivity in the previous week was 10.4 percent (Table 5-9) and was higher among females than males (13.8 percent vs. 7.3 percent). The prevalence was higher among black students than white students (15.3 percent vs. 9.3 percent) and among black females than white females (21.4 percent vs. 11.6 percent). Among female high school students, a substantial increase in inactivity was reported in the upper grades.

Thus the *Healthy People 2000* goal for inactivity has been met for adolescents overall but not for black females or for young adults.

## Vigorous Physical Activity

*Healthy People 2000* objective 1.4 (USDHHS 1990) proposes to increase to at least 75 percent the proportion of children and adolescents aged 6–17 years who engage in vigorous physical activity that promotes cardiorespiratory fitness 3 days or more per week for 20 minutes or more per occasion. In the 1992 NHIS-YRBS, 53.7 percent of 12- through 21-year-olds reported having exercised or taken part in sports that made them "sweat and breathe hard" during 3 or more of the 7 days preceding the survey (Table 5-10). However, one-fourth reported no vigorous activity during the same time period. Prevalences of vigorous activity were higher among males than females (60.2 percent vs. 47.2 percent) and among white youths than Hispanic youths (54.6 percent vs. 49.5 percent) (Table 5-10). Vigorous physical activity declined with age. Among males, the prevalence of vigorous activity was at least 60 percent for those aged 12–17 years but was lower at older ages (e.g., 42.2 percent among 21-year-olds). Among females aged 12–14 years, the prevalence was at least 60 percent but was lower at older ages (e.g., 30.2 percent among 21-year-olds). The prevalence of vigorous activity was associated positively with income and was higher during the spring than during other seasons.

In the 1995 YRBS, 63.7 percent of students in grades 9–12 reported having exercised or taken part in sports that made them "sweat and breathe hard" for at least 20 minutes during 3 or more of the 7 days

## Physical Activity and Health

Table 5-9. Percentage of young people reporting no participation in vigorous or moderate physical activity during any of the 7 days preceding the survey, by demographic group, 1992 National Health Interview Survey-Youth Risk Behavior Survey (NHIS-YRBS) and 1995 Youth Risk Behavior Survey (YRBS), United States

| Demographic group | 1992 NHIS-YRBS* | 1995 YRBS[†] |
|---|---|---|
| Overall | 13.7 (12.9, 14.5)[‡] | 10.4 (9.0, 11.9) |
| **Sex** | | |
| Males | 12.1 (11.0, 13.2) | 7.3 (6.5, 8.1) |
| Females | 15.3 (14.1, 16.5) | 13.8 (11.2, 16.3) |
| **Race/Ethnicity** | | |
| White, non-Hispanic | 13.4 (12.4, 14.5) | 9.3 (7.9, 10.7) |
| Males | 13.1 (11.7, 14.6) | 7.3 (6.4, 8.1) |
| Females | 13.7 (12.4, 15.1) | 11.6 (8.7, 14.4) |
| Black, non-Hispanic | 14.7 (12.7, 16.6) | 15.3 (12.4, 18.2) |
| Males | 9.2 (6.9, 11.5) | 8.1 (5.4, 10.7) |
| Females | 20.2 (17.0, 23.5) | 21.4 (16.9, 25.8) |
| Hispanic | 14.3 (12.4, 16.3) | 11.3 (8.6, 14.1) |
| Males | 11.1 (8.4, 13.8) | 7.5 (5.1, 9.9) |
| Females | 17.8 (14.9, 20.7) | 15.0 (10.6, 19.5) |

| Age (years) Males | 1992 NHIS-YRBS* | Grade in school Males | 1995 YRBS[†] |
|---|---|---|---|
| 12 | 7.7 (5.1, 10.2) | | |
| 13 | 6.0 (3.6, 8.3) | | |
| 14 | 3.6 (2.1, 5.1) | | |
| 15 | 6.3 (3.7, 8.9) | 9 | 6.0 (3.4, 8.7) |
| 16 | 9.6 (6.8, 12.4) | 10 | 5.2 (3.0, 7.4) |
| 17 | 10.5 (7.2, 13.9) | 11 | 7.9 (4.3, 11.4) |
| 18 | 18.8 (14.4, 23.3) | 12 | 10.0 (7.4, 12.5) |
| 19 | 18.6 (14.7, 22.5) | | |
| 20 | 22.3 (17.9, 26.8) | | |
| 21 | 18.1 (14.3, 21.9) | | |
| **Females** | | **Females** | |
| 12 | 8.4 (5.2, 11.5) | | |
| 13 | 6.8 (4.4, 9.2) | | |
| 14 | 8.3 (5.1, 11.5) | | |
| 15 | 9.8 (7.0, 12.6) | 9 | 8.7 (6.1, 11.3) |
| 16 | 14.4 (10.9, 17.9) | 10 | 9.2 (7.3, 11.0) |
| 17 | 16.8 (13.2, 20.3) | 11 | 17.8 (13.6, 22.0) |
| 18 | 18.7 (14.5, 22.8) | 12 | 18.5 (13.3, 23.7) |
| 19 | 22.3 (18.1, 26.5) | | |
| 20 | 25.0 (21.0, 28.9) | | |
| 21 | 19.6 (16.4, 22.9) | | |

| Annual family income | 1992 NHIS-YRBS* | |
|---|---|---|
| < $10,000 | 14.9 (12.6, 17.3) | |
| $10,000–19,999 | 16.0 (14.1, 17.9) | |
| $20,000–34,999 | 12.2 (10.6, 13.8) | |
| $35,000–49,999 | 13.8 (11.6, 15.9) | |
| $50,000+ | 11.2 (9.8, 12.7) | |

Sources: Centers for Disease Control and Prevention, National Center for Health Statistics, NHIS-YRBS, 1992 machine readable data file and documentation, 1993; Centers for Disease Control and Prevention, National Center for Chronic Disease Prevention and Health Promotion, YRBS 1995 data tape (in press).

*A national household-based survey of youths aged 12–21 years.
[†]A national school-based survey of students in grades 9–12.
[‡]95% confidence intervals.

Table 5-10. Percentage of young people reporting participation in vigorous physical activity during 3 or more of the 7 days preceding the survey, by demographic group, 1992 National Health Interview Survey-Youth Risk Behavior Survey (NHIS-YRBS) and 1995 Youth Risk Behavior Survey (YRBS), United States

| Demographic group | 1992 NHIS-YRBS* | 1995 YRBS[†] |
|---|---|---|
| Overall | 53.7 (52.5, 54.9)[‡] | 63.7 (60.4, 66.9) |
| **Sex** | | |
| Males | 60.2 (58.6, 61.8) | 74.4 (72.1, 76.6) |
| Females | 47.2 (45.6, 48.8) | 52.1 (47.5, 56.8) |
| **Race/Ethnicity** | | |
| White, non-Hispanic | 54.6 (53.2, 56.0) | 67.0 (62.6, 71.4) |
| Males | 60.2 (58.4, 62.0) | 76.0 (73.0, 78.9) |
| Females | 49.0 (46.8, 51.2) | 56.7 ( 50.0, 63.4) |
| Black, non-Hispanic | 52.6 (49.9, 55.3) | 53.2 (49.6, 56.8) |
| Males | 62.7 (58.8, 66.6) | 68.1 (62.8, 73.4) |
| Females | 42.3 (38.6, 46.0) | 41.3 (35.5, 42.1) |
| Hispanic | 49.5 (46.6, 52.4) | 57.3 (53.7, 60.9) |
| Males | 56.7 (52.6, 60.8) | 69.7 (64.9, 74.5) |
| Females | 41.7 (38.2, 45.2) | 45.2 (39.9, 50.6) |

| Age (years) | | Grade in school | |
|---|---|---|---|
| **Males** | | **Males** | |
| 12 | 70.8 (66.7, 74.9) | | |
| 13 | 73.7 (69.4, 78.0) | | |
| 14 | 76.1 (72.2, 80.0) | | |
| 15 | 72.6 (68.1, 71.1) | 9 | 80.8 (75.9, 85.6) |
| 16 | 65.6 (60.3, 70.9) | 10 | 75.9 (72.5, 79.3) |
| 17 | 60.2 (54.7, 65.7) | 11 | 70.2 (67.5, 72.9) |
| 18 | 48.4 (43.1, 53.7) | 12 | 66.9 (63.0, 70.7) |
| 19 | 44.1 (38.4, 49.8) | | |
| 20 | 43.4 (38.5, 48.3) | | |
| 21 | 42.2 (37.1, 47.3) | | |
| **Females** | | **Females** | |
| 12 | 66.2 (62.1, 70.3) | | |
| 13 | 63.1 (58.0, 68.2) | | |
| 14 | 63.1 (58.4, 67.8) | | |
| 15 | 56.6 (51.9, 61.3) | 9 | 60.9 (54.8, 67.0) |
| 16 | 50.9 (45.6, 56.2) | 10 | 54.4 (47.6, 61.3) |
| 17 | 43.6 (38.1, 49.1) | 11 | 44.7 (40.6, 48.9) |
| 18 | 37.5 (32.2, 42.8) | 12 | 41.0 (34.6, 47.5) |
| 19 | 32.6 (27.3, 37.9) | | |
| 20 | 28.2 (23.9, 32.5) | | |
| 21 | 30.2 (25.5, 34.9) | | |

| Annual family income | | |
|---|---|---|
| < $10,000 | 46.7 (43.2, 50.2) | |
| $10,000–19,999 | 48.5 (46.0, 51.1) | |
| $20,000–34,999 | 55.0 (52.5, 57.6) | |
| $35,000–49,999 | 58.4 (55.5, 61.3) | |
| $50,000+ | 60.2 (57.9, 62.6) | |

Sources: Centers for Disease Control and Prevention, National Center for Health Statistics, NHIS-YRBS, 1992 machine readable data file and documentation, 1993; Centers for Disease Control and Prevention, National Center for Chronic Disease Prevention and Health Promotion, YRBS 1995 data tape (in press).

*A national household-based survey of youths aged 12–21 years.
[†]A national school-based survey of students in grades 9–12.
[‡]95% confidence intervals.

191

preceding the survey (Table 5-10). However, 16.0 percent reported no vigorous physical activity during the same time period. Subgroup patterns were similar to those reported for the NHIS-YRBS. Vigorous physical activity was more common among male than female students (74.4 percent vs. 52.1 percent) and among white than black or Hispanic students (67 percent vs. 53.2 percent and 57.3 percent, respectively). Among both male and female students, vigorous activity was less common in the upper grades. From 1991 through 1995, the overall prevalence did not change significantly among students in grades 9–12 (data not shown).

NHIS-YRBS and YRBS data clearly show that the prevalence of vigorous physical activity among young people falls short of the *Healthy People 2000* goal of 75 percent.

## Other Physical Activity

*Healthy People 2000* objective 1.6 (USDHHS 1990) aims for at least 40 percent of people aged 6 and older to regularly perform physical activities that enhance and maintain muscular strength, muscular endurance, and flexibility. The 1992 NHIS-YRBS indicated that 45.6 percent of 12- through 21-year-olds had participated in strengthening or toning activities (e.g., push-ups, sit-ups, or weight lifting) during at least 3 of the 7 days preceding the survey (Table 5-11). These activities were more common among males than females (54.6 percent vs. 36.4 percent) and among white and Hispanic youths than black youths (46.4 percent and 45.4 percent, respectively, vs. 39.8 percent). Among both males and females, the prevalence of strengthening or toning activities decreased as age increased and was greater among young people living in households with higher incomes.

Similar to the NHIS-YRBS, the 1995 YRBS indicated that 50.3 percent of students in grades 9–12 had participated in strengthening or toning activities during at least 3 of the 7 days preceding the survey (Table 5-11). Subgroup patterns were similar to those reported for the 1992 NHIS-YRBS. Male students were more likely than female students to participate in strengthening or toning activities (59.1 percent vs. 41.0 percent), and white students were more likely than black students to do so (52.8 percent vs. 41.4 percent). Among female students, participation was greater among those in lower grades, but this practice

did not vary by grade among male students. Between 1991 and 1995, the overall prevalence of strengthening or toning activities among students in grades 9–12 did not change (data not shown).

In the 1992 NHIS-YRBS, 48.0 percent of 12- through 21-year-olds reported having participated in stretching activities (e.g., toe touching, knee bending, or leg stretching) during at least 3 of the 7 days preceding the survey. White and Hispanic youths were more likely than black youths to report this (49.2 percent and 48.5 percent, respectively, vs. 40.7 percent). Overall, the prevalence of stretching activities did not differ by sex, although these activities were more common among black males than among black females (44.9 percent vs. 36.5 percent). Among both males and females, the prevalence was higher in the younger age categories. Participation was also higher with higher family income.

In the 1995 YRBS, 53.0 percent of students in grades 9–12 reported having participated in stretching activities during at least 3 of the 7 days preceding the survey (Table 5-12). Subgroup patterns were generally similar to those reported for the NHIS-YRBS. Similar proportions of male and female students participated in stretching activities (55.5 percent and 50.4 percent, respectively), and white students were more likely than black students to do so (55.1 percent vs. 45.4 percent). Participation in stretching activities declined across grades for both male and female students. Between 1991 and 1995, the overall prevalence among students in grades 9–12 did not change significantly (data not shown).

Thus the *Healthy People 2000* objective for strengthening and stretching activities has been met overall among adolescents and young adults but not among all subgroups.

*Healthy People 2000* objective 1.3 (USDHHS 1990) proposes to increase to at least 30 percent the proportion of people aged 6 and older who engage regularly, preferably daily, in light to moderate physical activity for at least 30 minutes per day. Walking and bicycling can be used to measure light to moderate physical activity among young people. In the 1992 NHIS-YRBS, 26.4 percent of 12- through 21-year-olds reported having walked or bicycled for 30 minutes or more on at least 5 of the 7 days preceding the survey (Table 5-13). These activities were more common among males than females (29.1 percent vs. 23.7 percent) and among Hispanic youths than

Table 5-11. Percentage of young people reporting participation in strengthening or toning activities during 3 or more of the 7 days preceding the survey, by demographic group, 1992 National Health Interview Survey-Youth Risk Behavior Survey (NHIS-YRBS) and 1995 Youth Risk Behavior Survey (YRBS), United States

| Demographic group | 1992 NHIS-YRBS* | 1995 YRBS[†] |
|---|---|---|
| Overall | 45.6 (44.4, 46.8)[‡] | 50.3 (46.6, 54.0) |
| **Sex** | | |
| Males | 54.6 (53.0, 56.2) | 59.1 (56.1, 62.1) |
| Females | 36.4 (34.8, 38.0) | 41.0 (36.0, 46.0) |
| **Race/Ethnicity** | | |
| White, non-Hispanic | 46.4 (45.0, 47.8) | 52.8 (47.2, 58.4) |
| Males | 54.4 (52.6, 56.2) | 60.3 (56.4, 64.2) |
| Females | 38.4 (36.4, 40.4) | 44.4 (36.4, 2.4) |
| Black, non-Hispanic | 39.8 (37.5, 42.2) | 41.4 (37.9, 45.0) |
| Males | 53.2 (49.3, 57.1) | 54.2 (49.7, 58.6) |
| Females | 26.2 (23.1, 29.3) | 31.3 (26.7, 35.9) |
| Hispanic | 45.4 (42.5, 48.3) | 47.4 (41.8, 53.1) |
| Males | 53.3 (49.4, 57.2) | 57.8 (51.9, 63.8) |
| Females | 36.9 (33.2, 40.6) | 37.4 (29.6, 45.2) |

| Age (years) | 1992 NHIS-YRBS* | Grade in school | 1995 YRBS[†] |
|---|---|---|---|
| **Males** | | **Males** | |
| 12 | 59.4 (54.7, 64.1) | | |
| 13 | 66.3 (62.2, 70.4) | | |
| 14 | 61.1 (56.0, 66.2) | | |
| 15 | 66.6 (61.9, 71.3) | 9 | 65.3 (58.0, 72.5) |
| 16 | 61.3 (56.0, 66.6) | 10 | 60.0 (55.8, 64.2) |
| 17 | 53.9 (48.6, 59.2) | 11 | 55.9 (52.5, 59.2) |
| 18 | 46.0 (41.3, 50.7) | 12 | 54.7 (49.7, 59.7) |
| 19 | 45.2 (39.7, 50.7) | | |
| 20 | 42.0 (37.5, 46.5) | | |
| 21 | 40.5 (35.8, 45.2) | | |
| **Females** | | **Females** | |
| 12 | 43.9 (39.6, 48.2) | | |
| 13 | 46.9 (41.6, 52.2) | | |
| 14 | 47.6 (42.7, 52.5) | | |
| 15 | 44.0 (39.1, 48.9) | 9 | 51.3 (42.9, 59.8) |
| 16 | 38.1 (33.6, 42.6) | 10 | 45.6 (38.3, 53.0) |
| 17 | 37.1 (32.0, 42.2) | 11 | 31.0 (27.6, 34.3) |
| 18 | 31.1 (25.6, 36.6) | 12 | 30.0 (25.1, 34.9) |
| 19 | 26.4 (22.1, 30.7) | | |
| 20 | 26.3 (22.0, 30.6) | | |
| 21 | 23.2 (19.3, 27.1) | | |

| Annual family income | 1992 NHIS-YRBS* |
|---|---|
| <$10,000 | 36.4 (33.7, 39.1) |
| $10,000-$19,999 | 44.6 (41.9, 47.3) |
| $20,000-$34,999 | 46.5 (44.0, 49.1) |
| $35,000-$49,999 | 49.6 (46.7, 52.5) |
| $50,000+ | 51.4 (49.1, 53.8) |

Sources: Centers for Disease Control and Prevention, National Center for Health Statistics, NHIS-YRBS,1992 machine readable data file and documentation, 1993; Centers for Disease Control and Prevention, National Center for Chronic Disease Prevention and Health Promotion, YRBS 1995 data tape (in press).

*A national household-based survey of youths aged 12–21 years.
[†]A national school-based survey of students in grades 9–12.
[‡]95% confidence intervals.

# Physical Activity and Health

Table 5-12.   Percentage of young people reporting participation in stretching activities during 3 or more of the 7 days preceding the survey, by demographic group, 1992 National Health Interview Survey-Youth Risk Behavior Survey (NHIS-YRBS) and 1995 Youth Risk Behavior Survey (YRBS), United States

| Demographic group | 1992 NHIS-YRBS* | | 1995 YRBS[†] | |
|---|---|---|---|---|
| Overall | 48.0 | (46.8, 49.2)[‡] | 53.0 | (49.9, 56.2) |
| **Sex** | | | | |
| Males | 48.2 | (46.6, 49.8) | 55.5 | (52.3, 58.7) |
| Females | 47.9 | (46.3, 49.5) | 50.4 | (46.6, 54.3) |
| **Race/Ethnicity** | | | | |
| White, non-Hispanic | 49.2 | (47.8, 50.6) | 55.1 | (50.8, 59.3) |
| Males | 48.0 | (46.0, 50.0) | 56.1 | (52.1, 60.1) |
| Females | 50.4 | (48.4, 52.4) | 53.9 | (48.2, 59.5) |
| Black, non-Hispanic | 40.7 | (38.0, 43.4) | 45.4 | (41.7, 49.0) |
| Males | 44.9 | (41.0, 48.8) | 50.5 | (45.0, 55.9) |
| Females | 36.5 | (32.8, 40.2) | 41.5 | (36.6, 46.3 |
| Hispanic | 48.5 | (45.8, 51.2) | 49.1 | (45.0, 53.2) |
| Males | 49.9 | (46.0, 53.8) | 54.8 | (50.1, 59.6) |
| Females | 47.0 | (43.3, 50.7) | 43.5 | (37.6, 49.5) |

| Age (years) Males | | | Grade in school Males | | |
|---|---|---|---|---|---|
| 12 | 55.4 | (50.5, 60.3) | | | |
| 13 | 62.0 | (57.3, 66.7) | | | |
| 14 | 57.9 | (53.2, 62.6) | | | |
| 15 | 56.1 | (51.0, 61.2) | 9 | 65.7 | (58.9, 72.6) |
| 16 | 54.0 | (48.7, 59.3) | 10 | 51.1 | (47.8, 54.4) |
| 17 | 48.2 | (42.9, 53.5) | 11 | 52.9 | (48.1, 57.6) |
| 18 | 36.2 | (31.1, 41.3) | 12 | 49.8 | (42.0, 57.7) |
| 19 | 36.7 | (32.0, 41.4) | | | |
| 20 | 32.9 | (28.4, 37.4) | | | |
| 21 | 38.5 | (33.4, 43.6) | | | |
| Females | | | Females | | |
| 12 | 62.5 | (58.0, 67.0) | | | |
| 13 | 62.5 | (57.2, 67.8) | | | |
| 14 | 61.6 | (56.7, 66.5) | | | |
| 15 | 57.9 | (53.0, 62.8) | 9 | 59.9 | (52.8, 67.0) |
| 16 | 52.0 | (47.1, 56.9) | 10 | 55.8 | (49.6, 61.9) |
| 17 | 42.0 | (37.1, 46.9) | 11 | 39.5 | (33.7, 45.3) |
| 18 | 38.5 | (33.0, 44.0) | 12 | 38.4 | (32.7, 44.1) |
| 19 | 33.1 | (28.0, 38.2) | | | |
| 20 | 33.9 | (29.6, 38.2) | | | |
| 21 | 35.0 | (30.9, 39.1) | | | |

| Annual family income | | |
|---|---|---|
| < $10,000 | 40.8 | (37.7, 43.9) |
| $10,000–$19,999 | 44.5 | (41.8, 47.2) |
| $20,000–$34,999 | 48.2 | (45.9, 50.6) |
| $35,000–$49,999 | 51.9 | (49.2, 54.6) |
| $50,000+ | 54.2 | (51.7, 56.8) |

Sources: Centers for Disease Control and Prevention, National Center for Health Statistics, NHIS-YRBS, 1992 machine readable data file and documentation, 1993; Centers for Disease Control and Prevention, National Center for Chronic Disease Prevention and Health Promotion, YRBS 1995 data tape (in press).

*A national household-based survey of youths aged 12–21 years.
[†]A national school-based survey of students in grades 9–12.
[‡]95% confidence intervals.

Table 5-13. Percentage of young people reporting participation in walking or bicycling for 30 minutes or more during 5 or more of the 7 days preceding the survey, by demographic group, 1992 National Health Interview Survey-Youth Risk Behavior Survey (NHIS-YRBS) and 1995 Youth Risk Behavior Survey (YRBS), United States

| Demographic group | 1992 NHIS-YRBS* | | 1995 YRBS[†] |
|---|---|---|---|
| Overall | 26.4 (25.4, 27.4)[‡] | | 21.1 (18.7, 23.5) |
| **Sex** | | | |
| Males | 29.1 (27.5, 30.7) | | 21.6 (18.4, 24.8) |
| Females | 23.7 (22.3, 25.1) | | 20.5 (17.8, 23.2) |
| **Race/Ethnicity** | | | |
| White, non-Hispanic | 25.1 (23.9, 26.3) | | 18.3 (15.0, 21.6) |
| Males | 27.5 (25.7, 29.3) | | 19.7 (15.5, 23.8) |
| Females | 22.7 (21.1, 24.3) | | 16.8 (13.9, 19.8) |
| Black, non-Hispanic | 26.9 (24.6, 29.2) | | 27.0 (23.2, 30.9) |
| Males | 29.8 (26.7, 32.9) | | 27.2 (23.2, 31.2) |
| Females | 23.9 (20.2, 27.6) | | 26.4 (20.8, 32.0) |
| Hispanic | 32.3 (29.8, 34.9) | | 26.8 (22.6, 31.0) |
| Males | 35.5 (31.6, 39.4) | | 26.0 (19.9, 32.1) |
| Females | 28.8 (25.5, 32.1) | | 27.6 (23.8, 31.5) |

| Age (years) | | Grade in school | |
|---|---|---|---|
| **Males** | | **Males** | |
| 12 | 38.9 (34.6, 43.2) | | |
| 13 | 37.3 (32.4, 42.2) | | |
| 14 | 35.3 (31.2, 39.4) | | |
| 15 | 33.9 (29.0, 38.8) | 9 | 27.9 (22.1, 33.7) |
| 16 | 29.9 (25.6, 34.2) | 10 | 21.7 (17.8, 25.6) |
| 17 | 22.2 (17.7, 26.7) | 11 | 19.2 (16.2, 22.1) |
| 18 | 23.3 (18.6, 28.0) | 12 | 17.7 (13.1, 22.3) |
| 19 | 21.3 (17.2, 25.4) | | |
| 20 | 22.0 (17.9, 26.1) | | |
| 21 | 23.3 (19.0, 27.6) | | |
| **Females** | | **Females** | |
| 12 | 32.2 (28.1, 36.3) | | |
| 13 | 28.5 (24.0, 33.0) | | |
| 14 | 28.7 (23.8, 33.6) | | |
| 15 | 22.9 (18.8, 27.0) | 9 | 22.5 (18.5, 26.5) |
| 16 | 22.9 (18.8, 27.0) | 10 | 22.8 (18.5, 27.2) |
| 17 | 19.4 (15.5, 23.3) | 11 | 16.8 (13.3, 20.3) |
| 18 | 20.1 (16.0, 24.2) | 12 | 16.1 (11.6, 20.6) |
| 19 | 18.8 (14.5, 23.1) | | |
| 20 | 20.8 (16.7, 24.9) | | |
| 21 | 22.1 (18.4, 25.8) | | |

| Annual family income | | | |
|---|---|---|---|
| < $10,000 | 27.8 (25.1, 30.5) | | |
| $10,000–$19,999 | 29.5 (26.8, 32.2) | | |
| $20,000–$34,999 | 27.6 (25.2, 30.0) | | |
| $35,000–$49,999 | 25.5 (23.2, 27.9) | | |
| $50,000+ | 23.5 (21.5, 25.5) | | |

Sources: Centers for Disease Control and Prevention, National Center for Health Statistics, NHIS-YRBS, 1992 machine readable data file and documentation, 1993; Centers for Disease Control and Prevention, National Center for Chronic Disease Prevention and Health Promotion, YRBS 1995 data tape (in press).

*A national household-based survey of youths aged 12–21 years.
[†]A national school-based survey of students in grades 9–12.
[‡]95% confidence intervals.

## Physical Activity and Health

Table 5-14. Percentage of young people reporting participation in selected physical activities during 1 or more of the 7 days preceding the survey, by demographic group, 1992 National Health Interview Survey-Youth Risk Behavior Survey (NHIS-YRBS),* United States

| Demographic group | Aerobics or dancing | Baseball, softball, or Frisbee® | Basketball, football, or soccer |
|---|---|---|---|
| Overall | 38.2 (37.1, 39.2)[†] | 22.4 (21.4, 23.4) | 45.8 (44.6, 47.1) |
| **Sex** | | | |
| Males | 22.6 (21.3, 24.0) | 27.2 (25.7, 28.8) | 61.7 (60.1, 63.3) |
| Females | 53.9 (52.4, 55.5) | 17.5 (16.4, 18.7) | 29.7 (28.2, 31.3) |
| **Race/Ethnicity** | | | |
| White, non-Hispanic | 35.0 (33.7, 36.2) | 23.6 (22.3, 24.9) | 44.7 (43.1, 46.2) |
| Black, non-Hispanic | 49.4 (46.6, 52.1) | 16.6 (14.3, 18.9) | 49.5 (46.7, 52.3) |
| Hispanic | 42.0 (39.0, 45.0) | 23.4 (21.1, 25.7) | 47.1 (44.4, 49.8) |
| **Age (years)** | | | |
| **Males** | | | |
| 12 | 26.9 (22.5, 31.2) | 46.4 (41.6, 51.3) | 81.2 (77.4, 85.0) |
| 13 | 23.4 (19.6, 27.3) | 40.6 (35.8, 45.3) | 84.3 (80.8, 87.9) |
| 14 | 22.0 (18.4, 25.7) | 40.9 (36.6, 45.2) | 78.5 (74.3, 82.6) |
| 15 | 21.9 (17.7, 26.1) | 25.6 (21.0, 30.3) | 76.7 (72.5, 81.0) |
| 16 | 24.5 (20.2, 28.9) | 27.4 (22.9, 31.9) | 69.6 (64.5, 74.6) |
| 17 | 20.8 (16.8, 24.6) | 22.5 (18.1, 26.9) | 59.3 (54.2, 64.3) |
| 18 | 19.0 (14.9, 23.1) | 20.8 (16.3, 25.2) | 54.6 (49.1, 60.0) |
| 19 | 24.0 (19.6, 28.4) | 17.5 (13.8, 21.2) | 43.8 (38.5, 49.0) |
| 20 | 21.2 (17.2, 25.2) | 17.0 (13.3, 20.8) | 38.5 (33.9, 43.2) |
| 21 | 21.4 (17.2, 25.7) | 15.6 (12.1, 19.1) | 32.4 (27.6, 37.1) |
| **Females** | | | |
| 12 | 63.1 (58.7, 67.5) | 37.9 (33.4, 42.5) | 62.6 (57.6, 67.6) |
| 13 | 63.7 (59.5, 67.9) | 30.3 (26.2, 34.3) | 61.6 (56.9, 66.3) |
| 14 | 63.7 (59.0, 68.3) | 29.1 (24.7, 33.5) | 51.9 (46.8, 57.1) |
| 15 | 62.0 (57.5, 66.4) | 22.6 (18.3, 26.9) | 41.6 (37.2, 46.1) |
| 16 | 55.7 (50.5, 60.9) | 16.0 (12.3, 19.6) | 28.0 (23.3, 32.6) |
| 17 | 54.0 (48.8, 59.2) | 10.2 (7.4, 13.1) | 23.4 (19.0, 27.7) |
| 18 | 50.3 (45.2, 55.5) | 11.4 (7.3, 15.4) | 13.8 (10.2, 17.4) |
| 19 | 44.8 (39.1, 50.4) | 6.9 (4.4, 9.3) | 8.5 (6.0, 11.0) |
| 20 | 40.7 (36.2, 45.2) | 7.6 (4.8, 10.4) | 6.9 (4.7, 9.1) |
| 21 | 45.6 (41.0, 50.2) | 8.4 (5.9, 10.9) | 7.5 (5.2, 9.8) |

white or black youths (32.3 percent vs. 25.1 percent and 26.9 percent, respectively). Walking or bicycling decreased as age increased and was more prevalent in the fall than in other seasons.

In the 1995 YRBS, 21.1 percent of students in grades 9–12 reported having walked or bicycled for 30 minutes or more on at least 5 of the 7 days preceding the survey (Table 5-13). Male and female students reported similar prevalences of these activities. Black and Hispanic students were more likely

than white students to have walked or bicycled (27.0 percent and 26.8 percent, respectively, vs. 18.3 percent). Between 1993 and 1995, the overall prevalence among students in grades 9–12 did not change significantly (data not shown).

It thus appears that the *Healthy People 2000* objective for light to moderate physical activity has not been attained by adolescents and young adults.

The 1992 NHIS-YRBS provided information on participation in seven additional types of physical

**Table 5-14.** *Continued*

| House cleaning or yard work for ≥ 30 minutes | Running, jogging, or swimming | Skating, skiing, or skateboarding | Tennis, raquetball, or squash |
|---|---|---|---|
| 82.8 (81.7, 83.8) | 55.3 (54.1, 56.6) | 13.3 (12.5, 14.0) | 10.5 (9.8, 11.2) |
| 78.1 (76.6, 79.5) | 57.6 (55.9, 59.3) | 15.9 (14.8, 17.0) | 11.7 (10.7, 12.8) |
| 87.5 (86.3, 88.7) | 53.0 (51.4, 54.7) | 10.6 (9.6, 11.5) | 9.3 (8.4, 10.2) |
| 83.1 (81.9, 84.3) | 55.8 (54.3, 57.3) | 15.2 (14.2, 16.2) | 11.4 (10.6, 12.3) |
| 84.2 (81.9, 86.5) | 52.4 (49.5, 55.3) | 9.0 (7.3, 10.8) | 5.4 (4.2, 6.6) |
| 80.1 (77.9, 82.4) | 53.6 (50.9, 56.4) | 9.8 (8.2, 11.5) | 8.0 (6.7, 9.4) |
| 76.9 (72.9, 81.0) | 72.8 (68.3, 77.3) | 32.5 (27.8, 37.3) | 14.4 (10.8, 18.0) |
| 83.3 (80.1, 86.5) | 74.3 (70.1, 78.4) | 26.2 (22.1, 30.3) | 13.3 (10.3, 16.4) |
| 79.4 (75.5, 83.4) | 71.2 (66.8, 75.6) | 20.7 (16.9, 24.5) | 14.5 (11.3, 17.8) |
| 82.9 (79.3, 86.5) | 70.8 (66.5, 75.1) | 19.9 (15.9, 23.9) | 15.3 (11.7, 18.9) |
| 79.6 (75.7, 83.6) | 63.4 (58.8, 68.1) | 13.4 (10.0, 16.8) | 10.4 (7.4, 13.3) |
| 78.7 (74.5, 82.9) | 55.3 (49.9, 60.7) | 12.2 (8.6, 15.7) | 11.3 (8.0, 14.6) |
| 70.9 (65.9, 75.9) | 47.4 (42.2, 52.5) | 9.4 (6.3, 12.4) | 11.6 (8.3, 14.9) |
| 75.0 (69.6, 80.4) | 46.3 (41.3, 51.2) | 10.8 (7.7, 14.0) | 9.9 (6.9, 12.8) |
| 74.4 (70.3, 78.5) | 34.4 (29.9, 38.9) | 8.6 (6.1, 11.2) | 8.2 (5.5, 10.8) |
| 77.6 (73.7, 81.5) | 39.8 (34.1, 45.5) | 5.9 (3.8, 7.9) | 9.5 (6.5, 12.5) |
| 88.0 (84.8, 91.2) | 80.5 (76.4, 84.5) | 24.9 (20.5, 29.3) | 13.9 (10.5, 17.3) |
| 88.1 (85.1, 91.1) | 76.2 (72.1, 80.3) | 19.7 (16.1, 23.4) | 12.4 (9.2, 15.6) |
| 87.2 (83.9, 90.4) | 72.9 (68.6, 77.2) | 14.8 (11.6, 18.0) | 13.0 (10.0, 15.9) |
| 88.5 (85.3, 91.7) | 65.4 (60.7, 70.1) | 10.0 (7.0, 12.9) | 16.1 (12.6, 19.6) |
| 89.1 (85.7, 92.5) | 59.7 (54.8, 64.6) | 8.9 (6.2, 11.7) | 11.1 (8.0, 14.2) |
| 86.0 (82.6, 89.4) | 49.0 (43.5, 54.4) | 4.8 (2.7, 6.8) | 8.0 (5.4, 10.5) |
| 87.0 (83.4, 90.5) | 41.5 (35.8, 47.3) | 8.1 (5.5, 10.7) | 6.9 (4.4, 9.5) |
| 82.6 (78.1, 87.1) | 32.9 (27.8, 38.0) | 6.6 (4.1, 9.1) | 3.8 (2.1, 5.4) |
| 87.1 (83.0, 91.2) | 30.8 (25.8, 35.7) | 5.8 (3.5, 8.0) | 5.8 (3.6, 8.0) |
| 89.8 (86.2, 93.4) | 30.3 (26.0, 34.6) | 4.8 (3.1, 6.6) | 4.1 (2.2, 5.9) |

Source: Centers for Disease Control and Prevention, National Center for Health Statistics, NHIS-YRBS, 1992 machine readable data file and documentation, 1993.

*A national household-based survey of youths aged 12–21 years.
†95% confidence intervals.

activity during 1 or more of the 7 days preceding the survey: aerobics or dancing; baseball, softball, or Frisbee[1]; basketball, football, or soccer; house cleaning or yard work for at least 30 minutes; running, jogging, or swimming for exercise; skating, skiing, or skateboarding; and tennis, racquetball, or squash (Table 5-14). Among 12- through 21-year-olds, males were more likely than females to participate in baseball, softball, or Frisbee[®]; in basketball, football, or soccer; in running, jogging, or swimming for exercise; in skating, skiing, or skateboarding; and in tennis, racquetball, or squash.

[1]Use of trade names is for identification only and does not imply endorsement by the U.S. Department of Health and Human Services.

197

Table 5-15. Percentage of students in grades 9–12 reporting enrollment in physical education class, daily attendance in physical education class, and participation in exercise or sports for at least 20 minutes during an average physical education class, by demographic group, 1995 Youth Risk Behavior Survey (YRBS),[*] United States

| Demographic group | Enrolled in physical education | Attended physical education daily | Exercised or played sports $\geq$ 20 minutes per class[†] |
|---|---|---|---|
| Overall | 59.6 (48.6, 70.5)[‡] | 25.4 (15.8, 34.9) | 69.7 (66.4, 72.9) |
| **Sex** | | | |
| Males | 62.2 (52.5, 71.8) | 27.0 (16.8, 37.2) | 74.8 (71.8, 77.8) |
| Females | 56.8 (44.1, 69.6) | 23.5 (14.5, 32.4) | 63.7 (59.3, 68.1) |
| **Race/Ethnicity** | | | |
| White, non-Hispanic | 62.9 (49.8, 76.1) | 21.7 (9.9, 33.5) | 71.3 (67.0, 75.6) |
| Males | 64.2 (52.6, 75.8) | 23.3 (11.2, 35.3) | 74.8 (71.1, 78.5) |
| Females | 61.7 (46.4, 77.0) | 19.9 (8.0, 31.8) | 67.1 (60.5, 73.8) |
| Black, non-Hispanic | 50.2 (45.1, 55.3) | 33.8 (29.9, 37.8) | 59.0 (54.6, 63.3) |
| Males | 56.8 (50.6, 62.9) | 37.7 (32.3, 43.0) | 71.8 (65.9, 77.8) |
| Females | 44.4 (37.3, 51.5) | 30.1 (25.8, 34.5) | 46.6 (39.3, 53.8) |
| Hispanic | 51.0 (40.9, 61.2) | 33.1 (24.5, 41.8) | 68.5 (62.8, 74.1) |
| Males | 57.6 (48.6, 66.6) | 36.2 (28.8, 43.6) | 76.0 (67.0, 85.0) |
| Females | 44.6 (31.2, 58.0) | 30.1 (18.7, 41.5) | 59.0 (52.5, 65.6) |
| **Grade in school** | | | |
| **Males** | | | |
| 9 | 80.5 (75.1, 85.9) | 42.1 (23.3, 60.8) | 76.5 (72.2, 80.9) |
| 10 | 72.6 (62.3, 82.8) | 34.8 (18.9, 50.8) | 73.1 (67.9, 78.3) |
| 11 | 51.5 (32.8, 70.1) | 17.4 (9.3, 25.6) | 75.8 (70.3, 81.2) |
| 12 | 45.4 (29.0, 61.9) | 14.8 (9.2, 20.4) | 73.7 (68.1, 79.3) |
| **Females** | | | |
| 9 | 80.8 (73.8, 87.8) | 39.7 (21.5, 58.0) | 65.6 (57.2, 74.1) |
| 10 | 71.4 (59.3, 83.5) | 33.8 (17.4, 50.3) | 63.9 (58.8, 68.9) |
| 11 | 41.2 (22.8, 59.6) | 12.3 (7.6, 17.1) | 57.2 (48.4, 66.0) |
| 12 | 39.1 (20.9, 57.2) | 11.1 (6.5, 15.7) | 66.0 (59.7, 72.4) |

Source: Centers for Disease Control and Prevention, National Center for Chronic Disease Prevention and Health Promotion, YRBS 1995 data tape (in press).

[*]A national school-based survey of students in grades 9–12.
[†]Among students enrolled in physical education.
[‡]95% confidence intervals.

Females were more likely than males to participate in aerobics or dancing and in house cleaning or yard work for at least 30 minutes. White youths were more likely than black or Hispanic youths to participate in skating, skiing, or skateboarding and in tennis, racquetball, or squash. For both males and females, increasing age was associated with decreasing participation in baseball, softball, or Frisbee®; in basketball, football, or soccer; in running, jogging, or swimming for exercise; and in skating, skiing, or skateboarding. For females, participation in aerobics or dancing and in tennis, racquetball, or squash also decreased by age.

## Physical Education in High School

The YRBS provides data on enrollment and daily attendance in school physical education for students in grades 9–12. (See Chapter 6 for a discussion of the availability of physical education programs.) In 1995,

Table 5-16.  Percentage of students in grades 9–12 reporting participation on at least one sports team run by a
school or by other organizations during the year preceding the survey, by demographic group,
1995 Youth Risk Behavior Survey (YRBS),* United States

| Demographic group | Participation on sports team run by a school | Participation on sports team run by other organization |
|---|---|---|
| **Overall** | **50.3** (46.6, 54.0)† | **36.9** (34.4, 39.4) |
| **Sex** | | |
| Males | **57.8** (53.7, 62.0) | **46.4** (43.4, 49.3) |
| Females | **42.4** (38.6, 46.2) | **26.8** (24.2, 29.4) |
| **Race/Ethnicity** | | |
| White, non-Hispanic | **53.9** (49.6, 58.2) | **39.1** (35.7, 42.5) |
| Males | **59.9** (54.8, 65.0) | **47.2** (43.0, 51.4) |
| Females | **47.1** (43.0, 51.2) | **29.9** (26.8, 32.9) |
| **Black, non-Hispanic** | **45.0** (39.9, 50.2) | **32.4** (29.0, 35.9) |
| Males | **57.9** (52.6, 63.2) | **46.8** (42.4, 51.1) |
| Females | **34.9** (28.2, 41.7) | **21.1** (16.5, 25.8) |
| **Hispanic** | **37.8** (33.6, 42.0) | **32.0** (28.5, 35.6) |
| Males | **48.6** (44.0, 53.2) | **43.2** (37.9, 48.4) |
| Females | **27.3** (21.9, 32.7) | **21.2** (16.5, 25.9) |
| **Grade in school** | | |
| **Males** | | |
| 9 | **61.7** (54.0, 69.4) | **52.8** (47.0, 58.7) |
| 10 | **55.6** (50.1, 61.1) | **46.9** (42.4, 51.4) |
| 11 | **56.0** (49.7, 62.4) | **43.1** (40.6, 45.7) |
| 12 | **58.3** (52.0, 64.6) | **42.8** (39.2, 46.3) |
| **Females** | | |
| 9 | **43.7** (39.2, 48.2) | **32.0** (28.2, 35.9) |
| 10 | **47.9** (42.8, 53.0) | **32.4** (26.8, 38.0) |
| 11 | **39.4** (32.1, 46.7) | **23.8** (19.9, 27.6) |
| 12 | **38.8** (32.4, 45.1) | **19.8** (15.2, 24.3) |

Source: Centers for Disease Control and Prevention, National Center for Chronic Disease Prevention and Health Promotion, YRBS 1995 data
tape (in press).

*A national school-based survey of students in grades 9–12.
†95% confidence intervals.

59.6 percent of students in grades 9–12 were enrolled in physical education (Table 5-15). Enrollment did not vary by sex or race/ethnicity, but it decreased by grade. Between 1991 and 1995, overall enrollment in physical education among students in grades 9–12 did not change significantly (data not shown).

*Healthy People 2000* objective 1.8 (USDHHS 1990) recommends increasing to at least 50 percent the proportion of children and adolescents in grades 1–12 who participate in daily school physical education. The 1995 YRBS indicated that daily attendance in

physical education among high school students was 25.4 percent and did not vary by sex or race/ethnicity (Table 5-15). Daily attendance decreased with increasing grade for both male and female students. Between 1991 and 1995, overall daily attendance in physical education classes in grades 9–12 decreased significantly, from 41.6 percent to 25.4 percent (data not shown). Current trend data thus indicate that the *Healthy People 2000* goal of 50 percent has not been attained and is also becoming more distant.

*Healthy People 2000* objective 1.9 (USDHHS 1990) recommends that students be active for at least 50 percent of the class time they spend in physical education. In 1995, 69.7 percent of students in grades 9–12 who were taking physical education reported being physically active for at least 20 minutes, which is about half of a typical class period (Table 5-15). This active participation was more common among male students than female students (74.8 percent vs. 63.7 percent) and among white students than black students (71.3 percent vs. 59.0 percent). Between 1991 and 1995, the overall percentage of students in grades 9–12 taking physical education who reported being physically active for at least 20 minutes decreased from 80.7 percent to 69.7 percent (data not shown). Decreases between 1991 or 1993 and 1995 occurred for students in all grades. Thus a decreasing proportion of the high school students who are enrolled in physical education classes are meeting the *Healthy People 2000* goal for time spent being physically active in class.

Only 18.6 percent of all high school students were physically active for at least 20 minutes on a daily basis in physical education classes (data not shown).

### Sports Team Participation

The YRBS provides data on participation on sports teams during the 12 months preceding the survey for students in grades 9–12. In 1995, 50.3 percent of students participated on sports teams run by a school, and 36.9 percent participated on sports teams run by other organizations (Table 5-16). Participation on sports teams run by a school was more common among male students than female students (57.8 percent vs. 42.4 percent) and among white students than Hispanic students (53.9 percent vs. 37.8 percent). Between 1991 and 1995, participation on sports teams run by a school increased significantly among high school students overall, from 43.5 percent to 50.3 percent (data not shown). Specific increases were identified among female students, white and black students, and students in grades 11 and 12.

Participation on sports teams run by other organizations besides a school was more common among male students than female students (46.4 percent vs. 26.8 percent) and among white students than Hispanic students (39.1 percent vs. 32.0 percent).

Between 1991 and 1995, overall participation among students in grades 9–12 on sports teams run by other organizations did not change significantly (data not shown).

## Conclusions

### Adults

1. Approximately 15 percent of U.S. adults engage regularly (3 times a week for at least 20 minutes) in vigorous physical activity during leisure time.

2. Approximately 22 percent of adults engage regularly (5 times a week for at least 30 minutes) in sustained physical activity of any intensity during leisure time.

3. About 25 percent of adults report no physical activity in their leisure time.

4. Physical inactivity is more prevalent among women than men, among blacks and Hispanics than whites, among older than younger adults, and among the less affluent than the more affluent.

5. The most popular leisure-time physical activities among adults are walking and gardening or yard work.

### Adolescents and Young Adults

1. Only about one-half of U.S. young people (ages 12–21 years) regularly participate in vigorous physical activity. One-fourth report no vigorous physical activity.

2. Approximately one-fourth of young people walk or bicycle (i.e., engage in light to moderate activity) nearly every day.

3. About 14 percent of young people report no recent vigorous or light to moderate physical activity. This indicator of inactivity is higher among females than males and among black females than white females.

4. Males are more likely than females to participate in vigorous physical activity, strengthening activities, and walking or bicycling.

5. Participation in all types of physical activity declines strikingly as age or grade in school increases.

200

6. Among high school students, enrollment in physical education remained unchanged during the first half of the 1990s. However, daily attendance in physical education declined from approximately 42 percent to 25 percent.

7. The percentage of high school students who were enrolled in physical education and who reported being physically active for at least 20 minutes in physical education classes declined from approximately 81 percent to 70 percent during the first half of this decade.

8. Only 19 percent of all high school students report being physically active for 20 minutes or more in daily physical education classes.

## Research Needs

1. Develop methods to monitor patterns of regular, moderate physical activity.

2. Improve the validity and comparability of self-reported physical activity in national surveys.

3. Improve methods for identifying and tracking physical activity patterns among people with disabilities.

4. Routinely monitor the prevalence of physical activity among children under age 12.

5. Routinely monitor school policy requirements and of students' participation in physical education classes in elementary, middle, and high schools.

# Appendix A:
# Sources of National Survey Data

## National Health Interview Survey (NHIS)

This analysis used data from the 1991 NHIS to determine current prevalences of physical activity, and from 1985, 1990, and 1991 to determine physical activity trends, among U.S. adults aged 18 years and older (National Center for Health Statistics [NCHS] 1988, 1993; NCHS unpublished data). Since 1957, NCHS has been collecting year-round health data from a probability sample of the civilian, noninstitutionalized adult population of the United States. The design included oversampling of blacks to provide more precise estimates. For the 1985, 1990, and 1991 special supplement on health promotion and disease prevention, one adult aged 18 years or older was randomly selected from each family for participation from the total NHIS sample. Interviews were conducted in the homes; self-response was required for this special supplement, and callbacks were made as necessary. The sample was poststratified by the age, sex, and racial distribution of the U.S. population for the survey year and weighted to provide national estimates. The overall response rate for the NHIS has been 83 to 88 percent.

## Behavioral Risk Factor Surveillance System (BRFSS)

The Centers for Disease Control and Prevention (CDC) initiated the BRFSS in 1981 to help states obtain prevalence estimates of health behaviors, including physical activity, that were associated with chronic disease. The BRFSS conducts monthly, year-round, telephone interviews of adults aged 18 years of age and older sampled by random-digit dialing (Remington et al. 1988; Siegel et al. 1991; Frazier, Franks, Sanderson 1992). Physical activity questions have been consistent since 1986, except for a minor change from 1986 to 1987. In 1994, the most recent survey available, 49 states and the District of Columbia participated. Only 25 states and the District of Columbia have participated continuously since 1986. For 1986–1991, sample sizes ranged from approximately 35,000 to 50,000, and response rates from 62 to 71 percent; for 1992, the sample size was 96,343, and the response rate 71 percent; for 1994, the sample size was 106,030, and the response rate

70 percent. For examination of trends, analysis was restricted to the 25 states and the District of Columbia, that had consistently participated from 1986 through 1994. For 1992 cross-sectional analyses, data were included from all 48 states that had participated that year and from the District of Columbia. For 1994 cross-sectional analyses, data were included from the 49 participating states and from the District of Columbia.

## Third National Health and Nutrition Examination Survey (NHANES III)

NHANES III is the seventh in a series of national health examination surveys that began in the 1960s. The sample for NHANES III (NCHS 1994a) was selected from 81 counties across the United States. The survey period covered 1988–1994 and consisted of two phases of equal length and sample size. Both Phase I (1988–1991) and Phase II (1992–1994) used probability samples of the U.S. civilian noninstitutionalized population. Black and Mexican American populations were oversampled to obtain statistically reliable estimates for these minority groups. Phase II data were not available at the time this report was prepared. In Phase I, the selected population was 12,138 adults 18 years of age or older, of which 82 percent (9,901) underwent a home interview that included questions on physical activity. Participants in NHANES III also underwent a detailed medical examination in a mobile examination center. NHANES III data were weighted to the 1990 U.S. civilian noninstitutionalized population to provide national estimates.

## Youth Risk Behavior Survey (YRBS)

The CDC developed the YRBS (Kolbe 1990; Kolbe, Kann, Collins 1993) to measure six categories of priority health-risk behaviors among adolescents: 1) behaviors that contribute to intentional and unintentional injuries; 2) tobacco use; 3) alcohol and other drug use; 4) sexual behaviors that result in unintended pregnancy and sexually transmitted diseases, including HIV infection; 5) unhealthy dietary behaviors; and 6) physical inactivity. Data were collected through national, state, and local school-based surveys of high school students in grades 9–12 during the spring of odd-numbered years and through

a 1992 national household-based survey of young people aged 12–21 years. The 1991, 1993, and 1995 national school-based YRBS (Kann et al. 1993; CDC unpublished data) used three-stage cluster sample designs. The targeted population consisted of all public and private school students in grades 9–12 in the 50 states and the District of Columbia. Schools with substantial numbers of black and Hispanic students were sampled at relatively higher rates than all other schools.

Survey procedures were designed to protect student privacy and allow anonymous participation. The questionnaire was administered in the classroom by trained data collectors, and students recorded their responses on answer sheets designed for scanning by computer. The school response rates ranged from 70 to 78 percent, and the student response rate ranged from 86 to 90 percent. The total number of students who completed questionnaires was 12,272 in 1991, 16,296 in 1993, and 10,904 in 1995. The data were weighted to account for nonresponse and for oversampling of black and Hispanic students.

## National Health Interview Survey-Youth Risk Behavior Survey (NHIS-YRBS)

To provide more information about risk behaviors among young people, including those who do not attend school, the CDC added a youth risk behavior survey to the 1992 National Health Interview Survey (CDC 1993; NCHS 1994b). The survey was conducted as a follow-back from April 1992 through March 1993 among 12- through 21-year-olds from a national probability sample of households. School-aged youths not attending school were oversampled. NHIS-YRBS interviews were completed for 10,645 young people, representing an overall response rate of 74 percent.

The questionnaire for this survey was administered through individual portable cassette players with earphones. After listening to questions, respondents marked their answers on standardized answer sheets. This methodology was designed to help young people with reading problems complete the survey and to enhance confidentiality during household administration. Data from this report were weighted to represent the U.S. population of 12- through 21-year-olds.

# Appendix B:
# Measures of Physical Activity in Population Surveys

There is no uniformly accepted method of assessing physical activity. Various methods have been used (Stephens 1989); unfortunately, estimates of physical activity are highly dependent on the survey instrument. The specific problems associated with using national surveillance systems—such as those employed here—to monitor leisure-time physical activity have been reviewed previously (Caspersen, Merritt, Stephens 1994).

All of the population surveys cited have employed a short-term recall of the frequency, and in some cases the duration and intensity, of activities that either were listed for the participant to respond to or were probed for in an open-ended manner. The validity of these questions is not rigorously established. Estimates of prevalence of participation are influenced by sampling errors, seasons covered, and the number and wording of such questions; generally, the more activities offered, the more likely a participant will report some activity. Besides defining participation in any activity or in individual activities, many researchers have found it useful to define summary indices of regular participation in vigorous activity or moderate activity (Caspersen 1994; Caspersen, Merritt, Stephens 1994). These summary measures often require assumptions about the intensity of reported activities and the frequency and duration of physical activity required for health benefits.

## National Health Interview Survey (NHIS)

Participants in the NHIS were asked in a standardized interview whether they did any of 22 exercises, sports, or physically active hobbies in the previous 2 weeks: walking for exercise, jogging or running, hiking, gardening or yard work, aerobics or aerobic dancing, other dancing, calisthenics or general exercise, golf, tennis, bowling, bicycling, swimming or water exercises, yoga, weight lifting or training, basketball, baseball or softball, football, soccer, volleyball, handball or racquetball or squash, skating, and skiing (National Center for Health Statistics [NCHS] 1992). They were also asked, in an open-ended

fashion, for other unmentioned activities performed in the previous 2 weeks. For each activity, the interviewer asked the number of times, the average minutes duration, and the perceived degree to which heart rate or breathing increased (i.e., none or small, moderate, or large).

The physical activity patterns were scored by using data for frequency and duration derived directly from the NHIS. To estimate the regular, vigorous physical activity pattern, a previously proposed convention was followed (Caspersen, Pollard, Pratt 1987). One of two sex-specific regression equations was used to estimate the respondent's maximum cardiorespiratory capacity (expressed in metabolic equivalents [METs]) (Jones and Campbell 1982): $[60-0.55 \cdot \text{age (years)}]/3.5$ for men, and $[48-0.37 \cdot \text{age (years)}]/3.5$ for women. One MET is the value of resting oxygen uptake relative to total body mass and is generally ascribed the value of 3.5 milliliters of oxygen per kilogram of body mass per minute (for example, 3 METs equals 3 times the resting level; walking at 3 miles per hour on a level surface would be at about that intensity). Individual activity intensity was based on reported values (Taylor et al. 1978; Folsom et al. 1985; Stephens and Craig 1989).

The final activity intensity code for a specific activity was found by selecting one of three conditions corresponding to the perceived level of effort associated with usual participation. The perceived effort was associated with none or small, moderate, or large perceived increases in heart rate or breathing. For example, the activity intensity code for three levels of volleyball participation would be 5, 6, and 8 METs as the perceived effort progressed from none or small to large increases in heart rate or breathing. In some cases, a single intensity code was averaged for several types of activity participation that were not distinguished in the NHIS. This averaging was done for such activities as golf, calisthenics or general exercise, swimming or water exercises, skating, and skiing. To determine if an activity would qualify a person to meet the intensity criterion of vigorous physical activity, each intensity code had to meet or exceed 50 percent of the estimated age- and sex-specific maximum cardiorespiratory capacity.

For this report, three patterns of leisure-time activity were defined (Caspersen 1994):

- *No physical activity:* No reported activity during the previous 2 weeks.

- *Regular, sustained activity:* ≥ 5 times per week and ≥ 30 minutes per occasion of physical activity of any type and at any intensity.

- *Regular, vigorous activity:* ≥ 3 times per week and ≥ 20 minutes per occasion of physical activity involving rhythmic contractions of large muscle groups (e.g., jogging or running, racquet sports, competitive group sports) performed at ≥ 50 percent of estimated age- and sex-specific maximum cardiorespiratory capacity.

## Behavioral Risk Factor Surveillance System (BRFSS)

The BRFSS questionnaire first asks, "During the past month, did you participate in any physical activities or exercises such as running, calisthenics, golf, gardening, or walking for exercise?" If yes, participants were asked to identify their two most common physical activities and to indicate the frequency in the previous month and duration per occasion (Caspersen and Powell 1986; Caspersen and Merritt 1995). If running, jogging, walking, or swimming were mentioned, participants were also asked the usual distance covered.

The reported frequency and duration of activity were used for scoring. Intensity of physical activity was assigned by using the same intensity codes as the NHIS, and a correction procedure (explained later in this section) based on speeds of activities was used to create intensity codes for walking, running/jogging, and swimming (Caspersen and Powell 1986; Caspersen and Merritt 1995).

The estimate of speed was made by dividing the self-reported distance in miles by the duration in hours. The speed estimate was entered into specific regression equations to refine the intensity code for these four activities, because the application of a single intensity code is likely to underestimate or overestimate the intensity. Based on previously published formulae (American College of Sports Medicine 1988), five equations were constructed for predicting metabolic intensity of walking, jogging, and running at various calculated speeds:

| Equation 1 | METs = 1.80 (Speeds < 0.93 mph) |
| Equation 2 | METs = 0.72 x mph + 1.13 (Speeds ≥ 0.93 but < 3.75 mph) |
| Equation 3 | METs = 3.76 x mph - 10.20 (Speeds ≥ 3.75 but < 5.00 mph) |
| Equation 4 | METs = 1.53 x mph + 1.03 (Speeds ≥ 5.00 but < 12.00 mph) |
| Equation 5 | METs = 7.0 or 8.0 (Speeds ≥ 12.00 mph) |

Below 0.93 mph, an intensity code of 1.8 METs (Equation 1) was used, to be consistent with Montoye's intensity code for residual activities like those associated with slow movements (Montoye 1975). Equation 2 is extrapolated to include speeds as slow as 0.93 mph—the point at which metabolic cost was set at 1.8 METs. Persons whose calculated speeds fell between 0.93 and 12.0 mph were assigned an intensity from equations 2, 3, or 4, regardless of whether they said they walked, jogged, or ran. Equation 3 was created by simply connecting with a straight line the last point of equation 2 and the first point of equation 4. This interpolation was seen as a reasonable way to determine intensity within the range of speed where walking or jogging might equally occur. This assignment method was considered to be more objective, specific, and generally conservative than assigning an intensity code based solely on the self-reported type of activity performed. Thus, as a correction procedure for self-reported speeds judged likely to be erroneously high, an intensity of 2.5 METs was assigned for walking speeds above 5.0 mph, 7.0 METs for jogging speeds above 12.0 mph, and 8.0 METs for running speeds above 12.0 mph.

Another set of regression equations predicted metabolic intensity from swimming velocity:

| Equation 6 | METs = 1.80 (Speeds < 0.26 mph) |
| Equation 7 | METs = 4.19 x mph - 0.69 (Speeds ≥ 0.26 but < 2.11 mph) |
| Equation 8 | METs = 8.81 x mph - 9.08 (Speeds ≥ 2.11 but < 3.12 mph) |
| Equation 9 | METs = 5.50 (Speeds ≥ 3.12 mph) |

These equations were set forth in a Canadian monograph of energy expenditure for recreational activities (Groupe d'étude de Kino-Quebec sur le système de quantification de la dépense énergétique 1984). However, swimming speeds up to 3.12 mph for the crawl and backstroke, in the derivation of equations 7 and 8, were obtained from published research (Holmer 1974a; Holmer 1974b; Passmore and Durnin 1955). Default intensity codes were assigned as follows: 1.8 METs for swimming speeds less than 0.26 mph, and 5.5 METs for velocities greater than 3.12 mph, because such speeds are improbable and likely reflected errors in self-report.

Definitions used for leisure-time physical activity were the same as those described for the NHIS earlier in this appendix.

## Third National Health and Nutrition Examination Survey (NHANES III)

The NHANES III questions that addressed leisure-time physical activity (NCHS 1994a) were adapted from the NHIS. Participants first were asked how often they had walked a mile or more at one time in the previous month. They were then asked to specify their frequency of leisure-time physical activity during the previous month for the following eight activities: jogging or running, riding a bicycle or an exercise bicycle, swimming, aerobics or aerobic dancing, other dancing, calisthenics or exercises, gardening or yard work, and weight lifting. An open-ended question asked for information on up to four physical activities not previously listed. Information on duration of physical activity was not collected. Northern sites selected for NHANES III tended to be surveyed in warm rather than cold months, which might have led to a greater prevalence of reported physical activity than would otherwise be obtained from a year-round survey. No physical activity was defined as no reported leisure-time physical activity in the previous month. Regular, sustained activity and regular, vigorous activity were not defined for NHANES III because of the lack of information on activity duration.

## Youth Risk Behavior Survey (YRBS)

In the YRBS questionnaire (Kann et al. 1993), students in grades 9–12 were asked eight questions about physical activity. The question on vigorous physical activity asked, "On how many of the past 7 days did you exercise or participate in sports activities for at least 20 minutes that made you sweat and breathe hard, such as basketball, jogging, fast dancing, swimming laps, tennis, fast bicycling, or similar aerobic activities?" The questionnaire asked separately about the frequency of three specific activities in the previous 7 days: 1) stretching exercises, such as toe touching, knee bending, or leg stretching; 2) exercises to strengthen or tone the muscles, such as push-ups, sit-ups, or weight lifting; and 3) walking or bicycling for at least 30 minutes at a time. Participants were asked about physical education, "In an average week when you are in school, on how many days do you go to physical education (PE) classes?" and "During an average physical education (PE) class, how many minutes do you spend actually exercising or playing sports?" Students were also asked, "During the past 12 months, on how many sports teams run by your school did you play? (Do not include PE classes.)" and "During the past 12 months, on how many sports teams run by organizations outside of your school did you play?"

## National Health Interview Survey-Youth Risk Behavior Survey (NHIS-YRBS)

The NHIS-YRBS questionnaire (NCHS 1994b) ascertained the frequency of vigorous physical activity among U.S. young people aged 12–21 years by asking, "On how many of the past 7 days did you exercise or take part in sports that made you sweat and breathe hard, such as basketball, jogging, fast dancing, swimming laps, tennis, fast bicycling, or other aerobic activities?" Ten other questions asked about the previous 7 days' frequency of participating in the following specific activities: 1) stretching exercises, such as toe touching, knee bending, or leg stretching; 2) exercises to strengthen or tone muscles, such as push-ups, sit-ups, or weight lifting; 3) house cleaning or yard work for ≥ 30 minutes at a time; 4) walking or bicycling for ≥ 30 minutes at a time; 5) baseball, softball, or Frisbee®[1]; 6) basketball, football, or soccer; 7) roller skating, ice skating, skiing, or skateboarding; 8) running, jogging, or swimming for exercise; 9) tennis, racquetball, or squash; and 10) aerobics or dance. Questions about duration and intensity were not asked.

---

[1]Use of trade names is for identification only and does not imply endorsement by the U.S. Department of Health and Human Services.

# References

American College of Sports Medicine. *Guidelines for exercise testing and prescription.* 3rd ed. Philadelphia: Lea and Febiger, 1988:168–169.

Brener ND, Collins JL, Kann L, Warren CW, Williams BI. Reliability of the Youth Risk Behavior Survey questionnaire. *American Journal of Epidemiology* 1995;141:575–580.

Caspersen CJ. What are the lessons from the U.S. approach for setting targets. In: Killoran AJ, Fentem P, Caspersen C, editors. *Moving on: international perspectives on promoting physical activity.* London: Health Education Authority, 1994:35–55.

Caspersen CJ, Merritt RK. Physical activity trends among 26 states, 1986–1990. *Medicine and Science in Sports and Exercise* 1995;27:713–720.

Caspersen CJ, Merritt RK, Stephens T. International physical activity patterns: a methodological perspective. In: Dishman RK, editor. *Advances in exercise adherence.* Champaign, IL: Human Kinetics, 1994: 73–110.

Caspersen CJ, Pollard RA, Pratt SO. Scoring physical activity data with special consideration for elderly populations. In: Data for an aging population. *Proceedings of the 21st national meeting of the Public Health Conference on Records and Statistics.* Washington, DC: U.S. Government Printing Office, 1987:30–4. DHHS Publication No. (PHS)88–1214.

Centers for Disease Control. *1992 BRFSS Summary Prevalence Report.* Atlanta: U.S. Department of Health and Human Services, Public Health Service, Centers for Disease Control, National Center for Chronic Disease Prevention and Health Promotion, 1992.

Centers for Disease Control. Youth Risk Behavior Survey, 1991 data tape. Atlanta: U.S. Department of Health and Human Services, Public Health Service, Centers for Disease Control, National Center for Chronic Disease Prevention and Health Promotion, 1991. National Technical Information Service Order No. PB94–500121.

Centers for Disease Control and Prevention. *1994 BRFSS Summary Prevalence Report.* Atlanta: U.S. Department of Health and Human Services, Public Health Service, Centers for Disease Control and Prevention, National Center for Chronic Disease Prevention and Health Promotion, 1994.

Centers for Disease Control and Prevention. National Health Interview Survey—Youth Risk Behavior Survey, 1992 machine readable data file and documentation. Atlanta: U.S. Department of Health and Human Services, Public Health Service, Centers for Disease Control and Prevention, National Center for Health Statistics, 1993.

Centers for Disease Control and Prevention. Youth Risk Behavior Survey, 1993 data tape. Atlanta: U.S. Department of Health and Human Services, Public Health Service, Centers for Disease Control and Prevention, National Center for Chronic Disease Prevention and Health Promotion, 1993. National Technical Information Service Order No. PB95–503363.

Centers for Disease Control and Prevention. Youth Risk Behavior Survey, 1995 data tape. Atlanta: U.S. Department of Health and Human Services, Public Health Service, Centers for Disease Control and Prevention, National Center for Chronic Disease Prevention and Health Promotion (in press).

Folsom AR, Caspersen CJ, Taylor HL, Jacobs DR Jr, Luepker RV, Gomez-Marin O, et al. Leisure-time physical activity and its relationship to coronary risk factors in a population-based sample: the Minnesota Heart Survey. *American Journal of Epidemiology* 1985;121:570–579.

Frazier EL, Franks AL, Sanderson LM. Behavioral risk factor data. In: *Using chronic disease data: a handbook for public health practitioners.* Atlanta: U.S. Department of Health and Human Services, Public Health Service, Centers for Disease Control, National Center for Chronic Disease Prevention and Health Promotion, 1992:4-1–4-17.

Groupe d'étude de Kino-Quebec sur le système de quantification de la dépense énergétique (GSQ). Rapport final. Québec: Government du Québec, 1984.

Heath GW, Chang MH, Barker ND. Physical activity among persons with limitations—United States, 1991. Paper presented at the annual meeting of the Society for Disability Studies, June 17–19, 1995, Oakland, California.

Holmer I. Energy cost of arm stroke, leg kick, and the whole stroke in competitive swimming styles. *European Journal of Applied Physiology* 1974a;33:105–118.

Holmer I. Propulsive efficiency of breaststroke and freestyle swimming. *European Journal of Applied Physiology* 1974b;33:95–103.

Jacobs DR Jr, Hahn LP, Folsom AR, Hannan PJ, Sprafka JM, Burke GL. Time trends in leisure-time physical activity in the upper Midwest, 1957–1987: University of Minnesota Studies. *Epidemiology* 1991;2:8–15.

Jones NL, Campbell EJM. *Clinical exercise testing.* 2nd ed. Philadelphia: W.B. Saunders, 1982:249.

Kann L, Warren W, Collins JL, Ross J, Collins B, Kolbe LJ. Results from the national school-based 1991 Youth Risk Behavior Survey and progress toward achieving related health objectives for the nation. *Public Health Reports* 1993;108(Suppl 1):47–67.

Kolbe LJ. An epidemiological surveillance system to monitor the prevalence of youth behaviors that most affect health. *Health Education* 1990;21:44–48.

Kolbe LJ, Kann L, Collins JL. Overview of the Youth Risk Behavior Surveillance System. *Public Health Reports* 1993;108(Suppl 1):2–10.

Montoye HJ. *Physical activity and health: an epidemiologic study of an entire community.* Englewood Cliffs, NJ: Prentice Hall, 1975.

National Center for Health Statistics. *Plan and operation of the Third National Health and Nutrition Examination Survey, 1988–94.* Vital and Health Statistics, Series 1, No. 32. Hyattsville, MD: U.S. Department of Health and Human Services, Public Health Service, Centers for Disease Control and Prevention, National Center for Health Statistics, 1994a. DHHS Publication No. (PHS)94–1308 .

National Center for Health Statistics, Adams PF, Benson V. *Current estimates from the National Health Interview Survey, 1990.* Vital and Health Statistics, Series 10, No. 181. Hyattsville, MD: U.S. Department of Health and Human Services, Public Health Service, Centers for Disease Control, National Center for Health Statistics, 1991. DHHS Publication No. (PHS)92–1509.

National Center for Health Statistics, Benson V, Marano MA. *Current estimates from the National Health Interview Survey, 1992.* Vital and Health Statistics, Series 10, No. 189. Hyattsville, MD: U.S. Department of Health and Human Services, Public Health Service, Centers for Disease Control and Prevention, National Center for Health Statistics, 1994b. DHHS Publication No. (PHS)94–1517.

National Center for Health Statistics, Piani AL, Schoenborn CA. *Health promotion and disease prevention: United States, 1990.* Vital and Health Statistics, Series 10, No. 185. Hyattsville, MD: U.S. Department of Health and Human Services, Public Health Service, Centers for Disease Control and Prevention, National Center for Health Statistics, 1993. DHHS Publication No. (PHS)93–1513.

National Center for Health Statistics, Schoenborn CA. *Health promotion and disease prevention: United States, 1985.* Vital and Health Statistics, Series 10, No. 163. Hyattsville, MD: U.S. Department of Health and Human Services, Public Health Service, Centers for Disease Control, National Center for Health Statistics, 1988. DHHS Publication No. (PHS)88–1591.

Passmore R, Durnin JVGA. Human energy expenditure. *Physiological Reviews* 1955;35:801–840.

Remington PL, Smith MY, Williamson DF, Anda RF, Gentry EM, Hogelin GC. Design, characteristics, and usefulness of state-based behavioral risk factor surveillance: 1981–87. *Public Health Reports* 1988;103: 366–375.

Siegel PZ, Brackbill RM, Frazier EL, Mariolis P, Sanderson LM, Waller MN. Behavior Risk Factor Surveillance, 1986–1990. *Morbidity and Mortality Weekly Report* 1991; 40(No. SS–4):1–23.

Stephens T. Design issues and alternatives in assessing physical activity in general population surveys. In: Drury TF, editor. *Assessing physical fitness and physical activity in population-based surveys.* Hyattsville, MD: U.S. Department of Health and Human Services, Public Health Service, Centers for Disease Control, National Center for Health Statistics, 1989:197–210. DHHS Publication No. (PHS)89–1253.

Stephens T. Secular trends in adult physical activity: exercise boom or bust? *Research Quarterly for Exercise and Sport* 1987;58:94–105.

Stephens T, Caspersen CJ. The demography of physical activity. In: Bouchard C, Shephard RJ, Stephens T, editors. *Physical activity, fitness, and health: international proceedings and consensus statement.* Champaign, IL: Human Kinetics, 1994:204–213.

Stephens T, Craig CL. Fitness and activity measurement in the 1981 Canada Fitness Survey. In: Drury TF, editor. *Assessing physical fitness and physical activity in population-based surveys.* Hyattsville, MD: U.S. Department of Health and Human Services, Public Health Service, Centers for Disease Control, National Center for Health Statistics, 1989:401–32. DHHS Publication No. (PHS)89–1253.

Taylor HL, Jacobs DR Jr, Schucker B, Knudsen J, Leon AS, DeBacker G. A questionnaire for the assessment of leisure-time physical activities. *Journal of Chronic Diseases* 1978;31:741–755.

U.S. Department of Health and Human Services. *Healthy People 2000: national health promotion and disease prevention objectives—full report, with commentary.* Washington, DC: U.S. Department of Health and Human Services, Public Health Service, 1991. DHHS Publication No. (PHS)91–50212.

# CHAPTER 6

# UNDERSTANDING AND PROMOTING PHYSICAL ACTIVITY

## Contents

# Contents, *continued*

# UNDERSTANDING AND PROMOTING
# PHYSICAL ACTIVITY

## Introduction

As the benefits of moderate, regular physical activity have become more widely recognized, the need has increased for interventions that can promote this healthful behavior. Because theories and models of human behavior can guide the development and refinement of intervention efforts, this chapter first briefly examines elements of behavioral and social science theories and models that have been used to guide much of the research on physical activity. First for adults, then for children and adolescents, the chapter reviews factors influencing physical activity and describes interventions that have sought to improve participation in regular physical activity among these two age groups. To put in perspective the problem of increasing individual participation in physical activity, the chapter next examines societal barriers to engaging in physical activity and describes existing resources that can increase opportunities for activity. The chapter concludes with a summary of what is known about determinant and intervention research on physical activity and makes recommendations for research and practice.

## Theories and Models Used in Behavioral and Social Science Research on Physical Activity

Numerous theories and models have been used in behavioral and social science research on physical activity. These approaches vary in their applicability to physical activity research. Some models and theories were designed primarily as guides to understanding behavior, not as guides for designing interventions. Others were specifically constructed with a view toward developing interventions, and

some of these have been applied extensively in intervention research as well. Because most were developed to explain the behavior of individuals and to guide individual and small-group intervention programs, these models and theories may have only limited application to understanding the behavior of populations or designing communitywide interventions. Key elements most frequently used in the behavioral and social science research on physical activity are described below and summarized in Table 6-1.

## Learning Theories

Learning theories emphasize that learning a new, complex pattern of behavior, like changing from a sedentary to an active lifestyle, normally requires modifying many of the small behaviors that compose an overall complex behavior (Skinner 1953). Principles of behavior modification suggest that a complex-pattern behavior, such as walking continuously for 30 minutes daily, can be learned by first breaking it down into smaller segments (e.g., walking for 10 minutes daily). Behaviors that are steps toward a final goal need to be reinforced and established first, with rewards given for partial accomplishment if necessary. Incremental increases, such as adding 5 minutes to the daily walking each week, are then made as the complex pattern of behaviors is "shaped" toward the targeted goal. A further complication to the change process is that new patterns of physical activity behavior must replace or compete with former patterns of inactive behaviors that are often satisfying (e.g., watching television), habitual behaviors (e.g., parking close to the door), or behaviors cued by the environment (e.g., the presence of an elevator).

Reinforcement describes the consequences that motivate individuals either to continue or discontinue a behavior (Skinner 1953; Bandura 1986).

**Table 6-1. Summary of theories and models used in physical activity research**

| Theory/model | Level | Key concepts |
|---|---|---|
| Classic learning theories | Individual | Reinforcement<br>Cues<br>Shaping |
| Health belief model | Individual | Perceived susceptibility<br>Perceived severity<br>Perceived benefits<br>Perceived barriers<br>Cues to action<br>Self-efficacy |
| Transtheoretical model | Individual | Precontemplation<br>Contemplation<br>Preparation<br>Action<br>Maintenance |
| Relapse prevention | Individual | Skills training<br>Cognitive reframing<br>Lifestyle rebalancing |
| Social cognitive theory | Interpersonal | Reciprocal determinism<br>Behavioral capability<br>Self-efficacy<br>Outcome expectations<br>Observational learning<br>Reinforcement |
| Theory of planned behavior | Interpersonal | Attitude toward the behavior<br>  Outcome expectations<br>    Value of outcome expectations<br>Subjective norm<br>  Beliefs of others<br>    Motive to comply with others<br>Perceived behavioral control |
| Social support | Interpersonal | Instrumental support<br>Informational support<br>Emotional support<br>Appraisal support |
| Ecological perspective | Environmental | Multiple levels of influence<br>  Intrapersonal<br>  Interpersonal<br>  Institutional<br>  Community<br>  Public policy |

Source: Adapted from Glanz K and Rimer BK. *Theory at-a-glance: a guide for health promotion practice*, U.S. Department of Health and Human Services, 1995.

212

Most behaviors, including physical activity, are learned and maintained under fairly complex schedules of reinforcement and anticipated future rewards. Future rewards or incentives may include physical consequences (e.g., looking better), extrinsic rewards (e.g., receiving praise and encouragement from others, receiving a T-shirt), and intrinsic rewards (e.g., experiencing a feeling of accomplishment or gratification from attaining a personal milestone). It is important to note that although providing praise, encouragement, and other extrinsic rewards may help people adopt positive lifestyle behaviors, such external reinforcement may not be reliable in sustaining long-term change (Glanz and Rimer 1995).

## Health Belief Model
The health belief model stipulates that a person's health-related behavior depends on the person's perception of four critical areas: the severity of a potential illness, the person's susceptibility to that illness, the benefits of taking a preventive action, and the barriers to taking that action (Hochbaum 1958; Rosenstock 1960, 1966). The model also incorporates cues to action (e.g., leaving a written reminder to oneself to walk) as important elements in eliciting or maintaining patterns of behavior (Becker 1974). The construct of self-efficacy, or a person's confidence in his or her ability to successfully perform an action (discussed in more detail later in this chapter), has been added to the model (Rosenstock 1990), perhaps allowing it to better account for habitual behaviors, such as a physically active lifestyle.

## Transtheoretical Model
In this model, behavior change has been conceptualized as a five-stage process or continuum related to a person's readiness to change: precontemplation, contemplation, preparation, action, and maintenance (Prochaska and DiClemente 1982, 1984). People are thought to progress through these stages at varying rates, often moving back and forth along the continuum a number of times before attaining the goal of maintenance. Therefore, the stages of change are better described as spiraling or cyclical rather than linear (Prochaska, DiClemente, Norcross 1992). In this model, people use different processes of change as they move from one stage of change to another. Efficient self-change thus depends on doing the right

thing (processes) at the right time (stages) (Prochaska, DiClemente, Norcross 1992). According to this theory, tailoring interventions to match a person's readiness or stage of change is essential (Marcus and Owen 1992). For example, for people who are not yet contemplating becoming more active, encouraging a step-by-step movement along the continuum of change may be more effective than encouraging them to move directly into action (Marcus, Banspach, et al. 1992).

## Relapse Prevention Model
Some researchers have used concepts of relapse prevention (Marlatt and Gordon 1985) to help new exercisers anticipate problems with adherence. Factors that contribute to relapse include negative emotional or physiologic states, limited coping skills, social pressure, interpersonal conflict, limited social support, low motivation, high-risk situations, and stress (Brownell et al. 1986; Marlatt and George 1990). Principles of relapse prevention include identifying high-risk situations for relapse (e.g., change in season) and developing appropriate solutions (e.g., finding a place to walk inside during the winter). Helping people distinguish between a lapse (e.g., a few days of not participating in their planned activity) and a relapse (e.g., an extended period of not participating) is thought to improve adherence (Dishman 1991; Marcus and Stanton 1993).

## Theory of Reasoned Action and Theory of Planned Behavior
The theory of reasoned action (Fishbein and Ajzen 1975; Ajzen and Fishbein 1980) states that individual performance of a given behavior is primarily determined by a person's intention to perform that behavior. This intention is determined by two major factors: the person's attitude toward the behavior (i.e., beliefs about the outcomes of the behavior and the value of these outcomes) and the influence of the person's social environment or subjective norm (i.e., beliefs about what other people think the person should do, as well as the person's motivation to comply with the opinions of others). The theory of planned behavior (Ajzen 1985, 1988) adds to the theory of reasoned action the concept of perceived control over the opportunities, resources, and skills necessary to perform a behavior. Ajzen's concept of

perceived behavioral control is similar to Bandura's (1977a) concept of self-efficacy—a person's perception of his or her ability to perform the behavior (Ajzen 1985, 1988). Perceived behavioral control over opportunities, resources, and skills necessary to perform a behavior is believed to be a critical aspect of behavior change processes.

## Social Learning/Social Cognitive Theory

Social learning theory (Bandura 1977b), later renamed social cognitive theory (Bandura 1986), proposes that behavior change is affected by environmental influences, personal factors, and attributes of the behavior itself (Bandura 1977b). Each may affect or be affected by either of the other two. A central tenet of social cognitive theory is the concept of self-efficacy. A person must believe in his or her capability to perform the behavior (i.e., the person must possess self-efficacy) and must perceive an incentive to do so (i.e., the person's positive expectations from performing the behavior must outweigh the negative expectations). Additionally, a person must value the outcomes or consequences that he or she believes will occur as a result of performing a specific behavior or action. Outcomes may be classified as having immediate benefits (e.g., feeling energized following physical activity) or long-term benefits (e.g., experiencing improvements in cardiovascular health as a result of physical activity). But because these expected outcomes are filtered through a person's expectations or perceptions of being able to perform the behavior in the first place, self-efficacy is believed to be the single most important characteristic that determines a person's behavior change (Bandura 1986).

Self-efficacy can be increased in several ways, among them by providing clear instructions, providing the opportunity for skill development or training, and modeling the desired behavior. To be effective, models must evoke trust, admiration, and respect from the observer; models must not, however, appear to represent a level of behavior that the observer is unable to visualize attaining (Bandura 1986).

## Social Support

Often associated with health behaviors such as physical activity, social support is frequently used in behavioral and social research. There is, however, considerable variation in how social support is conceptualized and measured (Israel and Schurman 1990). Social support for physical activity can be instrumental, as in giving a nondriver a ride to an exercise class; informational, as in telling someone about a walking program in the neighborhood; emotional, as in calling to see how someone is faring with a new walking program; or appraising, as in providing feedback and reinforcement in learning a new skill (Israel and Schurman 1990). Sources of support for physical activity include family members, friends, neighbors, co-workers, and exercise program leaders and participants.

## Ecological Approaches

A criticism of most theories and models of behavior change is that they emphasize individual behavior change processes and pay little attention to sociocultural and physical environmental influences on behavior (McLeroy et al. 1988). Recently, interest has developed in ecological approaches to increasing participation in physical activity (McLeroy et al. 1988; CDC 1988; Stokols 1992). These approaches place the creation of supportive environments on a par with the development of personal skills and the reorientation of health services. Stokols (1992) and Simons-Morton and colleagues (CDC 1988; Simons-Morton, Simons-Morton, et al. 1988) have illustrated this concept of a health-promoting environment by describing how physical activity could be promoted by establishing environmental supports, such as bike paths, parks, and incentives to encourage walking or bicycling to work.

An underlying theme of ecological perspectives is that the most effective interventions occur on multiple levels. McLeroy and colleagues (1988), for example, have proposed a model that encompasses several levels of influences on health behaviors: intrapersonal factors, interpersonal and group factors, institutional factors, community factors, and public policy. Similarly, a model advanced by Simons-Morton and colleagues (CDC 1988) has three levels (individual, organizational, and governmental) in four settings (schools, worksites, health care institutions, and communities). Interventions that simultaneously influence these multiple levels and multiple settings may be expected to lead to greater and longer-lasting changes and maintenance of existing health-promoting habits. This is a promising area for the design of future intervention research to promote physical activity.

## Summary

Some similarities can be noted among the behavioral and social science theories and models used to understand and enhance health behaviors such as physical activity. Many of the theoretical approaches highlight the role of the perceived outcomes of behavior, although different terms are used for this construct, including perceived benefits and barriers (health belief model) and outcome expectations (social cognitive theory and theory of planned behavior) (Table 6-1). Several approaches also emphasize the influence of perceptions of control over behavior; this influence is given labels such as self-efficacy (health belief model, social cognitive theory) and perceived behavioral control (theory of planned behavior). Other theories and models feature the role of social influences, as in the concepts of observational learning (social cognitive theory), perceived norm (theory of reasoned action and theory of planned behavior), social support, and interpersonal influences (ecological perspective). Most of the theories and models, however, do not address the influence of the environment on health behavior.

# Behavioral Research on Physical Activity among Adults

Behavioral research in this area includes studies on both the factors influencing physical activity among adults (determinants research) and the effectiveness of strategies and programs to increase this behavior (interventions research). Although many of the key concepts presented in the preceding section are featured in both types of research presented here, neither area is limited to those concepts only.

## Factors Influencing Physical Activity among Adults

Research on the determinants of physical activity identifies those factors associated with, or predictive of, this behavior. This section reviews determinants studies in which the measured outcome was overall physical activity, adherence to or continued participation in structured physical activity programs, or movement from one stage of change to another (e.g.,

from contemplation to preparation). The section does not review studies in which the outcome measured was an intermediate measure of physical activity (e.g., intentions concerning future participation in physical activity). Although researchers have studied a wide array of potential influences on physical activity among adults, the section focuses on factors that can be modified, such as self-efficacy and social support, rather than on factors that cannot be changed, such as age, sex, and race/ethnicity.

### Modifiable Determinants

The modifiable determinants of adult physical activity include personal, interpersonal, and environmental factors (Table 6-1). Self-efficacy, a construct from social cognitive theory, has been consistently and positively associated with adult physical activity (Courneya and McAuley 1994; Desmond et al. 1993; Hofstetter et al. 1991; Yordy and Lent 1993), physical activity stage of change (Marcus, Eaton, et al. 1994; Marcus and Owen 1992; Marcus, Pinto, et al. 1994; Marcus, Selby, et al. 1992), and adherence to structured physical activity programs (DuCharme and Brawley 1995; Duncan and McAuley 1993; McAuley, Lox, Duncan 1993; Poag-DuCharme and Brawley 1993; Robertson and Keller 1992). The evidence is less conclusive, however, for the theory of planned behavior's construct of perceived behavioral control (Courneya 1995; Courneya and McAuley 1995; Godin et al. 1991, 1995; Godin, Valois, Lepage 1993; Kimiecik 1992; Yordy and Lent 1993).

Several studies have found no association between adult physical activity (whether physical activity, stage of change, or adherence) and either the health belief model's constructs of perceived benefits (Hofstetter et al. 1991; Mirotznik, Feldman, Stein 1995; Oldridge and Streiner 1990; Taggart and Connor 1995) and perceived barriers (Desmond et al. 1993; Godin et al. 1995; Neuberger et al. 1994; Oldridge and Streiner 1990; Taggart and Connor 1995) or the theory of reasoned action and theory of planned behavior's construct of attitude toward the behavior (Courneya and McAuley 1995; Godin, Valois, Lepage 1993; Hawkes and Holm 1993). Nonetheless, the cumulative body of evidence supports the conclusion that expectations of both positive (e.g., benefits) and negative (e.g., barriers) behavioral outcomes are associated with physical activity among adults. Expectation of positive outcomes or perceived benefits of physical activity has been consistently and positively associated with adult physical activity (Ali and Twibell 1995; Neuberger et al. 1994), physical activity stage of change (Booth et al. 1993; Calfas et al. 1994; Eaton et al. 1993; Marcus, Eaton, et al. 1994; Marcus and Owen 1992; Marcus, Pinto, et al. 1994; Marcus, Rakowski, Rossi 1992), and adherence to structured physical activity programs (Lynch et al. 1992; Robertson and Keller 1992). Conversely, the construct of perceived barriers to physical activity has been negatively associated with adult physical activity (Ali and Twibell 1995; Dishman and Steinhardt 1990; Godin et al. 1991; Hofstetter et al. 1991; Horne 1994), physical activity stage of change (Calfas et al. 1994; Lee 1993; Marcus, Eaton, et al. 1994; Marcus and Owen 1992; Marcus, Pinto, et al. 1994; Marcus, Rakowski, Rossi 1992), and adherence to structured physical activity programs (Howze, Smith, DiGilio 1989; Mirotznik et al. 1995; Robertson and Keller 1992). Additionally, attitude toward the behavior (outcome expectations and their values) has been consistently and positively related to physical activity (Courneya and McAuley 1994; Dishman and Steinhardt 1990; Godin et al. 1987, 1991; Kimiecik 1992; Yordy and Lent 1993) and stage of change (Courneya 1995).

Social support from family and friends has been consistently and positively related to adult physical activity (Felton and Parsons 1994; Horne 1994; Minor and Brown 1993; Sallis, Hovell, Hofstetter 1992; Treiber et al. 1991), stage of change (Lee 1993), and adherence to structured exercise programs (Duncan and McAuley 1993; Elward, Larson, Wagner 1992). Behavioral intention, a construct from the theory of reasoned action and the theory of planned behavior, also has consistently been associated with adult physical activity (Courneya and McAuley 1994; Godin et al. 1987, 1991; Godin, Valois, Lepage 1993; Kimiecik 1992; Yordy and Lent 1993), stage of change (Courneya 1995), and adherence to structured exercise programs (Courneya and McAuley 1995; DuCharme and Brawley 1995). Conversely, the construct of subjective norm from these theories has been both positively associated (Courneya 1995; Godin et al. 1987, 1991; Hawkes and Holm 1993; Kimiecik 1992; Yordy and Lent 1993) and not associated (Courneya and McAuley 1995; Godin et al. 1995; Hofstetter et al. 1991) with adult physical activity, stage of change, and adherence to structured exercise programs.

There is also mixed evidence regarding the positive relationship between the health belief model's construct of perceived severity of diseases and either physical activity (Godin et al. 1991) or adherence to structured exercise programs (Lynch et al. 1992; Mirotznik, Feldman, Stein 1995; Oldridge and Streiner 1990; Robertson and Keller 1992). Additionally, that model's construct of perceived susceptibility to illness has been unrelated to adult adherence to structured exercise programs (Lynch et al. 1992; Mirotznik et al. 1995; Oldridge and Streiner 1990).

The cumulative body of determinants research consistently reveals that exercise enjoyment is a determinant that has been positively associated with adult physical activity (Courneya and McAuley 1994; Horne 1994; McAuley 1991), stage of change (Calfas et al. 1994), and adherence to structured exercise programs (Wilson et al. 1994). Conversely, there has been no relationship between locus of control beliefs (i.e., perceptions of personal control over health, fitness, or physical activity) and either adult physical activity (Ali and Twibell 1995; Burk and Kimiecik 1994; Dishman and Steinhardt 1990; Duffy and MacDonald 1990) or adherence to structured exercise programs (Lynch et al. 1992; Oldridge and Streiner 1990). Although previous physical activity during adulthood has been consistently related to physical activity among adults (Godin et al. 1987, 1993; Minor and Brown 1993; Sharpe and Connell 1992) and stage of change (Eaton et al. 1993), history of physical activity during youth has been unrelated to adult physical activity (Powell and Dysinger 1987; Sallis, Hovell, Hofstetter 1992).

## Determinants for Population Subgroups

Few determinants studies of heterogeneous samples have examined similar sets of characteristics in subgroups. Self-efficacy is the variable with the strongest and most consistent association with physical activity in different subgroups from the same large study sample. Self-efficacy has been positively related to physical activity among men, women, younger adults, older adults (Sallis et al. 1989), Latinos (Hovell et al. 1991), overweight persons (Hovell et al. 1990), and persons with injuries or disabilities (Hofstetter et al. 1991). The generalizability of the self-efficacy associations is extended by studies of university students and alumni (Calfas et al. 1994; Courneya and McAuley 1994; Yordy and Lent 1993), employed women (Marcus, Pinto, et al. 1994), participants in structured exercise programs (Duncan and McAuley 1993; McAuley, Lox, Duncan 1993; Poag-DuCharme and Brawley 1993), and people with coronary heart disease (CHD) (Robertson and Keller 1992).

### Summary

Ideally, theories and models of behavioral and social science could be used to guide research concerning the factors that influence adult physical activity. In actuality, the application of these approaches to determinants research in physical activity has generally been limited to individual and interpersonal theories and models. Social support and some factors from social cognitive theory, such as confidence in one's ability to engage in physical activity (i.e., self-efficacy) and beliefs about the outcome of physical activity, have been consistently related to physical activity among adults. Factors from other theories and models, however, have received mixed support. Although perceptions of the benefits of, and barriers to, physical activity have been consistently related to physical activity among adults, other constructs from the health belief model, such as perceptions of susceptibility to, and the severity of, disease, have not been related to adult physical activity. Further, constructs from the theory of reasoned action and the theory of planned behavior, including intentions and beliefs about the outcomes of behavior, have been consistently related to adult physical activity, whereas there has been equivocal evidence of this relationship for normative beliefs and perceptions of the difficulty of engaging in the behavior. Exercise enjoyment, a determinant that does not derive directly from any of the behavioral theories and models, has been consistently associated with adult physical activity.

Few studies have specifically contrasted physical activity determinants among different sex, age, racial/ethnic, geographic location, or health status subgroups. Many studies contain relatively homogeneous samples of groups, such as young adults, elderly persons, white adults, participants in weight loss groups, members of health clubs, persons with heart disease, and persons with arthritis. Because the numbers of participants in the studies that include these subgroups are small, and because the studies evaluated different factors, making comparisons between studies is problematic.

## Interventions to Promote Physical Activity among Adults

This section reviews intervention studies in which the measured outcome was physical activity, adherence to physical activity, or movement in stage of change (Table 6-2). It does not include intervention studies designed to assess the effect of physical activity on health outcomes or risk factors (see Chapter 4). Further, this review places special emphasis on experimental and quasi-experimental studies, which are better able to control the influence of other factors and thus to determine if the outcomes were due to the intervention itself (Weiss 1972).

### Individual Approaches

Individual behavioral management approaches, including those derived from learning theories, relapse prevention, stages of change, and social learning theory, have been used with mixed success in numerous intervention studies designed to increase physical activity (Table 6-2). Behavioral management approaches that have been applied include self-monitoring, feedback, reinforcement, contracting, incentives and contests, goal setting, skills training to prevent relapse, behavioral counseling, and prompts or reminders. Applications have been carried out in person, by mail, one-on-one, and in group settings. Typically, researchers have employed these in combination with other behavioral management approaches or with those derived from other theories, such as social support, making it more difficult to ascertain their specific effects. In numerous instances, physical activity was only one of several behaviors addressed in an intervention, which also makes it difficult to determine the extent that physical activity was emphasized as an intervention component relative to other components.

Self-monitoring of physical activity behavior has been one of the most frequently employed behavioral management techniques. Typically, it has involved individuals keeping written records of their physical activity, such as number of episodes per week, time spent per episode, and feelings during exercising. In one study, women who joined a health club were randomly assigned to a control condition or one of two intervention conditions—self-monitoring of attendance or self-monitoring plus extra staff attention (Weber and Wertheim 1989). Overall, women in the

Table 6-2.  Studies of interventions to increase physical activity among adults

| Study | Design | Theoretical approach | Population |
|---|---|---|---|
| **Individual approaches** | | | |
| Weber and Wertheim (1989) | 3 month experimental | Self-monitoring | 55 women who joined a gym; mean age = 27 |
| King, Haskell, et al. (1995) | 2 year experimental | Behavioral management | 269 white adults aged 50–65 years |
| Lombard, Lombard, Winett (1995) | 24 week experimental | Stages of change | 155 university faculty and staff; mostly women |
| Cardinal and Sachs (1995) | 12 week experimental | Stages of change | 113 clerical staff at a university; mean age = 37; 63% black |
| Belisle (1987) | 10 week quasi-experimental with 3-month follow-up | Relapse prevention | 350 people enrolled in beginning exercise groups |
| Gossard et al. (1986) | 12 week experimental | Behavioral management | 64 overweight healthy men aged 40–60 years |
| King, Carl, et al. (1988) | 16 week pretest-posttest | Behavioral management | 38 blue-collar university employees; mean age = 45 |
| King and Frederiksen (1984) | 3 month experimental | Relapse prevention, social support, behavioral management | 58 college women aged 18–20 years |
| King, Taylor, et al. (1988) | Study 1: 6 month experimental | Relapse prevention, behavioral management | 152 Lockheed employees aged 42–55 years |
| | Study 2: 6 month experimental | Behavioral management | Lockheed employees from Study 1 |

I = intervention; C = control or comparison group.

| Intervention | Findings and comments |
|---|---|
| I-1: Self-monitoring of attendance, fitness exam<br>I-2: Self-monitoring, staff attention, fitness exam<br>C: Fitness exam | I-1 had better attendance than I-2 overall; interest in self-monitoring waned after 4 weeks |
| I-1: Self-monitoring, telephone contact, vigorous exercise at home<br>I-2: Self-monitoring, telephone contact, moderate exercise at home<br>I-3: Self-monitoring, vigorous exercise in group | Better exercise adherence at 1 year in home-based groups; at year 2 better adherence in vigorous home-based group; 5 times per week schedule may have been difficult to follow |
| I-1: Weekly calls, general inquiry<br>I-2: Weekly calls, structured inquiry<br>I-3: Call every 3 weeks, general inquiry<br>I-4: Call every 3 weeks, structured inquiry | Frequent call conditions had 63% walking compared with 26% and 22% in the infrequent condition; frequent call and structured inquiry had higher rate of walking than other groups |
| I-1: Mail-delivered lifestyle packet based on stages of change<br>I-2: Mail-delivered structured exercise packet with exercise prescription<br>C: Mail-delivered fitness feedback packet | No difference in stage of change status among or within groups |
| I: Exercise class and relapse prevention training<br>C: Exercise class<br>results across experimental groups | Higher attendance in relapse prevention group over 10 weeks and at 3 months; high attrition and inconsistent |
| I-1: Vigorous self-directed exercise, staff telephone calls, self-monitoring<br>I-2: Moderate self-directed exercise, staff telephone calls, self-monitoring<br>C: Staff telephone calls | Better adherence in the moderate-intensity group at 12 weeks compared with vigorous (96% vs. 90%) (no statistical tests reported); travel, work schedule conflicts, and weather were noted as barriers to physical activity |
| I: 90-minute classes 2 times/week after work, parcourse, self-monitoring, contests<br>C: None | Twofold increase in bouts of exercise compared with nonparticipants. Participants different from nonparticipants at baseline |
| I-1: Team building, relapse prevention training; group exercise<br>I-2: Team building, group exercise<br>I-3: Relapse prevention training and jogging alone<br>C: Jogging alone | I-2 and I-3 had twice the jogging episodes as I-1 and C at 5 weeks; at 3 months, 83% of I-3 were jogging compared with 38% of I-1 and I-2 and 36% of C |
| I-1: Home-based moderate exercise, self-monitoring with portable monitor, relapse prevention training, telephone calls from staff<br>I-2: Same as I-1 without telephone calls from staff | No difference in number of sessions and duration reported at 6-month follow-up |
| I-1: Daily self-monitoring<br>I-2: Weekly self-monitoring | I-1 had more exercise bouts per month (11 vs. 7.5) |

**Table 6-2.** *Continued*

| Study | Design | Theoretical approach | Population |
|-------|--------|----------------------|------------|
| Marcus and Stanton (1993) | 18 week experimental | Relapse prevention, social learning theory | 120 female university employees, mean age = 35 |
| McAuley et al. (1994) | 5 month experimental | Social learning theory | 114 sedentary middle-aged adults |
| Owen et al. (1987) | 12 week quasi-experimental | Behavioral management | 343 white-collar and professional workers, mean age = 36, mostly women |
| Robison et al. (1992) | 6 month quasi-experimental | Behavioral management, social support | 137 university staff at 6 campus worksites, mean age = 40 |
| **Interventions in health care settings** | | | |
| Logsdon, Lazaro, Meier (1989) (INSURE) | 1 year quasi-experimental | None mentioned | 2,218 patients from multi-specialty group practice sites |
| Calfas et al. (in press) | 2 week quasi-experimental | Stage of change | 212 patients |
| **Community approaches** | | | |
| Luepker et al. (1994) (Minnesota Heart Health Project) | 5 to 6 year quasi-experimental; 3 matchedpairs | Diffusion of innovations, social learning theory, community organization, communication theory | Community longitudinal cohort (n = 7,097), independent survey (n = 300–500) |
| Young et al. (in press) (Stanford Five-City Project) | 7 year quasi-experimental | Social learning theory, communication theory, community organization | 2 sets of paired, medium-sized cities (5th city used for surveillance only) |
| Macera et al. (1995) | 4 year quasi-experimental (2 matched communities) | None specified | Community residents ≥ 18 years; 24% African American (I), 35% African American (C) |
| Brownson et al. (1996) | 4 year quasi-experimental | Social learning theory, stage theory of innovation | Rural communities; largely African American |

I = intervention; C = control or comparison group.

| Intervention | Findings and comments |
|---|---|
| I-1: Relapse prevention training and exercise<br>I-2: Scheduled reinforcement for attendance and exercise<br>C: Exercise only | Better attendance in I-1 at 9 weeks; no difference at 18 weeks or 2-month follow-up |
| I: Modeling of exercise, provision of efficacy-based information (mastery accomplishments, social modeling, social persuasion, physiological response), walking program<br>C: Biweekly meetings on health information, walking program | Better class attendance (67% vs. 55%) and more minutes and miles walked among intervention group than controls |
| I: Self-management instruction, exercise class<br>C: Exercise class | No difference in activity levels at 6 months |
| I: Weekly group meetings, contracts, cash incentives, social support, exercise<br>C: Exercise, diary | Higher attendance among experimental groups than comparison groups (93–99% vs. 19%) |
| I: Screening and counseling from physicians who received continuing education; preventive visits at no charge | Increase in starting to exercise among intervention patients (34% to 24%) |
| I: Physician counseling; booster call from a health educator<br>C: Nothing | Intervention patients increased walking (37 minutes vs. 10 minutes per week) |
| I: Screening and education; mass media; community participation; environmental change; professional education; youth and adults<br>C: Nothing | Percent physically active higher in independent survey at 3 years; higher in the cohort at 7 years |
| I: Print materials; workshops and seminars; organized walking; organized walking events; "Heart & Sole" groups; worksite programs; TV spots | Men increased participation in vigorous activities; men and women in the intervention communities increased their overall number of physical activities; significant differences between intervention and comparison communities at baseline |
| I: Community cardiovascular risk reduction activities<br>C: None specified | No difference in physical activity prevalence, physican counseling for exercise, or exercise knowledge |
| I: Community organization; development of 6 coalitions; exercise classes and walking classes and walking clubs; demonstrations; sermons; newspaper articles; community improvements; $5,000 to each coalition from the state health department | Increased physical activity levels in coalition communities, declining levels in communities without; net effect was 7%. Planned Approach to Community Health education planning model |

**Table 6-2.** *Continued*

| Study | Design | Theoretical approach | Population |
|---|---|---|---|
| Marcus, Banspach, et al. (1992) (Pawtucket Heart Health Program: Imagine Action) | 6 week pretest-posttest uncontrolled | Stages of change | 610 sample of community residents, mean age = 42 |
| **Worksites** | | | |
| Blair et al. (1986) (Live for Life) | 2 year quasi-experimental | None | 4,300 Johnson & Johnson employees |
| Fries et al. (1993) | 24 month experimental | None | 4,712 Bank of America retirees |
| Heirich et al. (1993) | 3 year experimental | None specified | 1,300 automobile plant workers |
| **Communication** | | | |
| Osler and Jespersen (1993) | 2 year quasi-experimental | Social learning theory, communications (diffusion of innovations); community organization | Rural communities in Denmark (n = 8,000 [I]) |
| Owen et al. (1995) | 2 year pretest-posttest | Social learning theory, social marketing theory | 2 national physical activity campaigns in Australia |
| Brownell, Stunkard, Albaum (1980) | Study 1: 8 week quasi-experimental | None specified | 21,091 general public observations at a mall, train station, bus terminal |
| | Study 2: 4 month quasi-experimental | None specified | 24,603 general public observations at a train station |
| Blamey, Mutrie, Aitchison (1995) | 16 week quasi-experimental | None | 22,275 subway users observations |

I = intervention; C = control or comparison group.

| Intervention | Findings and comments |
|---|---|
| Written materials, resource manual, weekly fun walks, and activity nights | Participants more active after intervention with movement toward action and low relapse to earlier stage; suggests stage-based community intervention can result in movement toward action; study uncontrolled |
| I: Screening; lifestyle seminar; exercise programs; newsletters; contests; health communications; no smoking policies<br>C: Screening only | 20% of women and 30% of men began vigorous exercise of 2 years |
| I-1: Health risk appraisal; feedback letter; behavioral management materials; personalized health promotion program<br>I-2: Health risk appraisal; no feedback; full program in year 2<br>C: No intervention | No difference in physical activity year 1; I-1 greater physical activity in year 2 over I-2 |
| I-1: Fitness facility<br>I-2: Outreach and counseling to high risk employees<br>I-3: Outreach and counseling to all employees<br>C: Health education events | Percent exercising 3 times per week: I-1 = 30%, , I-2 = 44%, I-3 = 45%, C = 37% |
| I: Heart Week with assessments, health education, weekly community exercise, TV, radio, newspaper community messages<br>C: Not specified | No difference in self-reported physical activity, but intervention community expressed more interest in becoming active; low response rate to surveys (59%); became mainly a media campaign with little community involvement |
| I: Messages to promote walking and readiness to become active; modeling activity; radio and TV PSAs; T-shirts; special scripting of soap operas | 1st campaign—increase in percent who walked for exercise (70% to 74%), greatest impact on 50+ age group (twofold increase in reported walking—not significant)<br>2nd campaign—small declines in reported walking and in intentions to be more active |
| I: Sign reading "Your heart needs exercise— here's your chance" | Number of people using the stairs increased from 5% to 14% when sign was up. Use declined to 7% when sign was removed |
| I: Sign reading "Your heart needs exercise— here's your chance" | Number of people using the stairs increased from 12% to 18%; effect remained for 1 month after sign was removed |
| I: Sign reading "Stay Healthy, Save Time, Use the Stairs" | Baseline stair use increased to 15–17% when sign was up; persisted at 12 weeks after sign removal; larger increase among men |

223

**Table 6-2.** *Continued*

| Study | Design | Theoretical approach | Population |
|---|---|---|---|
| **Special populations: ethnic minorities** | | | |
| Heath et al. (1991) | 2 year quasi-experimental | None specified | 86 Native Americans with diabetes |
| Lewis et al. (1993) | 3 year quasi-experimental | Constituency-based model | African American residents of 6 public housing units |
| Nader et al. (1989) (San Diego Family Health Project) | 3 month experimental 9 month maintenance | Social learning theory | 623 Mexican and Anglo-American families with 5th grade children |
| Baranowski et al. (1990) | 14 weeks | None specified | 94 black families (63 adults, 64 children) |
| **Special populations: persons at risk for chronic disease** | | | |
| Perri et al. (1988) | 18 month experimental | Behavioral management | 123 overweight adults |
| Jeffery (1995) | 7 year uncontrolled | None mentioned | 280 community members trying to lose weight |
| King et al. (1989) | 2 year experimental | None mentioned | 96 men trying to maintain weight loss |
| **Special Populations: older adults** | | | |
| Mayer et al. (1994) | 2 year experimental | Social learning theory | 1,800 Medicare beneficiaries in HMO, mostly white, high SES |

I = intervention; C = control or comparison group.

| Intervention | Findings and comments |
|---|---|
| I: Exercise class<br>C: Nonparticipants | Participants in the exercise program lost 4 kg of weight on average, compared with 0.9 kg among nonparticipants; improvements occurred in fasting blood glucose levels and medication requirements |
| I-1: Basic exercise program<br>I-2: Basic exercise program; social; goal setting; attention; information; barrier reduction | Communities that were better organized and had more committed leaders had better program attendance and higher physical activity levels |
| I: Family newsletter; telephone; mail; personal contact; feedback; family behavior management; physical activity; nutrition education<br>C: Periodic evaluation | No difference in physical activity at 1 year |
| I: Individual counseling, small group education, aerobic activity, incentives (babysitting, transportation), telephone prompts, assessment<br>C: Assessment only | No difference in energy expenditure; low participation (20%) |
| I-1: Behavior therapy<br>I-2: Behavior therapy, maintenance<br>I-3: Behavior therapy, maintenance, social influence<br>I-4: Behavior therapy, maintenance, exercise<br>I-5: Behavior therapy, maintenance, exercise, social influence | Difference adherence in high exercise groups at 6 months; no differences at 12 and 18 months; high attrition (24%) |
| I-1: Diet management<br>I-2: Weight management, including exercise<br>I-3: Physical activity | I-2 resulted in greater weight loss at end, but no differences were observed at 1 year |
| I: Monthly mailings, advice and tips for coping, staff telephone calls<br>C: No intervention | Men who exercised and received the intervention regained less weight in year 2 than exercisers who did not get the intervention or dieters who were exposed to the intervention |
| I: Health risk appraisal, feedback, health education sessions, medical tests, immunizations, goal setting, self-monitoring<br>C: Not specified | No change in physical activity (3+ times a week) at 1 year, but 21% vs.14% moved from sedentary to active (no statistical test reported); attrition 16% in experimental group at 1 year |

self-monitoring group had significantly better adherence over 12 weeks than those in the self-monitoring plus attention or control groups; however, adherence over the last 6 weeks of the study was significantly better in the self-monitoring plus attention group. Actual differences were not large, amounting to 4 to 5 days of gym attendance over 3 weeks, compared with about 3 days among controls. In all three groups, adherence dropped off most sharply during the first 6 weeks of the study.

Classes, health clubs, and fitness centers are resources to promote physical activity, and numerous studies have been undertaken to improve attendance (Table 6-2). However, many people prefer to exercise on their own. Several studies have used behavioral management techniques to encourage people to do so on their own (Table 6-2). In some studies, training in behavioral management techniques has occurred in a group setting before the participants began exercising on their own; in others, information has been provided by mail. Results have been equivocal. King, Haskell, and colleagues (1995) assigned 50- through 65-year-old participants to one of three conditions: a vigorous, group-based program (three 60-minute sessions); a vigorous, home-based program (three 60-minute sessions); and a moderate, home-based program (five 30-minute sessions). At 1 year, adherence was significantly greater in both home-based programs than in the group-based program. At 2 years, however, the vigorous, home-based program had higher adherence than the other two programs. Researchers hypothesize that it was more difficult for the moderate group to schedule 5 days of weekly physical activity than for the vigorous group to schedule 3 days. Another study encouraged self-monitoring and social support (walking with a partner) and also tested a schedule of calling participants to prompt them to walk. Frequent calls (once a week) resulted in three times the number of reported episodes of activity than resulted from calling every 3 weeks (Lombard, Lombard, Winett 1995). Cardinal and Sachs (1995) randomly assigned 133 women to receive one of the three packets of information promoting physical activity: self-instructional packages that were based on stage of change and that provided tailored feedback; a packet containing a standard exercise prescription; and a packet providing minimal information about health status and

exercise status. No significant differences were observed among the three groups at baseline, 1 month, or 7 months.

The advent of interactive expert-system computer technologies has allowed for increased individualization of mailed feedback and other types of printed materials for health promotion (Skinner, Strecher, Hospers 1994). Whether these technologies can be shown to be effective in promoting physical activity at low cost is yet to be determined.

In summary, behavioral management approaches have been employed with mixed results. Where an effect has been demonstrated, it has often been small. Evidence of the effectiveness of techniques like self-monitoring, frequent follow-up telephone calls, and incentives appear to be generally positive over the short run, but not over longer intervals. Evidence on the relative effectiveness of interventions on adherence to moderate or vigorous activity is limited and unclear. Because of the small number of studies, the variety of outcome measures employed, and the diversity of settings examined, it is not clear under what circumstances behavioral management approaches work best.

In a number of studies, methodological issues, such as high attrition rates, short follow-up, small sample sizes, lack of control or comparison groups, incomplete reporting of data, or lack of clarity about how theoretical constructs were operationalized, also make it difficult to determine the effectiveness of behavioral management approaches or to generalize results to other settings or population groups. Stages of change theory suggests that people move back and forth across stages before they become able to sustain a behavior such as physical activity. The relatively short time frame of many studies and the use of outcome measures that are not sensitive to stages of change may have limited the ability to determine if and to what extent possessing behavioral management skills is useful in the maintenance of regular physical activity.

### Interventions in Health Care Settings
Health care settings offer an opportunity to individually counsel adults and young people about physical activity as well as other healthful behaviors, such as dietary practices (U.S. Preventive Services Task Force 1996). Approximately 80 percent of the

U.S. population see a physician during a 1-year period (National Center for Health Statistics 1991), but the extent to which physicians counsel their patients to be physically active is unclear. One survey of physicians found 92 percent reporting that they or someone in their practice counseled patients about exercise (Mullen and Tabak 1989), but in a more recent study, only 49 percent of primary care physicians stated they believed that regular daily physical activity was very important for the average patient (Wechsler et al. 1996). Counseling is likely to be brief, often less than 2 minutes (Wells et al. 1986), and ineffective counseling approaches are often employed (Orleans et al. 1985). Physicians may be less likely to counsel patients about health habits if their own health habits are poor (Wells et al. 1984).

Only three studies attempting to improve the physical activity counseling skills of primary care physicians have been reported in the literature; the results suggest small but generally positive effects on patients, with from 7 to 10 percent of sedentary persons starting to be physically active (Table 6-2). One feasibility trial of multiple risk factor reduction—the Industrywide Network for Social, Urban, and Rural Efforts (INSURE) Project—indicates that continuing medical education seminars, combined with reimbursement for prevention counseling and reminders to providers, can increase the percentage of these physicians' patients who subsequently start exercising (Logsdon, Lazaro, Meir 1989). The Physician-based Assessment and Counseling for Exercise (PACE) program incorporated social cognitive theory and the transtheoretical model to individualize brief (2–5 minutes) counseling messages for patients. Compared with patients who did not receive the program counseling, those who did had significantly greater improvements at 4–6 weeks in their reported stage of physical activity readiness, their reported amount of walking for exercise, and their scores from an activity monitor (Calfas et al. in press).

The Canadian Task Force on the Periodic Health Examination (1994) cited insufficient evidence as the reason for not making a recommendation regarding physical activity counseling. However, several other professional organizations have recently recommended routine physical activity counseling. The American Heart Association (Fletcher et al. 1992), the American Academy of Pediatrics (1994), the American Medical Association (1994), the President's Council on Physical Fitness and Sports (1992), and the U.S. Preventive Services Task Force (1989, 1996) all recommend including physical activity counseling as part of routine clinical preventive services for both adults and young people.

In summary, many providers do not believe that physical activity is an important topic to discuss with their patients, and many lack effective counseling skills. The studies that have attempted to increase provider counseling for physical activity demonstrate that providers can be effective in increasing physical activity among their patients. It is not known what alternative approaches to provider counseling can be used effectively in health care settings, although the work of Mayer and colleagues (1994) suggests that well-trained counselors conducting health education classes with patients may help older adults make changes in their stage of physical activity.

### Community Approaches

Communitywide prevention programs have evolved from the concept that a population, rather than an individual, approach is required to achieve primary prevention of disease through risk factor reduction (Luepker et al. 1994). Behaviors and lifestyle choices that contribute to an individual's risk profile are influenced by personal, cultural, and environmental factors (Bandura 1977b). Much of the current knowledge regarding community-based prevention strategies has been gained over the past 20 years from three U.S. research field trials for community-based health promotion—including physical activity promotion—to reduce cardiovascular disease (Table 6-2).

These three trials, which were funded by the National Heart, Lung, and Blood Institute during the 1980s, were the Minnesota Heart Health Program (MHHP) (Luepker et al. 1994), the Pawtucket Heart Health Program (PHHP) (Carleton et al. 1995), and the Stanford Five-City Project (SFCP) (Farquhar et al. 1990). The MHHP advocated regular physical activity as part of its broad effort to reduce risk for CHD in whole communities in the upper Midwest (Crow et al. 1986; Mittelmark et al. 1986). Three intervention communities received a 5- to 6-year program designed to reduce smoking, serum cholesterol, and blood pressure and to increase physical activity; three other communities served as comparison sites. Mass media were used to educate the public about the relationship

## Physical Activity and Health

between regular physical activity and reduced risk for CHD and to increase opportunities for physical activity. Health professionals promoted physical activity through their local organizations, through their advisory committees on preventive practice, and through serving as role models and opinion leaders. Systematic risk factor screening and education provided on-site measurement, education, and counseling aimed in part at increasing to 60 percent the prevalence of physical activity among the residents in the three intervention communities. The adult education component made available personal, intensive, and multiple-contact programs to increase physical activity;

this strategy focused on self-management and included changes in existing behaviors, in the meaning of those behaviors, and in the environmental cues that supported them. Direct education programs for school-aged children promoted physical activity in young people and their parents. The MHHP investigators reported small but significant effects for physical activity in the first 3 years among people in the cross-sectional study group; that effect disappeared with an increasing secular trend in physical activity in the comparison groups. The cohort group (followed over time) showed no intervention effect until the last follow-up survey (Figure 6-1).

**Figure 6-1.** Results of the Minnesota Heart Health Program on physical activity. Graph compares the percentage of respondents reporting regular physical activity in intervention cities and the secular trend estimated from control cities

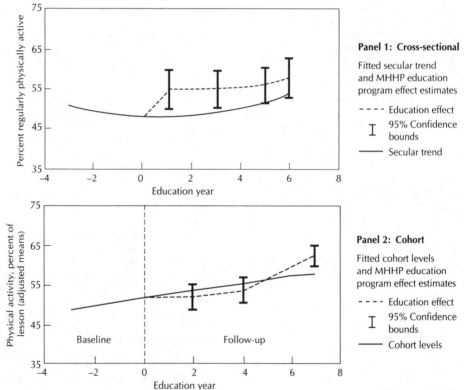

Source: Luepker RV et al. *American Journal of Public Health* 1994 (reprinted with permission).
Note: Adjusted for age, sex, and education.

The PHHP fostered community involvement in heart healthy behavior changes in Pawtucket, Rhode Island (Carleton et al. 1995). The focus was on grassroots organizing, volunteer delivery, and partnerships with existing organizations rather than on using electronic media (Lasater et al. 1986). In the area of physical activity promotion, the emphasis was on environmental and policy change through partnerships with city government and others. Working with the Department of Parks and Recreation, the PHHP was instrumental in establishing cardiovascular fitness trails in both of the city's parks. Early in its existence, the PHHP also helped that department place on the ballot and pass a large bond issue in return for renovations (e.g., lights, fencing to keep stray dogs out, resurfacing) to an existing quarter-mile track for walking. The Pawtucket 6-week Imagine Action Program, designed around the stages of change model, enrolled more than 600 participants, who subsequently reported being more active as a result of the program (Marcus, Banspach, et al. 1992). Results of this uncontrolled study suggest that a stage-based approach may be effective in moving people toward regular physical activity.

The SFCP included two intervention and two comparison communities in northern California (only morbidity and mortality data were monitored in the fifth city, and those results were not reported in this study). This project was designed to increase physical activity and weight control and to reduce plasma cholesterol levels, cigarette use, and blood pressure (Farquhar et al. 1990). Greater emphasis was placed on nutrition, weight control, and blood pressure than on physical activity. The program used concepts from social learning theory, diffusion theory, community organization, and social marketing in combination with a communication and behavior change model (Flora, Maccoby, Farquhar 1989). The program relied heavily on the use of electronic and print media for the delivery of health education information. General education was supplemented by four to five annual education campaigns targeting specific risk factors. Direct face-to-face activities included classes, contests, and school-based programs (Farquhar et al. 1990). Overall, the educational intervention had no significant impact on physical activity levels, knowledge, self-efficacy, or attitudes toward physical activity (Young et al., in press). In the cross-sectional sample, men in the experimental communities were significantly more

likely than those in the control communities to engage in at least one vigorous activity. For women in both the cross-sectional and cohort studies, a small but significant increase was observed in the number of moderate activities engaged in (Young et al., in press).

Among smaller-scale community studies, the results of efforts to promote physical activity have been mixed (Table 6-2). One exception was the community-based cardiovascular disease prevention program aimed at black residents in rural communities in the Missouri "Bootheel" (Brownson et al. 1996). In this 5-year, low-cost intervention project, educational efforts were combined with environmental changes. Local coalitions formed walking clubs, built walking trails, started exercise classes in churches, and organized special events to promote both physical activity and good nutrition. Although no difference in levels of physical inactivity was observed between the Bootheel and the rest of the state at follow-up, physical inactivity declined an average of 3 percent in Bootheel communities that had coalitions and increased an average of 3.8 percent in those without, for a net improvement of 6.8 percent.

In summary, results of community-based interventions to increase physical activity have been generally disappointing. Measurement of physical activity has varied across studies, making comparisons difficult. The presence of active community coalitions, widespread community involvement, and well-organized community efforts appear to be important, however, in increasing physical activity levels.

### Worksite Programs

Physical activity programs conducted on the worksite have the potential to reach a large percentage of the U.S. population (Bezold, Carlson, Peck 1986; National Center for Health Statistics 1987). As settings for physical activity promotion, many worksites have easy access to employees and supportive social networks and can make changes in the environment to help convey physical activity as an organizational norm (Shephard, in press).

The proportion of worksites offering physical activity and fitness programs has grown in recent years, from 22 percent in 1985 to 42 percent in 1992 (Table 6-3). For two groups of employers, those with 50–99 employees and those with 100–249

Table 6-3. Summary of progress toward *Healthy People 2000* objective 1.10

**"Increase the proportion of worksites offering employer-sponsored physical activity and fitness programs as follows:"**

| Year 2000 objective | 1985 | 1992 | Year 2000 target |
|---|---|---|---|
| Physical activity and fitness worksites with: | | | |
| 50–99 employees | 14% | 33% | 20% |
| 100–249 employees | 23% | 47% | 35% |
| 250–749 employees | 32% | 66% | 50% |
| 750+ employees | 54% | 83% | 80% |

Source: U.S. Department of Health and Human Services, 1992 National Survey of Worksite Health Promotion Activities, 1993.

employees, the percentage with exercise programs more than doubled over that time period. In each worksite size category, the percentage with exercise programs had already (i.e., in 1992) exceeded the year 2000 national objective for worksite health promotion listed in *Healthy People 2000* (USDHHS 1993). Generally, the extent of participation, effectiveness, and quality of those programs is unknown, for only a few worksite physical activity programs have been evaluated (Table 6-2).

In the Johnson & Johnson Live for Life program (Wilbur 1983), employees at four experimental sites participated in lifestyle seminars, contests, and exercise programs and received newsletters on health issues and other health communications. Experimental and control sites both received an annual health assessment. Overall, at the end of 2 years, 20 percent of women and 30 percent of men in the experimental sites reported beginning a vigorous exercise program; the prevalence at three comparison sites was 7 percent for women and 19 percent for men (Blair et al. 1986).

Fries and associates (1993) evaluated the effectiveness of a health promotion program that included physical activity for Bank of America retirees. In one intervention group, each participant paid $30 for a personalized, mail-delivered program that included a health risk appraisal and behavioral management books and other materials. A second group received a risk appraisal and nothing else for the first 12 months, after which it received the full intervention. A control group was monitored for claims data only. The first

intervention group did not differ from the second in self-reported physical activity at the end of year 1 but was significantly different in year 2.

Worksite programs less often attract sedentary, blue-collar, or less-educated employees, but interventions that are tailored to these persons' needs and interests (King, Carl, et al. 1988) and provide counseling and peer support (Heirich et al. 1993) show promise. In a controlled study, Heirich and colleagues (1993) compared different programs at four automotive manufacturing plants of like size and employee populations. The three approaches tested were 1) a staffed physical fitness facility, 2) one-to-one counseling and outreach with high-risk employees (i.e., those who had hypertension, were overweight, or smoked cigarettes), and 3) one-to-one counseling and outreach to all employees, peer support, and organizational change (e.g., the institution of nonsmoking areas). The fourth site, which served as a control, offered health education classes and special events. After 3 years, exercise prevalence at the four sites was lowest at the plant with the exercise facility. In the two counseling and outreach sites, nearly half of the employees reported exercising 3 times a week.

In summary, considerable progress has been made in meeting the *Healthy People 2000* goals for worksite physical activity programs. Too few studies exist to clearly determine what elements are required for physical activity programs at work to be effective in increasing physical activity levels among all employees, attracting diverse employee groups (such as blue-collar workers), or maintaining exercise levels over time. However, the limited research available suggests that widespread employee involvement and support coupled with organizational commitment evidenced by the presence of policies and programs may be important factors in increasing levels of physical activity. Existing controlled studies have been done in larger worksites; studies have not yet shown what might work in smaller worksites and in diverse worksites (e.g., where many employees travel or facilities may not exist).

## Communications Strategies

Communications strategies, both electronic and print, have the potential for reaching individuals and communities with a rapidity unmatched by other intervention strategies. For the general population, media can play several roles: to increase the perceived importance of physical activity as a health issue, to communicate the health and other benefits of physical activity, to generate interest in physical activity and awareness about available programs, to provide role models for physically active lifestyles, and to provide cues to action, such as getting people to request further information on physical activity, visit an exercise site, or begin exercising (Donovan and Owen 1994).

The effectiveness of different forms of media alone, including broadcast and print media, for promoting either initial adoption or subsequent maintenance of physical activity remains unclear because the few systematically evaluated interventions employing communications strategies have shown mixed results (Osler and Jespersen 1993; Booth et al. 1992; Owen et al. 1995; Luepker et al. 1994; Farquhar et al. 1990). The SFCP, discussed earlier, resulted in small increases in the number of moderate activities engaged in by women and vigorous activity engaged in by men. Two national mass media campaigns to increase physical activity, particularly walking, to prevent cardiovascular disease were conducted in Australia in 1990 and 1991 (Booth et al. 1992). Drawing on social marketing and social learning theories, both campaigns included paid advertisements on national television, public service announcements on radio, scripted episodes on two nationally broadcast television dramas, posters and leaflets, stickers, T-shirts and sweatshirts, magazine articles, distribution of a

professional article, soap operas specially scripted to feature physical activity, and publicity tours by two experts in heart health. The budgets and paid television coverage for the 1990 and 1991 campaigns were similar. Both campaigns were evaluated by one-on-one, home-based interviews with structured cross-sectional random samples of approximately 2,500 people 2 weeks before and 3 to 4 weeks after each campaign. Both campaigns resulted in significant differences in message awareness (46 percent vs. 71 percent in 1990; 63 percent vs. 74 percent in 1991). The 1990 postcampaign survey revealed significant increases in walking for exercise ($p < 0.01$) compared with the precampaign period, although the actual percentage increase was small (73.9 percent vs. 70.1 percent). In particular, adults over 50 years of age were nearly two times more likely to report walking at follow-up than before the campaign. The 1991 campaign produced different results. Evaluation showed that the percentage of persons reporting walking in the previous 2 weeks declined from precampaign levels among all adult age groups except people over 60 years of age. Intention to become more active also declined overall, from 26.3 percent to 24.8 percent (Owen et al. 1995).

Communications intended to serve as cues to action have been tested at places where people can choose whether to walk or ride. This approach involves placing signs to use the stairs near escalators in public places like train and bus stations or shopping malls (Brownell, Stunkard, Albaum 1980; Blamey, Mutrie, Aitchison 1995). For example, signs that said "Stay Healthy, Save Time, Use the Stairs" increased the percentage of people using stairs instead of an adjacent escalator from 8 percent to 15–17 percent (Blamey, Mutrie, Aitchison 1995). Twelve weeks after the sign was removed, the increase in stair use remained significant but showed a trend toward baseline.

In summary, communications strategies have had limited impact. It is not clear if communications approaches would be more effective in getting people to be regularly active if they were linked with opportunities to act on messages or if messages were tailored to stages of change or to the needs of subgroups in the population (Carleton et al. 1995; Donovan and Owen 1994; Young et al. in press).

Appropriately placed communications that serve as cues to action appear to increase the decision to use the stairs instead of ride the escalator.

### Special Population Programs

#### Racial and Ethnic Minorities

The few interventions studies that have been conducted with racial and ethnic minorities have produced mixed results. The Bootheel Project referred to earlier in this chapter found increased levels of physical activity in black communities with coalitions. The Physical Activity for Risk Reduction project (Lewis et al. 1993) was undertaken in black communities in Birmingham, Alabama, using a combination of behavioral management and community organization approaches. In the intervention groups, community members played roles in defining needs, identifying strategies, and conducting interventions. In those communities where strong organization, leadership, and commitment to the project were observed, statistically significant increases in physical activity were also noted.

Results of two family-based health promotion programs that used behavioral management approaches to promote physical activity showed no greater increase in physical activity among those participating in the programs than among those in a control group. Nader and colleagues (1989) conducted a nutrition and physical activity program for Anglo-American and Mexican American families with children in fifth and sixth grades; the program improved dietary habits but did not succeed in increasing physical activity levels, although participation in the program was high. Another family-based program, a 14-week intervention for African American families that included educational sessions and twice-weekly fitness center activities, had low attendance and did not increase physical activity (Baranowski et al. 1990).

The Indian Health Service undertook the community-based Zuni Diabetes Project to increase physical activity and decrease body weight among Zuni Indians in New Mexico who had non–insulin-dependent diabetes mellitus (NIDDM) (Leonard, Leonard, Wilson 1986). The exercise program consisted of several 1-hour aerobic sessions offered during the week. Zuni Indians who were trained in exercise and group leadership methods helped coordinate the program and build community ownership. After participating in aerobic sessions through the program, 43 percent of the participants began and maintained an at-home exercise program, whereas only 18 percent of a comparison group of previously sedentary nonparticipants with NIDDM did so (Heath et al. 1987).

#### People Who Are Overweight

Being overweight increases the risk of developing chronic diseases (see Chapter 4). Results of interventions to promote physical activity for weight loss have been mixed (Perri et al. 1988; Jeffery 1995; King et al. 1989).

The MHHP , one of the large community intervention trials discussed earlier in this chapter (Luepker et al. 1994), developed a series of component programs containing strategies to increase physical activity for losing weight or preventing weight gain (Jeffery 1995). The Building Your Fitness Futures program was a 4-week adult education class that focused on how to develop a regular exercise program. The Wise Weighs program was an 8-week adult education class that emphasized weight management strategies related to diet and exercise. The third MHHP intervention, a correspondence course, addressed diet and exercise through monthly newsletters and tested two levels of financial contract incentives ($5 and $60 dollars). Each of these programs was evaluated in the MHHP randomized trial. The Building Your Fitness Futures and the Wise Weighs programs resulted in only small weight loss that was not significant after 1 year. The correspondence course resulted in significantly greater weight loss among participants with $60 incentives than among those with $5 incentives.

Preventing weight gain may be easier than promoting weight loss. Wing (1995) suggests that there are three time periods during which interventions to prevent weight gain might be most effective: in the years between ages 25 and 35 years, in the peri-menopausal period for women, and in the year following successful weight loss. A fourth MHHP program that addressed physical activity, the Weight Gain Prevention Program, was a randomized trial of 211 community volunteers. The participants (approximately two-thirds women) were randomly assigned to either the intervention group (n = 103) or the no-contact control group (n = 108). This program was for normal-weight adults and included monthly newsletters and four classes emphasizing diet and regular exercise as well as a financial incentive component linked to weight maintenance. The intervention group lost 2 pounds on average over the course of the year and were significantly less likely to gain weight than the control group (82 percent vs. 56 percent) (Jeffery 1995).

*Older Adults*

Many of the diseases and disabling conditions associated with aging can be prevented, postponed, or ameliorated with regular physical activity (see Chapter 4). The few interventions that have been tested to increase physical activity levels among older adults show generally positive results. The 1990 Australian Heart Week campaign reviewed earlier resulted in a twofold increase in walking among adults over 50 years of age (Owen et al. 1995). Retirees in the study by Fries (1993), also discussed earlier, showed significantly greater improvements in physical activity in year 2 than did persons in the control group. Participants in a longitudinal study of Medicare recipients (n = 1,800) who belonged to a health maintenance organization were randomly assigned to a preventive care or a control group (Mayer et al. 1994). The intervention employed information and behavior modification approaches. Participants received recommended immunizations, completed a health risk appraisal, received face-to-face counseling that included goal setting, received follow-up telephone counseling, and participated in educational sessions on health promotion topics. A focus on physical activity was a priority in goal-setting discussions; 42 percent of participants selected increasing physical activity as their goal. Members of both groups were largely white, well educated, and generally had above-average incomes. The prevalence of physical activity was high in both groups at baseline; approximately 60 percent reported getting regular exercise. At 1 year, the intervention group showed a significant 7 percent increase in self-reported physical activity.

Much of the published research on physical activity describes researcher-initiated interventions. However, individuals and small groups of people often initiate physical activity on their own, independent of any formal program. A qualitative research study by Duncan, Travis, and McAuley (1995) used observations and in-depth interviews to examine motivation for initiating and maintaining mall walking by older persons in rural West Virginia. Most participants in this study reported becoming physically active at the urging of their physicians; several others were motivated by personal interest in health maintenance, and some were encouraged by family members. Mall walkers maintained a regular routine, showing up at the same time each day, walking in pairs or small groups, and then adjourning to a mall eatery for coffee or breakfast. Interviews revealed that participants perceived mall walking as meaningful "work" to be doing during retirement. A need for socializing with others, a sense of belonging to a community of mall walkers, and the safe environment of the mall were other factors contributing to adherence. Study researchers recommended that community-based physical activity programs try to replicate various aspects of work, such as keeping attendance records and providing occasional recognition or acknowledgment of a job well done (such as pins, certificates, or celebrations).

*People with Disabilities*

People with disabilities have similar health promotion and disease prevention needs as persons without disabilities. Interventions to promote physical activity for risk reduction among persons with mobility, visual, hearing, mental, or emotional impairments are largely absent from the literature. Physical activity interventions for managing chronic conditions, on the other hand, have led to enhanced cardiorespiratory fitness and improved skeletal muscle function in persons with multiple sclerosis (Ponichtera-Mulcare 1993), increased walking capacity and reduction in pain for patients with low back pain (Frost et al. 1995), and improvements in endurance among patients with chronic obstructive pulmonary disease (Atkins and Robert 1984).

In summary, interventions that have been successful in increasing physical activity among minorities have employed community organization strategies, such as coalition building and community engagement at all levels. Family-oriented interventions in community centers that have employed behavioral management approaches have not resulted in increases in physical activity. Physical activity interventions incorporating incentives show promise for promoting weight loss or preventing weight gain. Although there are a limited number of studies, positive effects have been shown for interventions and communications strategies promoting physical activity in older adult populations, at least among older white adults with moderate incomes and education levels. What is not well known is what interventions may be effective with racial or ethnic minority older adults who may face barriers such as language, transportation, income, education, or disability. It is not clear what interventions might be effective to promote physical activity, other than for disease management, among people with disabilities, or what strategies might assist with the management of pain, periods of illness, environmental barriers, or other circumstances to improve adherence with physical activity recommendations.

### Summary

The review of adult intervention research literature provides limited evidence that interventions to promote physical activity can be effective in a variety of settings using a variety of strategies. Controlled interventions that have been effective at the workplace, in health care settings, and in communities have resulted in increased physical activity, although effects have tended to be small, in the range of 5–10 percent, and short-lived. Multiple interventions conducted over time may need to be employed to sustain physical activity behavior. Most experimental and quasi-experimental intervention research has been theory-based, much if not most relying largely on behavioral management strategies, often in combination with other approaches, such as communications and social support. Mixed results have made it impossible to determine what theory or theories alone or in combination have most relevance to physical activity. Research strategies that appear promising include the tailoring of interventions to people's needs, experiences, and stages of change; the timing of intervention strategies to reinforce new behaviors and prevent relapse (such as through frequent follow-up telephone calls); peer involvement and support; and an engaged community at all levels. It is not known if interventions could be strengthened by combining them with policy approaches (Luepker 1994; Winkleby 1994).

Intervention studies with adults were often conducted over a brief period of time, had little or no follow-up, and focused on the endpoint of specified vigorous physical activity rather than on moderate-intensity physical activity or total amount of activity. Studies used different endpoints, such as class participation versus specified changes in behavior, making them difficult to compare. Because physical activity interventions were often only one component of an intervention to reduce multiple risk factors, they may not have been robust enough to result in much or any increase in physical activity. Few if any studies compared their results to a standard of effectiveness, such as recommended frequency or duration of moderate or vigorous physical activity, or clearly stated the extent of stage-based change.

## Behavioral Research on Physical Activity among Children and Adolescents

Behavioral research in this area includes studies on the factors influencing physical activity among young people as well as studies examining the effectiveness of interventions to increase this behavior. This research, however, is more limited than the determinants and interventions literature for adults.

### Factors Influencing Physical Activity among Children and Adolescents

The emphasis in this section is on factors that influence unstructured physical activity during free time among youths rather than on supervised physical activity, such as physical education classes. Studies of organized youth sports have also been excluded. Only studies with some measure of physical activity as the outcome, however, are included in this review. For example, studies that investigated attitudes toward physical activity and did not relate those to a measure of physical activity were excluded. As was the case in the adult section, this section focuses on studies that address modifiable determinants of physical activity, such as self-efficacy, rather than on studies that examine factors that cannot be altered to influence participation in physical activity, such as age, sex, and race/ethnicity.

### Modifiable Determinants

The modifiable determinants of youth physical activity include personal, interpersonal, and environmental factors (Table 6-1). Self-efficacy, a construct from social cognitive theory, has been positively associated with physical activity among older children and adolescents (Reynolds et al. 1990; Trost et al. 1996; Zakarian et al. 1994). Similarly, perceptions of physical or sports competence (Biddle and Armstrong 1992; Biddle and Goudas 1996; Dempsey, Kimiecik, Horn 1993; Ferguson et al. 1989; Tappe, Duda, Menges-Ehrnwald 1990) also have been positively associated with physical activity among older children and adolescents.

Expectations about the outcomes of physical activity are associated with physical activity among preadolescents and adolescents. Perceived benefits have been positively associated (Ferguson et al. 1989; Tappe, Duda, Menges-Ehrnwald 1990; Zakarian et al. 1994), whereas perceived barriers have been negatively associated (Stucky-Ropp and DiLorenzo 1993; Tappe, Duda, Menges-Ehrnwald 1990; Zakarian et al. 1994). Intention to be active, a construct from the theory of reasoned action and the theory of planned behavior, has been consistently and positively related to physical activity among older children and adolescents (Biddle and Goudas 1996; Ferguson et al. 1989; Godin and Shephard 1986; Reynolds et al. 1990) .

Enjoyment, the major reason young people engage in physical activity (Borra et al. 1995), has been positively associated with physical activity among both children and adolescents (Stucky-Ropp and DiLorenzo 1993; Tinsley et al. 1995). Favorable attitudes toward physical education also have been positively related to adolescent participation in physical activity (Ferguson et al. 1989; Zakarian et al. 1994).

Social influences—such as physically active role models and support for physical activity—are important determinants of physical activity among young people (Tinsley et al. 1995). Parental activity (Moore et al. 1991; Poest et al. 1989; Sallis, Patterson, McKenzie et al. 1988) is positively related to physical activity among preschoolers. Studies reveal no relationship between parental physical activity and physical activity among elementary school children (McMurray et al. 1993; Sallis, Alcaraz, et al. 1992), and either no relationship (Biddle and Goudas 1996; Garcia et al. 1995; Stucky-Ropp and DiLorenzo 1993; Sallis, Patterson, Buono, et al. 1988) or positive relationships (Anderssen and Wold 1992; Butcher

1985; Gottlieb and Chen 1985; Stucky-Ropp and DiLorenzo 1993; Sallis, Patterson, Buono, et al. 1988) to the physical activity of middle school students (grades 5–8). Parental physical activity is positively related to physical activity among older adolescents (Reynolds et al. 1990; Zakarian et al. 1994). The physical activity of friends (Anderssen and Wold 1992; Stucky-Ropp and DiLorenzo 1993; Zakarian et al. 1994) and siblings (Perusse et al. 1989; Sallis, Patterson, Buono, et al. 1988) also is positively associated with physical activity among older children and adolescents.

Parental encouragement is positively related to physical activity among preschoolers (McKenzie, Sallis, et al. 1991; Klesges et al. 1984, 1986; Sallis et al. 1993), and parental or adult support for physical activity is positively associated with physical activity among adolescents (Anderssen and Wold 1992; Biddle and Goudas 1996; Butcher 1985; Zakarian et al. 1994). Friends' support for physical activity (Anderssen and Wold 1992; Zakarian et al. 1994) also is positively related to physical activity among adolescents.

Direct help from parents, such as organizing exercise activities (Anderssen and Wold 1992) or providing transportation (Sallis, Alacraz, et al. 1992), is positively related to physical activity among older children and younger adolescents. Access to play spaces and facilities (Garcia et al. 1995; Sallis et al. 1993; Zakarian et al. 1994) is positively related to physical activity among youths of all ages. The availability of equipment has been positively related to physical activity among preadolescent and adolescent girls (Butcher 1985; Stucky-Ropp and DiLorenzo 1993). Further, two studies of young children have demonstrated that time spent outdoors is a positive correlate of physical activity level (Klesges et al. 1990; Sallis et al. 1993).

### Determinants for Population Subgroups

Among the limited number of subgroup-specific determinants studies, sex-specific differences are investigated most frequently. In two studies of adolescents (Kelder et al. 1995; Tappe, Duda, Menges-Ehrnwald 1990), competition motivated boys more than girls, and weight management motivated girls more than boys. Additionally, boys have higher levels of self-efficacy than girls (Trost et al. 1996) and higher levels of perceived competence (Tappe, Duda, Menges-Ehrnwald 1990) for physical activity.

## Summary

Few studies of the factors that influence physical activity among children and adolescents have applied the theories and models of behavioral and social science. The research reviewed in this section, however, has revealed that many of the factors that influence physical activity among adults are also determinants of physical activity among children and adolescents. Older children's and adolescents' intentions to engage in physical activity, as well as their perceptions of their ability to engage in such activity (i.e., self-efficacy and perceived competence), are positively related to their participation in physical activity. Social influences, such as parental and peer engagement in, and support for, physical activity, also are positively related to physical activity among young people. Further, exercise enjoyment and positive attitudes toward physical education have been positively associated with physical activity among older children and adolescents. Research is limited, however, on patterns of determinants for population subgroups, such as girls, ethnic minorities, and children with disabilities or chronic health conditions (e.g., asthma).

## Interventions to Promote Physical Activity among Children and Adolescents

The most extensive and promising research on interventions for promoting physical activity among young people has been conducted with students in schools, primarily at the elementary school level. Although many school-based studies have focused on short-term results, a few studies have also examined long-term behavioral outcomes. There is limited evidence concerning the effectiveness of school-community programs, interventions in health care settings, family programs, and programs for special populations. In this section, the emphasis is on interventions designed to promote both unstructured physical activity during free time and supervised physical activity, such as physical education classes. Interventions designed to increase participation in, or adherence to, organized youth sports have been excluded from this review. The review places special emphasis on experimental studies, which feature random assignment of individuals or groups

to intervention (experimental) or comparison (control) conditions, or quasi-experimental studies, which feature intervention and comparison groups.

## School Programs

Because most young people between the ages of 6 and 16 years attend school, schools offer an almost populationwide setting for promoting physical activity to young people, primarily through classroom curricula for physical education and health education. The CDC (in press) recommends that comprehensive school and community health programs promoting physical activity among children and adolescents be developed to increase knowledge about physical activity and exercise, develop behavioral and motor skills promoting lifelong physical activity, foster positive attitudes toward physical activity, and encourage physical activity outside of physical education classes. CDC's 1994 School Health Policies and Programs Study (Kann et al. 1995) examined the current nationwide status of policies and programs for multiple components of a school health program. The study examined kindergarten through 12th-grade health education and physical education at state, district, school, and classroom levels (Errecart et al. 1995). Results from the health education component of this study revealed that physical activity and fitness instruction were required in 65 percent of states and 82 percent of districts and were included in a required health education course in 78 percent of schools. Only 41 percent of health education teachers provided more than one class period of instruction on these physical activity topics during the school year (Collins et al. 1995).

Results from the physical education component of the School Health Policies and Program Study revealed that physical education instruction is required by most states (94 percent) and school districts (95 percent) (Pate, Small, et al. 1995). These policies, however, do not require students to take physical education every year. For instance, although most middle and junior high schools (92 percent) and most senior high schools (93 percent) require at least one physical education course, only half of these middle and junior high schools and only 26 percent of these senior high schools require the equivalent of at least 3 years of physical education. Additionally, only 26 percent of all states require schools to offer a course at the senior high school level in lifetime physical activity (i.e., physical activity that can be practiced throughout one's lifetime) (Pate, Small, et al. 1995). The School Health Policies and Programs Study also revealed that instructional practices in physical education often do not reflect the emphasis on lifetime physical activity that is recommended in the national objectives in *Healthy People 2000* (USDHHS 1990), in the National Physical Education Standards (National Association for Sport and Physical Education 1995), and in the CDC's *Guidelines for School and Community Health Programs to Promote Physical Activity Among Youth* (in press). More than half of physical education teachers devoted multiple class periods to traditional sports activities, such as basketball (87 percent), volleyball (82 percent), and baseball/softball (82 percent), whereas much smaller proportions of teachers devoted multiple class periods to lifetime physical activities, such as jogging (47 percent), aerobic

dance (30 percent), and swimming (14 percent) (Pate, Small, et al. 1995) (Table 6-4). Additionally, only 15 percent of all physical education teachers required students to develop individualized fitness programs (Pate, Small, et al. 1995). Despite current guidelines' emphasis on lifetime physical activity, during the 2 years preceding the study only 22 percent of physical education teachers received in-service training on developing individualized fitness programs, and only 13 percent received training on increasing students' physical activity outside of physical education class (Pate, Small, et al. 1995).

Detailed findings from the School Health Policies and Programs Study are important because school-based physical education may be the most widely available resource for promoting physical activity among young people in the United States. For physical education to meet public health goals, it should provide all students with recommended amounts of weekly physical activity (USDHHS 1990).

Table 6-4. Percentage of all physical education courses in which more than one class period was devoted to each activity, by activity, School Health Policies and Programs Study, 1994

| Activity | Percentage of all courses |
|---|---|
| Basketball | 86.8 |
| Volleyball | 82.3 |
| Baseball/softball | 81.5 |
| Flag/touch football | 68.5 |
| Soccer | 65.2 |
| Jogging | 46.5* |
| Weight lifting or training | 37.3* |
| Tennis | 30.3* |
| Aerobic dance | 29.6* |
| Walking quickly | 14.7* |
| Swimming | 13.6* |
| Handball | 13.2* |
| Racquetball | 4.9* |
| Hiking/backpacking | 3.0* |
| Bicycling | 1.3* |

Source: Adapted from Pate RP et al. School physical education. *Journal of School Health* 1995 (reprinted with permission).
*Lifetime physical activities

Ironically, observations of physical education classes indicate that insufficient class time is spent actually engaging in physical activity (McKenzie et al. 1995; McKenzie et al., in press; Simons-Morton et al. 1991, 1993, 1994).

The School Health Policies and Programs Study provided a national overview of the status of school health programs (Kann et al. 1995). Intervention research has been reported from several studies (Table 6-5). Most of the early research in schools focused on knowledge-based health education classroom lessons; these studies generally reported positive changes in knowledge and attitudes but not in behaviors. Summarized in review articles (Sallis, Simons-Morton, et al. 1992; Simons-Morton, Parcel, O'Hara et al. 1988), these studies suffered from methodological problems, such as small samples and measurement limitations. Contemporary programs emphasize the importance of multicomponent interventions that address both the individual and the environmental level to support engagement in physical activity among youths (Kelder, Perry, Klepp 1993; Luepker et al. 1996; McKenzie et al., in press; Perry et al. 1990, 1992; Simons-Morton, Parcel, O'Hara 1988; Stone et al. 1995).

The Know Your Body (KYB) program (Williams, Carter, Eng 1980) has been the focus of three school-based cardiovascular risk reduction studies (Bush, Zuckerman, Taggart, et al. 1989; Bush, Zuckerman, Theiss, et al. 1989; Resnicow et al. 1992; Walter 1989). This program includes health screening, behavior-oriented health education curricula, and special interventions for students with one or more cardiovascular disease risk factors (e.g., hypercholesterolemia, hypertension, obesity, lack of exercise, cigarette smoking) (Williams, Carter, Eng 1980). Although this program was designed to improve students' knowledge, attitudes, and behaviors related to physical activity, nutrition, and cigarette use, the measurement and reporting of physical activity behavior has been inconsistent among the three studies. In the first study, the measure for self-reported physical activity was found to be unreliable, and the results related to this measure were not reported (Walter 1989). In the second KYB study, students' physical activity behavior was not assessed (Resnicow et al. 1992). The third study was a 5-year, randomized cardiovascular risk reduction trial among 1,234 African American students in grades four

through six from nine schools stratified for socio-economic status (Bush, Zuckerman, Taggart, et al. 1989; Bush, Zuckerman, Theiss, et al. 1989). This project included the KYB health education curriculum, health screening, parent education, and KYB advisory boards for parents, community members, students, and physicians. After 4 years, students from both the intervention and control schools had significant increases in health knowledge at posttest, and intervention students had significantly better gains in health knowledge (Bush, Zuckerman, Theiss, et al. 1989). Physical activity, however, decreased significantly among students from both the intervention and control schools, and there was no difference in physical activity between the intervention and control schools.

The Stanford Adolescent Heart Health Program (Killen et al. 1988) was a classroom-based randomized cardiovascular disease risk reduction trial for 1,447 tenth graders from four matched high schools within two school districts. One school within each district was designated at random to receive a 20-week risk reduction intervention, and the other school served as the control. The classroom-based intervention focused on three cardiovascular risk factors, including physical activity. At the 2-month follow-up, students from the intervention schools had significantly higher gains in knowledge about physical activity than did students in the control schools. Among students not regularly exercising at baseline, those in the intervention schools had significantly greater increases in physical activity than did those in control schools. Additionally, students who received the intervention had significantly lower resting heart rates and subscapular and triceps skinfold measures. The long-term effectiveness of this program was not reported.

An Australian study (Dwyer et al. 1979, 1983) was one of the first randomized trials that investigated the effects of daily physical activity on the health of elementary school students. The study included 513 fifth-grade students from seven Adelaide metropolitan schools. Three classes from each school participated in the study and were randomly assigned to one of three conditions: fitness, skills, or control. Students in the control condition received the usual three 30-minute physical education classes per week. The students in both intervention conditions received 75 minutes of daily physical education: one condition emphasized fitness activities featuring high levels of physical activity, and the other emphasized skill development activities without special emphasis on the intensity or duration of physical activity. With the class as the unit of analysis, the fitness condition led to significantly greater increases in endurance fitness and decreases in skinfold measurements. Although this study did not evaluate the impact of increased physical education on students' engagement in physical activity outside of class, it showed that academic test scores did not differ between the intervention and control groups, despite the additional 275 minutes of class time the intervention groups spent on physical education rather than on traditional academic subjects.

Go For Health (GFH) was a 3-year school health project designed to promote healthful diet and exercise behaviors among elementary school students (Parcel et al. 1987; Simons-Morton, Parcel, O'Hara 1988; Simons-Morton et al. 1991). This project involved four elementary schools (kindergarten through fourth grade) from the Texas City Independent School District. Two schools were assigned to serve as controls, and the other two were designated as GFH intervention schools. The intervention was based on social cognitive theory and included a GFH health education curriculum, physical education classes that focused on vigorous physical activity, and lower-fat school lunches. The physical activity results revealed a significant increase from pretest to posttest (2 years) in the percentage of physical education class time that students in the intervention schools were engaged in moderate-to-vigorous physical activity. Additionally, posttest values were significantly greater than those for the control schools (Simons-Morton et al. 1991). Although this study did not examine changes in physical activity outside of physical education classes, it highlighted the importance of organizational changes to promote physical activity among students.

The Sports, Play, and Active Recreation for Kids (SPARK) study, conducted in San Diego, California, tested the effects of combining a health-related physical education curriculum and in-service programs on the quantity and quality of physical education classes in elementary schools (McKenzie et al. 1993). In a single school district, 28 fourth-grade classes in seven schools were randomly assigned to one of three conditions: 10 classes were taught in their usual manner by classroom teachers (control group); 10 classes were taught the SPARK program by classroom teachers who had received in-service training and follow-up consultations; and 8 classes were taught the SPARK program by physical education specialists hired by the research project. Direct observation found that students assigned to either of the two intervention groups engaged in significantly more weekly physical activity during physical education classes than did controls. Teachers who received the new physical education curriculum and in-service training provided significantly higher-quality instruction than did teachers in the control group, although the trained classroom teachers' instruction did not match the quality of the instruction provided by the physical education specialists. This study demonstrated that an improved physical education curriculum, combined with well-designed training for physical education specialists and classroom teachers, can substantially increase the amount of physical activity children receive in school (McKenzie et al. 1993) and can help ensure that the resulting physical education classes are enjoyable (McKenzie et al. 1994).

The Child and Adolescent Trial for Cardiovascular Health (CATCH) study was a multicenter, randomized trial to test the effectiveness of a cardiovascular health promotion program in 96 schools in four states (Luepker et al. 1996; Perry et al. 1990, 1992; Stone 1994). A major component of CATCH was an innovative health-related physical education program, beginning at the third grade, for elementary school students. For 2.5 years, randomly assigned schools received a standardized physical education intervention, including new curriculum, staff development, and follow-up consultations. In these intervention schools, observed participation in moderate-to-vigorous activity during physical education classes increased from 37.4 percent of class time at baseline to 51.9 percent (Luepker et al. 1996). This increase represented an average of 12 more minutes of daily vigorous physical activity in physical education classes than was observed among children in control schools (Luepker et al. 1996; McKenzie et al. 1995). Figure 6-2 shows the effect of CATCH on physical activity during physical education class. The CATCH study showed that children's

Table 6-5. Studies of interventions to increase physical activity among children and adolescents

| Study | Design | Theoretical approach | Population |
|---|---|---|---|
| **School programs** | | | |
| Bush, Zuckerman, Taggart, et al. (1989), Bush, Zuckerman, Theiss, et al. (1989) (Know Your Body) | 4 year experimental | Social learning theory | 1,234 students initially in grades 4–6, follow-up in grades 7–9 |
| Killen et al. (1988) (Stanford Adolescent Heart Health Program) | 7 week experimental 2-month follow-up | Social cognitive theory | 1,447 students in grade 10 |
| Dwyer et al. (1983) | 14 week experimental | None | 513 students in grade 5 |
| Simons-Morton et al. (1991) (Go For Health) | 3 year quasi-experimental | Social cognitive theory | 409 grades 3 and 4 PE classes |
| McKenzie et al. (1993) (SPARK) | 8 month experimental | | 112 PE lessons |
| Luepker et al. (1996); McKenzie (in press); Edmundson et al. (1996) (CATCH) | 3 year experimental | Social cognitive theory | 96 schools; 3,239 students initially in grade 3, follow-up at grade 5 |
| **School-community programs** | | | |
| Kelder, Perry, Klepp (1993) (Minnesota Heart Health Program: Class of 1989 Study) | 7 year quasi-experimental | Social learning theory | Students in grade 6 from 2 Minnesota Heart Health Program communities |

I = intervention; C = control or comparison; HE = health education; PE = physical education.

| Intervention | Findings and comments |
|---|---|
| I-1: 45 minutes, 2 times/week, Know Your Body HE curriculum; health screening and results<br>I-2: 45 minutes, 2 times/week, Know Your Body HE curriculum; health screening<br>C: Health screening | Decrease in physical activity for both groups between pretest and follow-up. No difference in physical activity between groups at posttest. Increase in posttest knowledge by each group. Great increases in knowledge by intervention groups at posttest, 18% response rate at 4-year follow-up |
| I: 20 classroom PE sessions, 50 minutes each, 3 times/week, HE risk reduction curriculum<br>C: No intervention | Intervention groups compared with control had a higher proportion of nonexercisers at baseline exercising at follow-up |
| I-1: 75 minutes daily PE, fitness curriculum<br>I-2: 75 minutes daily PE, skill curriculum<br>C: 30 minutes PE 3 times/week, standard curriculum | Physical activity not assessed; no differences in academic achievement between intervention and control groups despite additional 275 minutes of time spent in PE by intervention groups |
| I: 6 behaviorally based HE modules; five 6- to 8-week modules of PE, children's active PE curriculum; reduced fat and sodium school lunch<br>C: No intervention | Increase from pretest to posttest in the percent of PE class time intervention school students spent in moderate-to-vigorous physical activity; higher percentage of PE class time spent in moderate-to-vigorous physical activity by intervention schools compared with controls in posttest |
| I-1: PE provided by PE specialists<br>I-2: PE provided by "specially trained" classroom teachers<br>C: PE provided by classroom teachers | At posttest PE specialists spent more minutes per lesson on very active physical activity and fitness activities than specially trained classroom teachers and classroom teachers; specially trained classroom teachers spent more minutes per lesson on very active physical activity and fitness activities than classroom teachers |
| I-1: HE curricula; PE featuring enjoyable moderate-to-vigorous physical activity; EAT SMART school food service intervention<br>I-2: Same as I-1 with family involvement<br>C: No intervention | Intervention schools compared to control schools provided a greater percentage of PE time spent in moderate to vigorous physical activity at posttest; family involvement had no effect on physical activity and psychosocial outcomes; data from the intervention groups combined for comparison with the control groups; intervention students were not different from control students in total daily physical activity at posttest; intervention students spent 12 more minutes per day engaged in vigorous physical activity than controls; pretest-to-posttest increases in students' perceptions of self-efficacy for exercise and positive social reinforcement for exercise among both intervention and control students; intervention students' posttest scores on these and other psychosocial measures were not different from those of control students |
| I: Peer-led physical activity challenge at grade 8; 10 lesson Slice of Life HE curriculum at grade 10<br>C: No intervention | At 7-year follow-up students from schools in intervention community had higher levels of physical activity than students from schools in control community, particularly among girls; 45% response rate at 7-year follow-up |

**Figure 6-2. Moderate-to-vigorous and vigorous physical activity observed during Child and Adolescent Trial for Cardiovascular Health (CATCH) physical education classes**

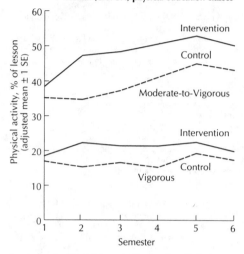

Source: Luepker RV et al. *Journal of the American Medical Association* 1996 (reprinted with permission).

Note: Observed at six time points, 1991 through 1994. The CATCH intervention, introduced during semester 2, increased the percentage of time spent in moderate-to-vigorous and vigorous activity as measured by the System for Observing Fitness Instruction Time classroom observation system. Intervention and control curves diverged significantly according to repeated-measures analysis of variance with the class session as the unit of analysis: for moderate-to-vigorous activity, $P = 2.17$, $df = 5$, 1979, $P = .02$; for vigorous activity, $F = 2.95$, $df = 5$, 1979, $P = .04$. Analysis controlled for CATCH site, the location of the lesson, the specialty of the teacher, and random variation among schools and weeks of observation.

physical activity can be increased by a standardized intervention applied to existing physical education programs in four geographically and ethnically diverse regions. Although the intervention students showed significant pretest to follow-up increases in their perceptions of positive social reinforcement and self-efficacy for exercise (Edmundson et al. 1996), these psychosocial determinants were not significantly more prevalent than those observed among the control groups at follow-up (Luepker et al. 1996). Although the family intervention component produced no additional increase in physical activity among students (Luepker et al. 1996), the

CATCH physical education and classroom programs successfully increased moderate-to-vigorous physical activity in physical education class and increased students' daily participation in vigorous physical activity.

### School-Community Programs

The Class of 1989 Study (Kelder, Perry, Klepp 1993; Kelder et al. 1995), an ancillary study of the MHHP (Luepker et al. 1994), tested the efficacy of a school-based health promotion program. One of three MHHP intervention communities and its matched pair were involved in the Class of 1989 Study. The intervention cities were engaged in an extensive communitywide intervention program designed to improve eating, exercise, and smoking patterns for the entire population. The physical activity intervention included a peer-led physical activity challenge, in which students were encouraged to engage in out-of-school exercise activities. The program's assessment included annual measurements collected from a large number of students (baseline n = 2,376) for 7 years, beginning in the sixth grade. Throughout most of the follow-up period, physical activity levels were significantly higher among female students in the intervention community than among those in the control community. For male students, the levels did not differ significantly between the communities. Results suggest that at least among female students, a multicomponent intervention that includes peer-led behavioral education in schools and complementary communitywide strategies can increase levels of regular physical activity (Kelder, Perry, Klepp 1993; Kelder et al. 1995).

### Interventions in Health Care Settings

Health professionals also have a potential role in promoting physical activity, healthy eating, and other health behaviors among children and adolescents (American Medical Association 1994; U.S. Preventive Services Task Force 1996). Results of a national survey of pediatricians showed that one-half of respondents believed that regular exercise during childhood is important in preventing cardiovascular disease in adulthood (Nader et al. 1987). However, only one-fourth believed they would be effective in counseling their young patients to get regular vigorous exercise. The American Medical Association's Guidelines for Adolescent Preventive Health Services (1994) is one example of practical counseling recommendations that have been developed for those who provide health services to adolescents.

### Special Population Programs

Physical activity can assist in the treatment or rehabilitation of several diseases that occur during youth (Rowland 1990; Greenan-Fowler 1987); however, relatively few interventions have been conducted to examine how to promote physical activity among young people with special needs. The most extensive study is a series of randomized investigations of children who are overweight (Epstein, Wing, Valoski 1985; Epstein, McCurley, et al. 1990; Epstein, Valoski, et al. 1990; Epstein et al.1994). In this series, family-based treatments of 5- to 12-year-old obese children incorporated both physical activity and nutrition interventions, and the programs were based specifically on principles of behavior modification. Parents were trained to improve their children's physical activity by setting behavioral change goals with their children, by identifying effective reinforcers (e.g., spending time with parents), and by reinforcing children when goals were met. Ten-year follow-ups of children in these four randomized studies revealed that 30 percent of children receiving family-based interventions were no longer obese, and 20 percent had decreased their percentage overweight by 20 percent or more (Epstein et al. 1994). The 10-year follow-up investigation also revealed that the percentage of overweight children in each study decreased most when the intervention involved both the parent and the child or when a change in lifestyle exercise was emphasized. Epstein and colleagues (1994) also compared the effectiveness of three forms of physical activity interventions: lifestyle physical activity, in which activity was incorporated into daily routines; structured aerobic exercise; and calisthenics. At the 10-year follow-up, the lifestyle group had lost the most weight, and both the lifestyle group and the aerobic exercise group had greater weight-loss results than the calisthenics group (Epstein et al. 1994).

### Summary

The preceding review of the research literature on interventions among young people reveals that school-based approaches have had consistently strong effects on increasing physical activity in elementary school students when the intervention orients the physical education program toward delivering moderate-to-vigorous physical activity. Further, social learning theory appears to have had the widest application to this interventions research. Much research has taken place at the elementary school level; very little is known about increasing children's physical activity in middle and high school physical education classes or in settings other than school physical education classes. It seems likely that these interventions would be strengthened by designing programs that combine school and community policy with health education and physical education. Data are lacking on ways to tailor interventions to the needs and interests of young people and to prevent the rapid decline in physical activity that occurs during late childhood and adolescence, especially among girls. Additionally, few physical activity interventions and research studies encompass populations particularly characterized by race/ethnicity, socioeconomic status, risk factor status, disabilities, or geographic location.

## Promising Approaches, Barriers, and Resources

Many questions remain about how best to promote physical activity in the general population of young people and adults, as well as in clinical populations and other subgroups. Policy initiatives, the provision of more physical activity facilities and programs, and media campaigns are promising, but studies testing their effects are limited. The following two sections describe existing policy and program approaches[1] that have the potential to increase population levels of physical activity but have received little or no evaluation. They are reviewed separately from the previously discussed, better-documented research studies.

[1]Descriptions of specific physical activity programs across the United States can be found in the Combined Health Information Database, a computerized bibliographic database of health information and health promotion resources developed and managed by several federal agencies, including the CDC, the National Institutes of Health, the Department of Veterans Affairs, and the Health Resources and Services Administration. Intended for all health professionals who need to locate health information for themselves or their clients, this resource is available in many libraries, state agencies, and federal agencies.

## Environmental and Policy Approaches

Most interventions that have been evaluated in research studies are discrete programs targeting population subgroups (e.g., employees, schoolchildren) or communities. Interventions have shown some success in promoting physical activity, but their results have been inconsistent. A possible reason for limited results is a lack of concomitant support from the larger environment within which such interventions take place. Many physical activity researchers believe that environmental and policy interventions must occur to complement interventions that focus on behavior change among individuals or small groups. This larger perspective recognizes the powerful moderating effect that environment has on individual volition. As King, Jeffery, and colleagues (1995) observe, "Environmental and policy interventions are based on the recognition that people's health is integrally connected to their physical and social environments" (p. 501).

Two premises underlie environmental and policy approaches. First, interventions addressing chronic disease risk factors, such as physical inactivity, require comprehensive, population-based approaches that incorporate both individual and societal-level strategies (Green and Simons-Morton 1996; Schmid, Pratt, Howze 1995). Second, strategies should not rely solely on active approaches requiring individual initiative, such as enrolling in exercise classes, but should also incorporate passive approaches, such as providing walking trails or policies that permit employees to exercise during work hours (Schmid, Pratt, Howze 1995). An example of intervention elements combining passive and active approaches is a school board policy that permits school facilities to remain open before and after school for community use, together with health communications that make citizens aware of these facilities and encourage their use.

As presented previously, ecological models of health behavior (McLeroy et al. 1988; CDC 1988; Stokols 1992) provide frameworks for conceptualizing what the role of policy approaches is to health promotion and how individuals interact with their social, institutional, cultural, and physical environments. The concept of the health-promoting environment suggests that communities and other settings can facilitate healthy behaviors by providing environmental inducements to be active, such as by offering safe, accessible, and attractive trails for walking and biking.

National objectives and recommendations have encouraged the development of policies, programs, and surveillance strategies that would help create an environment that promotes physical activity (USDHHS 1990; Pate, Pratt, et al. 1995; National Association for Sport and Physical Education 1995; U.S. Department of Transportation [USDOT] 1994). Increasing national levels of physical activity and of cardiorespiratory fitness has also been targeted as a priority health objective in *Healthy People 2000* (USDHHS 1990) and the *Dietary Guidelines for Americans* (U.S. Department of Agriculture and USDHHS 1995).

Many efforts to raise public awareness and promote physical activity are under way. In 1994, the American Heart Association, the American College of Sports Medicine, and the American Alliance for Health, Physical Education, Recreation and Dance formed a National Coalition for Promoting Physical Activity. The coalition's goals are to increase public awareness of the benefits of physical activity, provide an opportunity for forming effective partnerships, and enhance delivery of consistent messages about physical activity (National Coalition for Promoting Physical Activity 1995). The CDC has established guidelines for promoting physical activity and healthy eating among young people (CDC 1996; CDC in press) and has initiated a public education effort to encourage active lifestyles and healthy eating among Americans. The National Institutes of Health (NIH) has used national campaigns to promote messages to both the general public and patients on the importance of physical activity and a heart healthy diet. The NIH also sponsors research on physical activity in special populations, including women from diverse economic backgrounds, and in various settings, such as worksites, schools, and health care institutions. In 1995, the NIH sponsored the Consensus Development Conference on Physical Activity and Cardiovascular Health, which recommended regular physical activity for most persons aged 2 years and older (see Appendix B in Chapter 2). The President's Council on Physical Fitness and Sports works with a broad range of partners in private industry, voluntary organizations, and the media to promote physical activity, fitness, and sports participation by Americans of all ages. As part of the midcourse review of the physical activity and fitness objectives of *Healthy People 2000*, the council presented a synopsis of ongoing grassroots activities by Healthy People 2000 Consortium members in support of increasing participation in physical activity and improvement in fitness (USDHHS 1995). The President's Council on Physical Fitness and Sports is also an advisory body to the President and to the Secretary of the DHHS on matters involving physical activity, fitness, and sports that enhance and improve health. Thirty-nine Governor's Councils on Physical Fitness and Sports stimulate state and local activities and program development; these efforts target fitness promotion for school-aged youths, older adults, working adults, and families (National Association of Governor's Councils on Physical Fitness and Sports 1996).

## Community-Based Approaches

Community-based programs can be tailored to meet the needs of their specific populations. More collaborative work is under way between state and local governments, community groups, and businesses to reduce risk factors among employees and residents. Two-year follow-up data from one such effort in Smyth County, Virginia, suggested that 40 percent of school system employees had increased their physical activity participation during the program period (CDC 1992).

Two large subpopulations may be especially important to address in community-based programs: young people and older adults. Communities will face a growing need to provide a supportive environment for their children and adolescents. Between 1995 and 2020, the number of young people under 18 years old will increase by an estimated 13 percent, from 69 million to 78 million (Bureau of the Census 1996). The framework for community-level physical activity programs for young people is already in place: millions of American youths participate in sports sponsored by community leagues, religious organizations, social service organizations, and schools. In addition to organized sports, communities need to provide recreational programs and opportunities for all young people in a community, because such programs may encourage a lifetime habit of physical activity as well as other immediate community benefits. According to The Trust for Public Land, arrests among young people in one community decreased by 28 percent

after the community instituted an academic and recreational support program for teenagers (National Park Service 1994). In another community, juvenile crime dropped 55 percent when community recreational facilities stayed open until 2 a.m. (National Park Service 1994).

Communities will also need to meet the challenges of a growing population of older adults. Between 1995 and 2020, the number of people over the age of 60 will increase by 43 percent, from 44 to 63 million (Bureau of the Census 1996). Programs and facilities designed to meet the needs of aging baby boomers and older adults can help ensure that these rapidly growing segments of the population obtain the health benefits of regular, moderate physical activity. In one community, 35 age-peer exercise instructors for older adults were recruited and trained by a local university as volunteers to conduct age-appropriate physical activity programs on a regular basis at sites such as libraries, senior centers, and nursing homes in their neighborhoods. Because they were age peers, the instructors were sensitive to many of the concerns that older adults had about physical activity, such as fear of falling and fracturing a hip. Over the following year, instructors conducted more than 1,500 half-hour exercise programs for more than 500 older adults at 20 sites (DiGilio, Howze, Shack 1992 ).

Places of worship represent a potentially effective site for physical activity promotion programs in communities, since these settings can provide the impetus for starting—and the social support for maintaining—behavioral regimens (Eng, Hatch, Callan 1985; Eng and Hatch 1991) such as regular physical activity. Among the advantages of such settings are a history of participating in a range of community health and social projects; large memberships, including families; a presence in virtually every U.S. community; and connections to minority and low-income communities typically underserved by health promotion programs (King 1991). The Fitness Through Churches Project promoted aerobic exercise in conjunction with other health behaviors to African American residents of Durham, North Carolina (Hatch et al. 1986). The results from this pilot program suggest that physical activity programs offered at places of worship are feasible and attractive to clergy and their congregations. Another project, the Health and Religion Project (HARP) of

Rhode Island (Lasater et al. 1986), found that volunteers can be trained to provide heart health programs, including physical activity, in church settings (DePue et al. 1990).

## Societal Barriers

The major barrier to physical activity is the age in which we live. In the past, most activities of daily living involved significant expenditures of energy. In contrast, the overarching goal of modern technology has been to reduce this expenditure through the production of devices and services explicitly designed to obviate physical labor. From the days of hunting and gathering to turn-of-the-century farming practices and early industrial labor, the process of earning a living was once a strenuous activity. Today, many Americans engage in little or no physical activity in the course of a working day typically spent sitting at a desk or standing at a counter or cash register. A large part of many people's time is spent inside buildings where elevators or escalators are prominent features and stairs are difficult to find and may seem unsafe. Motorized transportation carries millions of Americans to and from work and on almost every errand. These inactive daily expeditions occur virtually door-to-door, with the help of parking lots built as near to destinations as possible to minimize walking and increase convenience and safety. Whereas older cities and towns were built on the assumption that stores and services would be within walking distance of local residents, the design of most new residential areas reflects the supposition that people will drive from home to most destinations. Thus work, home, and shopping are often separated by distances that not only discourage walking but may even necessitate commuting by motorized transportation.

Television viewing, video games, and computer use have contributed substantially to the amount of time people spend in sedentary pursuits (President's Council on Physical Fitness and Sports and Sporting Goods Manufacturers Association 1993). Next to sleeping, watching TV occupies the greatest amount of leisure time during childhood (Dietz 1990). Preschoolers exhibit the highest rate of TV watching (27–28 hours per week). By the time a person graduates from high school, he or she will likely have spent 15,000–18,000 hours in front of a television—and 12,000 hours in school (Strasburger 1992).

In the face of these powerful societal inducements to be inactive, efforts must be made to encourage physical activity within the course of the day and to create environments in communities, schools, and workplaces that afford maximum opportunity to be active. Policy interventions can address public concerns about safety, financial costs, and access to indoor and outdoor facilities. Such interventions also can address the concerns of employers and governments about liability in the event of injury. At the state and local level, governments determine building codes and public safety, traffic, and zoning statutes that have potential bearing on physical activity opportunities in communities.

Concerns about crime can be a major barrier to physical activity for both adults and young people. In a national survey of parents, 46 percent believed their neighborhood was not very safe from crime for their children (Princeton Survey Research Associates 1994). Minority parents were about half as likely as white parents to report that their neighborhoods were safe. Successful implementation of policy interventions may help address such concerns. For example, decisions to put more police on a beat in a high-crime area may help residents feel safer going outside to walk. Similarly, neighborhood watch groups formed to increase safety and reduce crime may be a vehicle for promoting physical activity. Opening schools for community recreation and malls for walking can provide safe and all-weather venues that enable all members of the community to be active.

Transportation, health, and community planners as well as private citizens can help ensure that children living in areas near schools can safely walk or bike to school and that adults can walk or bike to work. Fear of traffic is one of the most frequently cited reasons for not bicycling (USDOT 1993). Adult pedestrians and bicyclists account for 14 percent of yearly traffic fatalities (USDOT 1994). In a survey of adults, those who rode a bicycle in the preceding year were asked whether they would commute to work by bicycle under specific conditions. Fifty-three percent said they would do so if safe, separate, designated paths existed; 47 percent would if their employer offered financial or other incentives; 46 percent would if safe bike lanes were available; and 45 percent would if their workplace had showers, lockers, and a secure area for bike storage (USDOT 1994). More than half the respondents indicated they would walk, or walk more, if there were safe pathways (protected from automobile hazards) and if crime were not a consideration. A majority also wanted their local government to provide better opportunities to walk and bicycle.

These percentages stand in sharp relief against current practice: only 4.5 percent of Americans commute to work by bicycle or on foot (USDOT 1994). Even in such comparatively small numbers, these people are estimated to save as much as 1.3 billion gallons of gasoline yearly and to prevent 16.3 million metric tons of exhaust emissions (USDOT 1994). Every mile walked or cycled for transportation saves 5 to 22 cents that would have been spent for a mile by automobile, including reduced cost from pollution and oil imports (USDOT 1994). The Intermodal Surface Transportation Efficiency Act, passed in 1991, promotes alternatives to automobile use by making funds available for states to construct or improve bicycling facilities and pedestrian walkways (USDOT 1993). Decisions on how these funds are used are made locally, and organizations such as local transportation, health, and parks departments can promote the use of these funds in ways that increase the prevalence of physical activity in their communities.

In a growing number of communities, concerns about environmental quality have led to zoning restrictions that protect open spaces and other areas that can subsequently be used for recreational pursuits. Such greenways, or linear open space, can connect neighborhoods and foster the use of bicycling and walking for transportation (Indianapolis Department of Parks and Recreation 1994).

## Societal Resources

Although there is no comprehensive listing of physical activity resources in the United States, such a document would be extensive. Millions of Americans have sports supplies, bicycles, and exercise machines in their homes or have access to public and private resources such as tennis courts, parks, playgrounds, and health clubs. Numerous organizations promote physical activity as part of their mission or in fund-raising efforts such as walks or runs. In addition, TV programs, magazines, books, videos, and CD-ROMs on physical activity are marketed. Although using a computer is a sedentary activity, physical activity interest and advocacy groups are on the Internet, and the World Wide Web contains information about many organizations and resources related to physical activity. The multitude of physical education teachers, aerobics instructors, dance instructors, recreation leaders, coaches, and personal trainers constitute an energetic pool of physical activity advocates and role models.

Ensuring the availability and accessibility of environments and facilities conducive to exercise is central to seeing that the public has the opportunity to obtain regular physical activity. Facilities should be convenient, affordable, comfortable, and safe (King et al. 1992). Many communities offer sufficient facilities, but unless they are also accessible and affordable, people may not use them (Sallis et al. 1990). Walking for exercise needs no more equipment than a comfortable pair of shoes, but it does require a safe environment. Other activities vary widely in the resources they require—specialized clothing and equipment, playgrounds, bicycle lanes, swimming pools, fields for outdoor games, courts for indoor games, fitness facilities for weight lifting and aerobic exercise, studios for dancing, to mention a few.

Proximity of resources to home or worksites is particularly important (Sallis et al. 1990). In a telephone survey, 72 percent of respondents indicated that there was a park or playground within walking distance of their home, and 75 percent of these persons had used them (Godbey et al. 1992). Rural residents are less likely to have such access (Godbey et al.1992), but they may have open spaces of other kinds. In addition, large indoor areas, such as shopping malls and schools, have become popular venues for individuals and for walking groups and clubs. In some communities, schools stay open before or after the school day so community residents can use them for hall walking (King, Jeffery, et al. 1995). Results from a survey of exercise facilities in San Diego, California, suggest that schools may be the most available yet least-used resource for physical activity among community residents (Sallis et al. 1990).

## Summary

The scope, quality, and effectiveness of the wide range of policies and programs described in this section have the potential to foster more physically active lifestyles in the U.S. population. These efforts could be targeted to meet the needs of population subgroups and could be designed to use effective strategies. Public health goals for physical activity and fitness are more likely to be achieved if policies and programs are guided by approaches known to be effective and tailored to meet the needs of all members of the community. Policies and programs should be periodically evaluated to learn how they can be improved to promote physical activity.

The discussion of existing barriers and resources makes it clear that attention should be given to addressing not only the challenges of individual behavior change but also the environmental barriers that inhibit a populationwide transition from a sedentary to an active lifestyle. Expenditure of resources for bike paths, parks, programs, and law enforcement to make playgrounds and streets safer will encourage physical activity in daily living and should thus be viewed as contributing to the health of all Americans. At the same time, evaluations of such changes can occur and more research accordingly conducted to clarify how much the availability of community spaces, facilities, and programs might encourage physical activity. Such information would better inform specific public policy decisions about providing environmental supports and resources to promote physical activity.

Behavioral and social scientists, exercise specialists, recreation specialists, health professionals, architects, city planners, and engineers—all these disciplines need to work together to engage communities, schools, and worksites in creating opportunities and removing barriers to physical activity. To create lasting behavior change in communities, policies as well as individuals must change. Interventions that simultaneously influence individuals, community organizations, and government policies should lead to greater and longer-lasting changes.

# Chapter Summary

This chapter has reviewed approaches taken by researchers to understand and encourage physical activity among adults, children, and adolescents living in a technologically advanced society. Behavioral and social science research on physical activity is a relatively recent endeavor, and many questions remain to be answered about not only increasing but also sustaining physical activity. Several factors seem to be key influences on physical activity levels for both adults and young people. Having confidence in one's ability to be active (self-efficacy); enjoying physical activity; receiving support from family, friends, or peers; and perceiving that the benefits of physical activity outweigh its barriers or costs appear to be central determining factors influencing activity levels across the life span.

For adults, some interventions in communities, in health care settings, in worksites, and at home have resulted in small increases in physical activity, which if widely applied could create significant public health benefits. Among young people, school-based programs are the most widely available resource for promoting physical activity and have the potential for reaching large numbers of children and adolescents. Research indicates that children's levels of physical activity in physical education class are greater when physical education teachers are specially trained in methods to increase the time their students spend engaging in moderate-to-vigorous physical activity. Few studies, however, have been conducted at middle and high school levels—a time when most adolescents decrease their physical activity.

Only limited information exists about the needs of population subgroups of all ages and how determinants of physical activity may change over the life span because of puberty, the normal aging process, health conditions, type of occupation, and other biological, social, and environmental influences. Effective approaches for weight gain prevention are few, especially in light of the recently observed trend of increasing weight among U.S. adults and children (Kuczmarski et al. 1994; Troiano et al. 1995). Although recommendations given by health care providers can increase physical activity among adults, a similar effect of counseling for children and adolescents has not been examined. It is unclear what approaches can help people recover from relapses into inactivity—whether from illness, the weather, demands at work or at home, or other reasons—and sustain the habit of regular physical activity over time. Questions also remain about how to address barriers to physical activity and how to more effectively use resources in communities, schools, and worksites to increase physical activity. Recent research and promising approaches have begun to address some of these questions and provide direction for future research and interventions to promote physical activity among all Americans.

## Conclusions

1. Consistent influences on physical activity patterns among adults and young people include confidence in one's ability to engage in regular physical activity (e.g., self-efficacy), enjoyment of physical activity, support from others, positive beliefs concerning the benefits of physical activity, and lack of perceived barriers to being physically active.

2. For adults, some interventions have been successful in increasing physical activity in communities, worksites, health care settings, and at home.

3. Interventions targeting physical education in elementary school can substantially increase the amount of time students spend being physically active in physical education class.

## Research Needs

### Determinants of Physical Activity

1. Assess the determinants of various patterns of physical activity among those who are sedentary, intermittently active, routinely active at work, and regularly active.

2. Assess determinants of physical activity for various population subgroups (e.g., by age, sex, race/ethnicity, socioeconomic status, health/disability status, geographic location).

3. Examine patterns and determinants of physical activity at various developmental and life transitions, such as from school to work, from one job or city to another, from work to retirement, and from health to chronic illness.

4. Evaluate the interactive effects of psychosocial, cultural, environmental, and public policy influences on physical activity.

### Physical Activity Interventions

1. Develop and evaluate the effectiveness of interventions that include policy and environmental supports.

2. Develop and evaluate interventions designed to promote adoption and maintenance of moderate physical activity that addresses the specific needs and circumstances of population subgroups, such as racial/ethnic groups, men and women, girls and boys, the elderly, the disabled, the overweight, low-income groups, and persons at life transitions, such as adolescence, early adulthood, family formation, and retirement.

3. Develop and evaluate the effectiveness of interventions to promote physical activity in combination with healthy dietary practices that can be broadly disseminated to reach large segments of the population and can be sustained over time.

## References

Ajzen I. *Attitudes, personality, and behavior.* Chicago: Dorsey Press, 1988.

Ajzen I. From intentions to actions: a theory of planned behavior. In: Kuhl J, Beckman J, editors. *Action-control: from cognition to behavior.* New York: Springer, 1985:11–39.

Ajzen I, Fishbein M. *Understanding attitudes and predicting social behavior.* Englewood Cliffs, NJ: Prentice-Hall, 1980.

Ali NS, Twibell RK. Health promotion and osteoporosis prevention among postmenopausal women. *Preventive Medicine* 1995;24:528–534.

American Academy of Pediatrics, Committee on Sports Medicine and Fitness. Assessing physical activity and fitness in the office setting. *Pediatrics* 1994;93:686–689.

American Medical Association, Elster AB, Kuznets NJ. *AMA guidelines for adolescent preventive services (GAPS): recommendations and rationale.* Baltimore: Williams and Wilkins, 1994.

Anderssen N, Wold B. Parental and peer influences on leisure-time physical activity in young adolescents. *Research Quarterly for Exercise and Sport* 1992;63:341–348.

Atkins CJA, Robert M. Behavioral exercise programs in the management of chronic obstructive pulmonary disease. *Journal of Consulting and Clinical Psychology* 1984;52:591–603.

Bandura A. Self-efficacy: toward a unifying theory of behavioral change. *Psychological Review* 1977a;84:191–215.

Bandura A. *Social foundations of thought and action: a social-cognitive theory*. Englewood Cliffs, NJ: Prentice-Hall, 1986.

Bandura A. *Social learning theory*. Englewood Cliffs, NJ: Prentice-Hall, 1977b.

Baranowski T, Simons-Morton B, Hooks P, Henske J, Tiernan K, Dunn JK, et al. A center-based program for exercise change among Black-American families. *Health Education Quarterly* 1990;17:179–196.

Becker MH, editor. The health belief model and personal health behavior. *Health Education Monographs* 1974;2:324–373.

Belisle M. Improving adherence to physical activity. *Health Psychology* 1987:6:159–172.

Bezold C, Carlson RJ, Peck JC. *The future of work and health*. Dover, MA: Auburn House Publishing, 1986.

Biddle S, Armstrong N. Children's physical activity: an exploratory study of psychological correlates. *Social Science and Medicine* 1992;34:325–331.

Biddle S, Goudas M. Analysis of children's physical activity and its association with adult encouragement and social cognitive variables. *Journal of School Health* 1996;66:75–78.

Blair SN, Piserchia PV, Wilbur CS, Crowder JH. A public health intervention model for worksite health promotion: impact on exercise and physical fitness in a health promotion plan after 24 months. *Journal of the American Medical Association* 1986;255:921–926.

Blamey A, Mutrie N, Aitchison T. Health promotion by encouraged use of stairs. *British Medical Journal* 1995;311:289–290.

Booth M, Bauman A, Oldenburg B, Owen N, Magnus P. Effects of a national mass-media campaign on physical activity participation. *Health Promotion International* 1992;7:241–247.

Booth ML, Macaskill P, Owen N, Oldenburg B, Marcus BH, Bauman A. Population prevalence and correlates of stages of change in physical activity. *Health Education Quarterly* 1993;20:431–440.

Borra ST, Schwartz NE, Spain CG, Natchipolsky MM. Food, physical activity, and fun: inspiring America's kids to more healthful lifestyles. *Journal of the American Dietetic Association* 1995;7:816–818.

Brownell KD, Marlatt AG, Lichtenstein E, Wilson GT. Understanding and preventing relapse. *American Psychologist* 1986;41;765–782.

Brownell KD, Stunkard AJ, Albaum JM. Evaluation and modification of exercise patterns in the natural environment. *American Journal of Psychiatry* 1980;137:1540–1545.

Brownson RC, Smith CA, Pratt M, Mack NE, Jackson-Thompson J, Dean CG, et al. Preventing cardiovascular disease through community-based risk reduction: the Bootheel Heart Health Project. *American Journal of Public Health* 1996;86:206–213.

Bureau of the Census. *Current population reports: population projections of the United States by age, sex, race, and Hispanic origin: 1995–2050*. Washington, DC: U.S. Department of Commerce, Economics and Statistics Administration, Bureau of the Census, 1996.

Burk C, Kimiecik J. Examining the relationship among locus of control, value, and exercise. *Health Values* 1994;18:14–23.

Bush PJ, Zuckerman AE, Taggart VS, Theiss PK, Peleg EO, Smith SA. Cardiovascular risk factor prevention in black schoolchildren: the Know Your Body evaluation project. *Health Education Quarterly* 1989;16:215–227.

Bush PJ, Zuckerman AE, Theiss PK, Taggart VS, Horowitz C, Sheridan MJ, et al. Cardiovascular risk factor prevention in black schoolchildren: two-year results of the Know Your Body program. *American Journal of Epidemiology* 1989;129:466–482.

Butcher J. Longitudinal analysis of adolescent girls' participation in physical activity. *Sociology of Sport Journal* 1985;2:130–143.

Calfas KJ, Long BJ, Sallis JF, Wooten WJ, Pratt M, Patrick K. A controlled trial of physician counseling to promote the adoption of physical activity. *Preventive Medicine* (in press).

Calfas KJ, Sallis JF, Lovato CY, Campbell J. Physical activity and its determinants before and after college graduation. *Medicine, Exercise, Nutrition, and Health* 1994;3:323–334.

Canadian Task Force on the Periodic Health Examination. *The Canadian guide to clinical preventive health care*. Ottawa, Canada: Canada Communication Group, 1994.

Cardinal BJ, Sachs ML. Prospective analysis of stage-of-exercise movement following mail-delivered, self-instructional exercise packets. *American Journal of Health Promotion* 1995;9:430–432.

Carleton RA, Lasater TM, Assaf AR, Feldman HA, McKinlay S, Pawtucket Heart Health Program Writing Group. The Pawtucket Heart Health Program: community changes in cardiovascular risk factors and projected disease risk. *American Journal of Public Health* 1995;85:777–785.

Centers for Disease Control and Prevention. Guidelines for school and community health programs to promote physical activity among youth. Atlanta: U.S. Department of Health and Human Services, Public Health Service, Centers for Disease Control and Prevention. *Morbidity and Mortality Weekly Report* (in press).

Centers for Disease Control and Prevention. Guidelines for school health programs to promote lifelong healthy eating. *Morbidity and Mortality Weekly Report* 1996;45 (No. RR-9):1–42.

Centers for Disease Control. *Promoting physical activity among adults; a CDC community intervention handbook*. Atlanta: U.S. Department of Health and Human Services, Public Health Service, Centers for Disease Control,1988.

Centers for Disease Control and Prevention. Worksite and community health promotion/risk reduction project-Virginia, 1987–1991. *Morbidity and Mortality Weekly Report* 1992;41:55–57.

Collins JL, Small ML, Kann L, Pateman BC, Gold RS, Kolbe LJ. School health education. *Journal of School Health* 1995;65:302–311.

Courneya KS. Understanding readiness for regular physical activity in older individuals: an application of the theory of planned behavior. *Health Psychology* 1995;14:80–87.

Courneya KS, McAuley E. Are there different determinants of the frequency, intensity, and duration of physical activity? *Behavioral Medicine* 1994;20:84–90.

Courneya KS, McAuley E. Cognitive mediators of the social influence-exercise adherence relationship: a test of the theory of planned behavior. *Journal of Behavioral Medicine* 1995;18:499–515.

Crow R, Blackburn H, Jacobs D, Hannan P, Pirie P, Mittelmark M, et al. Population strategies to enhance physical activity: the Minnesota Heart Health Program. *Acta Medica Scandinavica Supplementum* 1986;711:93–112.

Dempsey JM, Kimiecik JC, Horn TS. Parental influence on children's moderate to vigorous physical activity participation: an expectancy-value approach. *Pediatric Exercise Science* 1993;5:151–167.

DePue JD, Wells BL, Lasater TM, Carleton RA. Volunteers as providers of heart health programs in churches: a report on implementation. *American Journal of Health Promotion* 1990;4:361–366.

Desmond AW, Conrad KM, Montgomery A, Simon KA. Factors associated with male workers' engagement in physical activity. *AAOHN Journal* 1993;41:73–83.

Dietz WH. Children and television. In: Green M, Hagerty RJ, editors. *Ambulatory pediatrics* IV. Philadelphia: W.B. Saunders, 1990:39–41.

DiGilio DA, Howze EA, Schack FK. The cost-effectiveness of peer-led exercise programs. In: Harris S, Harris R, Harris WS, editors. *Physical activity, aging, and sports. Vol. 2. Practice, program, and policy*. Albany, NY: Center for the Study of Aging, 1992:226–231.

Dishman RK. Increasing and maintaining exercise and physical activity. *Behavior Therapy* 1991;22:345–378.

Dishman RK, Steinhardt M. Health locus of control predicts free-living, but not supervised, physical activity: a test of exercise-specific control and outcome-expectancy hypotheses. *Research Quarterly for Exercise and Sport* 1990;61:383–394.

Donovan RJ, Owen N. Social marketing and population interventions. In: Dishman RK, editor. *Advances in exercise adherence*. Champaign, IL: Human Kinetics, 1994:249–290.

DuCharme KA, Brawley LR. Predicting the intentions and behavior of exercise initiates using two forms of self-efficacy. *Journal of Behavioral Medicine* 1995;18:479–497.

Duffy ME, MacDonald E. Determinants of functional health of older persons. *Gerontologist* 1990;30:503–509.

Duncan HH, Travis SS, McAuley WJ. An emergent theoretical model for interventions encouraging physical activity (mall walking) among older adults. *Journal of Applied Gerontology* 1995;34:64–77.

Duncan TE, McAuley E. Social support and efficacy cognitions in exercise adherence: a latent growth curve analysis. *Journal of Behavioral Medicine* 1993;16:199–218.

Dwyer T, Coonan WE, Leitch DR, Hetzel BS, Baghurst RA. An investigation of the effects of daily physical activity on the health of primary school students in South Australia. *International Journal of Epidemiology* 1983;12:308–313.

## Physical Activity and Health

Dwyer T, Coonan WE, Worsley A, Leitch DR. An assessment of the effects of two physical activity programmes on coronary heart disease risk factors in primary school children. *Community Health Studies* 1979;III:196–202.

Eaton CB, Reynes J, Assaf AR, Feldman H, Lasater T, Carleton RA. Predicting physical activity change in men and women in two New England communities. *American Journal of Preventive Medicine* 1993;9: 209–219.

Edmundson E, Parcel GS, Perry CL, Feldman HA, Smyth M, Johnson CC, et al. The effects of the Child and Adolescent Trial for Cardiovascular Health intervention on psychosocial determinants of cardiovascular disease risk behavior among third-grade students. *American Journal of Health Promotion* 1996;10:217–225.

Elward K, Larson E, Wagner E. Factors associated with regular aerobic exercise in an elderly population. *Journal of the American Board of Family Practice* 1992;5: 467–474.

Eng E, Hatch J, Callan A. Institutionalizing social support through the church and into the community. *Health Education Quarterly* 1985;12:81–92.

Eng E, Hatch JW. Networking between agencies and black churches: the lay health advisor model. *Prevention in Human Services* 1991;10:123–146.

Epstein LH, McCurley J, Wing RR, Valoski A. Five-year follow-up of family-based behavioral treatments for childhood obesity. *Journal of Consulting and Clinical Psychology* 1990;58:661–664.

Epstein LH, Valoski A, Wing RR, McCurley J. Ten-year follow-up of behavioral, family-based treatment for obese children. *Journal of the American Medical Association* 1990;264:2519–2523.

Epstein LH, Valoski A, Wing RR, McCurley J. Ten-year outcomes of behavioral family-based treatment for childhood obesity. *Health Psychology* 1994;13: 373–383.

Epstein LH, Wing RR, Valoski A. Childhood obesity. *Pediatric Clinics of North America* 1985;32:363–379.

Errecart MT, Ross JG, Robb W, Warren CW, Kann L, Collins JL, et al. Methodology. *Journal of School Health* 1995;65:295–301.

Farquhar JW, Foartmann SP, Flora JA, Taylor CB, Haskell WL, Williams PT, Maccoby N, Wood PD. Effects of communitywide education on cardiovascular disease risk factors; the Stanford Five-City Project. *Journal of the American Medical Association* 1990;264:359–365.

Felton GM, Parsons MA. Factors influencing physical activity in average-weight and overweight young women. *Journal of Community Health Nursing* 1994;11:109–119.

Ferguson KJ, Yesalis CE, Pomrehn PR, Kirkpatrick MB. Attitudes, knowledge, and beliefs as predictors of exercise intent and behavior in schoolchildren. *Journal of School Health* 1989;59:112–115.

Fishbein M, Ajzen I. *Belief, attitude, intention, and behavior: an introduction to theory and research.* Boston: Addison-Wesley, 1975.

Fletcher GF, Blair SN, Blumenthal J, Caspersen C, Chaitman B, Epstein S, et al. Benefits and recommendations for physical activity programs for all Americans. A statement for health professionals by the Committee on Exercise and Cardiac Rehabilitation of the Council on Clinical Cardiology, American Heart Association. *Circulation* 1992;96:340–344.

Flora JA, Maccoby N, Farguhar JW. Communication campaign to prevent cardiovascular disease: the Stanford Community Studies. In: Rice RD, Atkin, CK, editors. *Public communication campaigns.* 2nd ed. Newbury Park, CA: Sage Publications 1989:233–252.

Fries JF, Bloch DA, Harrington H, Richardson N, Beck R. Two-year results of a randomized controlled trial of a health promotion program in a retiree population: the Bank of America study. *American Journal of Medicine* 1993;94:455–462.

Frost H, Moffett JAK, Moser JS, Fairbank JCT. Randomised controlled trial for evaluation of fitness programme for patients with chronic low back pain. *British Medical Journal* 1995;310:151–154.

Glanz K, Rimer BK. *Theory at a glance: a guide for health promotion practice.* Bethesda, MD: U.S. Department of Health and Human Services, Public Health Service, National Institutes of Health, National Cancer Institute, July 1995.

Garcia AW, Broda MAN, Frenn M, Coviak C, Pender NJ, Ronis DL. Gender and developmental differences in exercise beliefs among youth and prediction of their exercise behavior. *Journal of School Health* 1995;65: 213–219.

Godbey G, Graefe A, James SW. *The benefits of local recreation and park services: a nationwide study of the perceptions of the American public.* Arlington, VA: National Recreation and Park Association, 1992.

Godin G, Desharnais R, Valois P, Bradet R. Combining behavioral and motivational dimensions to identify and characterize the stages in the process of adherence to exercise. *Psychology and Health* 1995;10:333–344.

Godin G, Shephard RJ. Psychosocial factors influencing intentions to exercise of young students from grades 7 to 9. *Research Quarterly for Exercise and Sport* 1986;57:41–52.

Godin G, Desharnais R, Jobin J, Cook J. The impact of physical fitness and health-age appraisal upon exercise intentions and behavior. *Journal of Behavioral Medicine* 1987;10:241–250.

Godin G, Valois P, Jobin J, Ross A. Prediction of intention to exercise of individuals who have suffered from coronary heart disease. *Journal of Clinical Psychology* 1991;47:762–772.

Godin G, Valois P, Lepage L. The pattern of influence of perceived behavioral control upon exercising behavior: an application of Ajzen's theory of planned behavior. *Journal of Behavioral Medicine* 1993;16:81–102.

Gossard D, Haskell WL, Taylor CB, Mueller JK, Rogers F, Chandler M, et al. Effects of low- and high-intensity home-based exercise training on functional capacity in healthy middle-aged men. *American Journal of Cardiology* 1986;57:446–449.

Gottlieb NH, Chen M. Sociocultural correlates of childhood sporting activities: their implications for heart health. *Social Science and Medicine* 1985;21:533–539.

Green LW, Simons-Morton DG. Education and life-style determinants of health and disease. In: Holland WW, Detels R, Knox G, editors. *Oxford textbook of public health.* 2nd ed. Vol. I: *Influences of public health.* New York: Oxford University Press, 1996:181–195.

Greenan-Fowler E, Powell C, Varni JW. Behavioral treatment of adherence to therapeutic exercise by children with hemophilia. *Archives of Physical Medicine and Rehabilitation* 1987;68:846–849.

Hatch JW, Cunningham AC, Woods WW, Snipes FC. The Fitness Through Churches project: description of a community-based cardiovascular health promotion intervention. *Hygie* 1986;5:9–12.

Hawkes JM, Holm K. Gender differences in exercise determinants. *Nursing Research* 1993;42:166–172.

Heath GW, Leonard BE, Wilson RH, Kendrick JS, Powell KE. Community-based exercise intervention: Zuni Diabetes Project. *Diabetes Care* 1987;10:579–583.

Heath GW, Wilson RH, Smith J, Leonard BE. Community-based exercise and weight control: diabetes risk reduction and glycemic control in Zuni Indians. *American Journal of Clinical Nutrition* 1991;53:1642S–1646S.

Heirich MA, Foote A, Erfurt JC, Konopka B. Work-site physical fitness programs: comparing the impact of different program designs on cardiovascular risks. *Journal of Occupational Medicine* 1993;35:510–517.

Hochbaum GM. *Public participation in medical screening programs: a sociopsychological study.* Washington, DC: U.S. Public Health Service, 1958. Publication No. (PHS)572.

Hofstetter CR, Hovell MF, Macera C, Sallis JF, Spry V, Barrington E, et al. Illness, injury, and correlates of aerobic exercise and walking: a community study. *Research Quarterly for Exercise and Sport* 1991;62:1–9.

Horne TE. Predictors of physical activity intentions and behaviour for rural homemakers. *Canadian Journal of Public Health* 1994;85:132–135.

Hovell MF, Barrington E, Hofstetter R, Sallis JF, Rauh M, Black D. Correlates of physical activity in overweight and not overweight persons: an assessment. *Perspectives in Practice* 1990;90:1260.

Hovell M, Sallis J, Hofstetter R, Barrington E, Hackley M, Elder J, et al. Identification of correlates of physical activity among Latino adults. *Journal of Community Health* 1991;16:23–36.

Howze EH, Smith M, DiGilio DA. Factors affecting the adoption of exercise behavior among sedentary older adults. *Health Education Research, Theory and Practice* 1989;4:173–180.

Indianapolis Department of Parks and Recreation. *Indianapolis greenways plan.* Indianapolis: Indianapolis Department of Parks and Recreation, 1994.

Israel BA, Schurman SJ. Social support, control, and the stress process. In: Glanz K, Lewis FM, Rimer BK, editors. *Health behavior and health education: theory, research, and practice.* San Francisco: Jossey-Bass Publishers, 1990:187–215.

Jeffery RW. Community programs for obesity prevention: the Minnesota Heart Health Program. *Obesity Research* 1995;3 Supplement:283s–288s.

Kann L, Collins JL, Pateman BC, Small ML, Ross JC, Kolbe LJ. The School Health Policies and Programs Study (SHPPS): rationale for a nationwide status report on school health programs. *Journal of School Health* 1995; 65:291–294.

## Physical Activity and Health

Kelder SH, Perry CL, Klepp KI. Community-wide youth exercise promotion: long-term outcomes of the Minnesota Heart Health Program and the Class of 1989 Study. *Journal of School Health* 1993;63:218–223.

Kelder SH, Perry CL, Peters RJ Jr, Lytle LL, Klepp KI. Gender differences in the Class of 1989 Study: the school component of the Minnesota Heart Health Program. *Journal of Health Education* 1995;26 (Supplement):S36–S44.

Killen JD, Telch MJ, Robinson TN, Maccoby N, Taylor CB, Farquhar JW. Cardiovascular disease risk reduction for tenth graders: a multiple-factor school-based approach. *Journal of the American Medical Association* 1988;260:1728–1733.

Kimiecik J. Predicting vigorous physical activity of corporate employees: comparing the theories of reasoned action and planned behavior. *Journal of Sport and Exercise Psychology* 1992;14:192–206.

King AC. Community intervention for promotion of physical activity and fitness. *Exercise and Sport Sciences Reviews* 1991;19:211–259.

King AC, Blair SN, Bild DE, Dishman RK, Dubbert PM, Marcus BH, et al. Determinants of physical activity and interventions in adults. *Medicine and Science in Sports and Exercise* 1992;24:S221–S223.

King AC, Carl F, Birkel L, Haskell WL. Increasing exercise among blue-collar employees: the tailoring of worksite programs to meet specific needs. *Preventive Medicine* 1988;17:357–365.

King AC, Frederiksen LW. Low-cost strategies for increasing exercise behavior; relapse preparation training and social support. *Behavior Modification* 1984;8:3–21.

King AC, Frey-Hewitt B, Dreon DM, Wood PD. Diet vs exercise in weight maintenance: the effects of minimal intervention strategies on long-term outcomes in men. *Archives of Internal Medicine* 1989;149:2741–2746.

King AC, Haskell WL, Young DR, Oka RK, Stefanick ML. Long-term effects of varying intensities and formats of physical activity on participation rates, fitness, and lipoproteins in men and women aged 50 to 65 years. *Circulation* 1995;91:2596–2604.

King AC, Jeffery RW, Fridinger F, Dusenbury L, Provence S, Hedlund S, et al. Environmental and policy approaches to cardiovascular disease prevention through physical activity: issues and opportunities. *Health Education Quarterly* 1995;22:499–511.

King AC, Taylor CB, Haskell WL, Debusk RF. Strategies for increasing early adherence to and long-term maintenance of home-based exercise training in healthy middle-aged men and women. *American Journal of Cardiology* 1988;61:628–632.

Klesges RC, Coates TJ, Moldenhauer-Klesges LM, Holzer B, Gustavson J, Barnes J. The fats: an observational system for assessing physical activity in children and associated parent behavior. *Behavioral Assessment* 1984;6:333–345.

Klesges RC, Eck LH, Hanson CL, Haddock CK, Klesges LM. Effects of obesity, social interactions, and physical environment on physical activity in preschoolers. *Health Psychology* 1990;9:435–449.

Klesges RC, Malcott JM, Boschee PF, Weber JM. The effects of parental influences on children's food intake, physical activity, and relative weight. *International Journal of Eating Disorders* 1986;5:335–346.

Kuczmarski RJ, Flegal KM, Campbell SM, Johnson CL. Increasing prevalence of overweight among US adults. The National Health and Nutrition Examination Surveys, 1960 to 1991. *Journal of the American Medical Association* 1994;272:205–211.

Lasater TM, Wells BL, Carleton RA, Elder JP. The role of churches in disease prevention research studies. *Public Health Reports* 1986;101:125–131.

Lee C. Attitudes, knowledge, and stages of change: a survey of exercise patterns in older Australian women. *Health Psychology* 1993;12:476–480.

Leonard B, Leonard C, Wilson R. Zuni Diabetes Project. *Public Health Reports* 1986;101:282–288.

Lewis CE, Raczynski JM, Heath GW, Levinson R, Hilyer JC Jr, Cutter GR. Promoting physical activity in low-income African-American communities: the PARR project. *Ethnicity and Disease* 1993;3:106–118.

Logsdon DN, Lazaro CM, Meier RV. The feasibility of behavioral risk reduction in primary medical care. *American Journal of Preventive Medicine* 1989;5:249–256.

Lombard DN, Lombard TN, Winett RA. Walking to meet health guidelines: the effect of prompting frequency and prompt structure. *Health Psychology* 1995;14:164–170.

Luepker RV. Community trials. *Preventive Medicine* 1994;23:602–605.

Luepker RV, Murray DM, Jacobs DR Jr, Mittelmark MB, Bracht N, Carlaw R, et al. Community education for cardiovascular disease prevention: risk factor changes in the Minnesota Heart Health Program. *American Journal of Public Health* 1994;84:1383–1393.

Luepker RV, Perry CL, McKinlay SM, Nader PR, Parcel GS, Stone EJ, et al. Outcomes of a field trial to improve children's dietary patterns and physical activity: the Child and Adolescent Trial for Cardiovascular Health (CATCH). *Journal of the American Medical Association* 1996;275:768–776.

Lynch DJ, Birk TJ, Weaver MT, Gohara AF, Leighton RF, Repka FJ, et al. Adherence to exercise interventions in the treatment of hypercholesterolemia. *Journal of Behavioral Medicine* 1992;15:365–377.

Macera CA, Croft JB, Brown DR, Ferguson JE, Lane MJ. Predictors of adopting leisure-time physical activity among a biracial community cohort. *American Journal of Epidemiology* 1995;142:629–635

Marcus BH, Banspach SW, Lefebvre RC, Rossi JS, Carleton RA, Abrams DB. Using the stages of change model to increase the adoption of physical activity among community participants. *American Journal of Health Promotion* 1992;6:424–429.

Marcus BH, Eaton CA, Rossi JS, Harlow LL. Self-efficacy, decision-making, and stages of change: an integrative model of physical exercise. *Journal of Applied Social Psychology* 1994;24:489–508.

Marcus BH, Owen N. Motivational readiness, self-efficacy, and decision making for exercise. *Journal of Applied Social Psychology* 1992;22:3–16.

Marcus BH, Pinto BM, Simkin LR, Audrain JE, Taylor ER. Application of theoretical models to exercise behavior among employed women. *American Journal of Health Promotion* 1994;9:49–55.

Marcus BH, Rakowski W, Rossi JS. Assessing motivational readiness and decision making for exercise. *Health Psychology* 1992;11:257–261.

Marcus BH, Selby VC, Niaura RS, Rossi JS. Self-efficacy and the stages of exercise behavior change. *Research Quarterly for Exercise and Sport* 1992;63:60–66.

Marcus BH, Stanton AL. Evaluation of relapse prevention and reinforcement interventions to promote exercise adherence in sedentary females. *Research Quarterly for Exercise and Sport* 1993;64:447–452.

Marlatt GA, George WH. Relapse prevention and the maintenance of optimal health In: Shumaker SA, Schron EB, Ockene, editors. *The Handbook of Health Behavior Change*, New York: Springer Publishing Company, 1990: 44–63.

Marlatt GA, Gordon JR. *Relapse prevention: maintenance strategies in the treatment of addictive behaviors.* New York: Guilford Press, 1985.

Mayer JA, Jermanovich A, Wright BL, Elder JP, Drew JA, Williams SJ. Changes in health behaviors of older adults: the San Diego Medicare Preventive Health Project. *Preventive Medicine* 1994;23:127–133.

McAuley E. Efficacy, attributional, and affective responses to exercise participation. *Journal of Sport & Exercise Psychology* 1991;13:382–393.

McAuley E, Courneya KS, Rudolph DL, Lox CL. Enhancing exercise adherence in middle-aged males and females. *Preventive Medicine* 1994;23:498–506.

McAuley E, Lox C, Duncan TE. Long-term maintenance of exercise, self-efficacy, and physiological change in older adults. *Journal of Gerontology* 1993;48:218–224.

McKenzie TL, Feldman H, Woods SE, Romero KA, Dahlstrom V, Stone EJ, et al. Children's activity levels and lesson context during third-grade physical education. *Research Quarterly for Exercise and Sport* 1995;66:184–193.

McKenzie TL, Nader PR, Strikmiller PK, Yang M, Stone EJ, Perry CL, et al. School physical education: effect of the Child and Adolescent Trial for Cardiovascular Health (CATCH). *Preventive Medicine* (in press).

McKenzie TL, Sallis JF, Faucette N, Roby JJ, Kolody B. Effects of a curriculum and inservice program on the quantity and quality of elementary physical education classes. *Research Quarterly for Exercise and Sport* 1993;64:178–187.

McKenzie TL, Sallis JF, Nader PR, Patterson TL, Elder, JP, Berry CC, Ruff JW, Atkins CJ, Buono MJ, Nelson JA. Beaches: an observational system for assessing children's eating and physical activity behavior and associated events. *Journal of Applied Behavior Analysis* 1991; 24: 141–151.

McKenzie TL, Strikmiller PK, Stone EJ, Woods SE, Ehlinger S, Romero KA, et al. CATCH: physical activity process evaluation in a multicenter trial. *Health Education Quarterly* 1994;21(2 Suppl):S73–S89.

McLeroy KR, Bibeau D, Steckler A, Glanz K. An ecological perspective on health promotion programs. *Health Education Quarterly* 1988;15:351–377.

McMurray RB, Bradley CB, Harrell JS, Bernthal PR, Frauman AC, Bangdiwala SI. Parental influences on childhood fitness and activity patterns. *Research Quarterly for Exercise and Sport* 1993;64:249–255.

Minor MA, Brown JD. Exercise maintenance of persons with arthritis after participation in a class experience. *Health Education Quarterly* 1993;20:83–95.

## Physical Activity and Health

Mirotznik J, Feldman L, Stein R. The health belief model and adherence with a community center-based, supervised coronary heart disease exercise program. *Journal of Community Health* 1995;20:233–247.

Mittelmark MB, Luepker RV, Jacobs DR, Bracht NF, Carlaw RW, Crow RS, et al. Community-wide prevention of cardiovascular disease: education strategies of the Minnesota Heart Health Program. *Preventive Medicine* 1986;15:1–17.

Moore LL, Lombardi DA, White MJ, Campbell JL, Oliveria SA, Ellison C. Influence of parents' physical activity levels on activity levels of young children. *Journal of Pediatrics* 1991;118:215–219.

Mullen PD, Tabak ER. Patterns of counseling techniques used by family practice physicians for smoking, weight, exercise, and stress. *Medical Care* 1989;27:694–704.

Nader PR, Sallis JF, Patterson TL, Abramson IS, Rupp JW, Senn KL, et al. A family approach to cardiovascular risk reduction: results from the San Diego Family Health Project. *Health Education Quarterly* 1989;16:229–244.

Nader PR, Taras HL, Sallis JF, Patterson TL. Adult heart disease prevention in childhood: a national survey of pediatricians' practices and attitudes. *Pediatrics* 1987;79:843–850.

National Association for Sport and Physical Education. *Moving into the future: national physical education standards—a guide to content and assessment.* New York: Mosby, 1995.

National Association of Governor's Councils on Physical Fitness and Sports. *Information brochure.* Indianapolis: National Association of Governor's Councils on Physical Fitness and Sports, 1996.

National Center for Health Statistics. *Health, United States, 1990.* Hyattsville, MD: U.S. Department of Health and Human Services, Public Health Service, Centers for Disease Control, National Center for Health Statistics, 1991.

National Center for Health Statistics, Kovar MG, LaCroix AZ. Aging in the eighties: ability to perform work-related activities. Data from the supplement on aging to the National Health Interview Survey: United States, 1984. *Advance data from Vital and Health Statistics, No. 136.* Hyattsville, MD: U.S. Department of Health and Human Services, Public Health Service, National Center for Health Statistics, May 8, 1987. DHHS Publication No. (PHS)87-1250.

National Coalition for Promoting Physical Activity. National Coalition for Promoting Physical Activity sets its sites (sic) on motivating America (press release). May 31, 1995.

National Park Service. *An Americans' network of parks and open space: creating a conservation and recreation legacy.* Washington, DC: U.S. Department of the Interior, National Park Service, National Park System Advisory Board, 1994.

Neuberger GB, Kasal S, Smith KV, Hassanein R, DeViney S. Determinants of exercise and aerobic fitness in outpatients with arthritis. *Nursing Research* 1994;43:11–17.

Oldridge NB, Streiner DL. The health belief model: predicting compliance and dropout in cardiac rehabilitation. *Medicine and Science in Sports and Exercise* 1990;22:678–683.

Orleans CT, George LK, Houpt JL, Brodie KH. Health promotion in primary care: a survey of U.S. family practitioners. *Preventive Medicine* 1985;14:636–647.

Osler M, Jespersen NB. The effect of a community-based cardiovascular disease prevention project in a Danish municipality. *Danish Medical Bulletin* 1993;40:485–489.

Owen N, Bauman A, Booth M, Oldenburg B, Magnus P. Serial mass-media campaigns to promote physical activity: reinforcing or redundant? *American Journal of Public Health* 1995;85:244–248.

Owen N, Lee C, Naccarella L, Haag K. Exercise by mail: a mediated behavior-change program for aerobic exercise. *Journal of Sport Psychology* 1987;9:346–357.

Parcel GS, Simons-Morton BG, O'Hara NM, Baranowski T, Kolbe LJ, Bee DE. School promotion of healthful diet and exercise behavior: an integration of organizational change and social learning theory interventions. *Journal of School Health* 1987;57:150–156.

Pate RR, Pratt M, Blair SN, Haskell WL, Macera CA, Bouchard C, et al. Physical activity and public health: a recommendation from the Centers for Disease Control and Prevention and the American College of Sports Medicine. *Journal of the American Medical Association* 1995;273:402–407.

Pate RR, Small ML, Ross JG, Young JC, Flint KH, Warren CW. School physical education. *Journal of School Health* 1995;65:312–318.

Perri MG, McAllister DA, Gange JJ, Jordan RC, McAdoo WG, Nezu AM. Effects of four maintenance programs on the long-term management of obesity. *Journal of Consulting and Clinical Psychology* 1988;56:529–534.

Perry CL, Parcel GS, Stone E, Nader P, McKinlay SM, Luepker RV, Webber LS. The Child and Adolescent Trial for Cardiovascular Health (CATCH): overview of the intervention program and evaluation methods. *Cardiovascular Risk Factors* 1992;2:36–44.

Perry CL, Stone EJ, Parcel GS, Ellison RC, Nader PR, Webber LS, et al. School-based cardiovascular health promotion: the Child and Adolescent Trial for Cardiovascular Health (CATCH). *Journal of School Health* 1990;60:406–413.

Perusse L, Tremblay A, Leblanc C, Bouchard C. Genetic and environment influences on level of habitual physical activity and exercise participation. *American Journal of Epidemiology* 1989;129:1012–1022.

Poag-DuCharme KA, Brawley LR. Self-efficacy theory: use in the prediction of exercise behavior in the community setting. *Journal of Applied Sport Psychology* 1993;5:178–194.

Poest CA, Williams JR, Witt DD, Atwood ME. Physical activity patterns of preschool children. *Early Childhood Research Quarterly* 1989;4:367–376.

Ponichtera-Mulcare JA. Exercise and multiple sclerosis. *Medicine and Science in Sports and Exercise* 1993;25:451–465.

Powell KE, Dysinger W. Childhood participation in organized school sports as precursors of adult physical activity. *American Journal of Preventive Medicine* 1987;3:276–281.

President's Council on Physical Fitness. *The physician's Rx: exercise.* Washington, DC: President's Council on Physical Fitness and Sports, 1992.

President's Council on Physical Fitness and Sports and Sporting Goods Manufacturers Association. *American attitudes toward physical activity and fitness: a national survey.* Washington, DC: President's Council on Physical Fitness and Sports, 1993.

Princeton Survey Research Associates. Prevention magazines children's health index. *Prevention* 1994 Sep.

Prochaska JO, DiClemente CC. *The transtheoretical approach: crossing traditional boundaries of change.* Homewood, IL: Dorsey Press, 1984.

Prochaska JO, DiClemente CC. Transtheoretical therapy: toward a more integrative model of change. *Psychotherapy: Theory, Research, and Practice* 1982;20:161–173.

Prochaska JO, DiClemente CC, Norcross JC. In search of how people change: applications to addictive behaviors. *American Psychologist* 1992;47:1102–1114.

Resnicow K, Cohn L, Reinhardt J, Cross D, Futterman R, Kirschner E, et al. A three-year evaluation of the Know Your Body program in inner-city schoolchildren. *Health Education Quarterly* 1992;19:463–480.

Reynolds KD, Killen JD, Bryson SW, Maron DJ, Taylor CB, Maccoby N, et al. Psychosocial predictors of physical activity in adolescents. *Preventive Medicine* 1990;19:541–551.

Robertson D, Keller C. Relationships among health beliefs, self-efficacy, and exercise adherence in patients with coronary artery disease. *Heart and Lung* 1992;21:56–63.

Robison JI, Rogers MA, Carlson JJ, Mavis BE, Stachnik T, Stoffelmayr B, et al. Effects of a 6-month incentive-based exercise program on adherence and work capacity. *Medicine and Science in Sports and Exercise* 1992;24:85–93.

Rosenstock IM. The health belief model: explaining health behavior through expectancies. In: *health behavior and health education. Theory, research, and practice.* San Francisco: Jossey-Bass Publishers, 1990:39–62.

Rosenstock IM. What research in motivation suggests for public health. *American Journal of Public Health* 1960;50:295–301.

Rosenstock IM. Why people use health services. *Milbank Memorial Fund Quarterly* 1966;44(Suppl):94–124.

Rosenstock IM, Strecher VJ, Becker MH. Social learning theory and the health belief model. *Health Education Quarterly* 1988;15:175–183.

Rowland TW. *Exercise and children's health.* Champaign, IL: Human Kinetics, 1990.

Sallis JF, Alcaraz JE, McKenzie TL, Hovell MF, Kolody B, Nader PR. Parental behavior in relation to physical activity and fitness in 9-year-old children. *American Journal of Diseases of Children* 1992;146:1383–1388.

Sallis JF, Hovell MF, Hofstetter CR. Predictors of adoption and maintenance of vigorous physical activity in men and women. *Preventive Medicine* 1992;21:237–251.

Sallis JF, Hovell MF, Hofstetter CR, Elder JP, Hackley M, Caspersen CJ, et al. Distance between homes and exercise facilities related to frequency of exercise among San Diego residents. *Public Health Reports* 1990;105:179–185.

Sallis JF, Hovell MF, Hofstetter CR, Faucher P, Elder JP, Blanchard J, et al. A multivariate study of determinants of vigorous exercise in a community sample. *Preventive Medicine* 1989;18:20–34.

Sallis JF, McKenzie TL, Alcaraz JE. Habitual physical activity and health-related physical fitness in fourth-grade children. *American Journal of Diseases of Children* 1993;147:890–896.

## Physical Activity and Health

Sallis JF, Nader PR, Broyles SL, Berry CC, Elder JP, McKenzie TL, et al. Correlates of physical activity at home in Mexican-American and Anglo-American preschool children. *Health Psychology* 1993;12:390–398.

Sallis JF, Patterson TL, Buono MJ, Atkins CJ, Nader PR. Aggregation of physical activity habits in Mexican-American and Anglo families. *Journal of Behavioral Medicine* 1988;11:31–41.

Sallis JF, Patterson TL, McKenzie TL, Nader PR. Family variables and physical activity in preschool children. *Journal of Developmental and Behavioral Pediatrics* 1988;9:57–61.

Sallis JF, Simons-Morton BG, Stone EJ, Corbin CB, Epstein LH, Faucette N, et al. Determinants of physical activity and interventions in youth. *Medicine and Science in Sports and Exercise* 1992;24(6 Suppl):S248–S257.

Schmid TL, Pratt M, Howze E. Policy as intervention: environmental and policy approaches to the prevention of cardiovascular disease. *American Journal of Public Health* 1995;85:1207–1211.

Sharp PA, Connell CM. Exercise beliefs and behaviors among older employees: a health promotion trial. *Gerontologist* 1992:32;444-449.

Shephard RJ. Worksite fitness and exercise programs: a review of methodology and health impact. *American Journal of Health Promotion* (in press).

Simons-Morton BG, Parcel GS, Baranowski T, Forthofer R, O'Hara NM. Promoting physical activity and a healthful diet among children: results of a school-based intervention study. *American Journal of Public Health* 1991;81:986–991.

Simons-Morton BG, Parcel GS, O'Hara NM. Implementing organizational changes to promote healthful diet and physical activity at school. *Health Education Quarterly* 1988;15:115–130.

Simons-Morton BG, Parcel GS, O'Hara NM, Blair SN, Pate RR. Health-related physical fitness in childhood: status and recommendations. *Annual Review of Public Health* 1988;9:403–425.

Simons-Morton BG, Taylor WC, Snider SA, Huang IW. The physical activity of fifth-grade students during physical education classes. *American Journal of Public Health* 1993;83:262–264.

Simons-Morton BG, Taylor WC, Snider SA, Huang IW, Fulton JE. Observed levels of elementary and middle school children's physical activity during physical education classes. *Preventive Medicine* 1994;23:437–441.

Simons-Morton DB, Simons-Morton BG, Parcel GS, Bunker JF. Influencing personal and environmental conditions for community health: a multilevel intervention model. *Community Health* 1988;11:25–35.

Skinner BF. *Science and human behavior.* New York: Free Press, 1953.

Skinner CS, Strecher VJ, Hospers H. Physicians' recommendations for mammography: do tailored messages make a difference? *American Journal of Public Health* 1994;84:43–49.

Stokols D. Establishing and maintaining healthy environments: toward a social ecology of health promotion. *American Psychologist* 1992;47:6–22.

Stone EJ. Foreword to process evaluation in the Multicenter Child and Adolescent Trial for Cardiovascular Health (CATCH). *Health Education Quarterly* 1994;21(2 Suppl):S3–S4.

Stone EJ, Baranowski T, Sallis JF, Cutler JA. Review of behavioral research for cardiopulmonary health: emphasis on youth, gender, and ethnicity. *Journal of Health Education* 1995;26(Suppl):S9–S17.

Strasburger VC. Children, adolescents, and television. *Pediatrics in Review* 1992;13:144–151.

Stucky-Ropp RC, DiLorenzo TM. Determinants of exercise in children. *Preventive Medicine* 1993;22:880–889.

Taggart HM, Connor SE. The relation of exercise habits to health beliefs and knowledge about osteoporosis. *Journal of American College Health* 1995;44:127–130.

Tappe MK, Duda JL, Menges-Ehrnwald P. Personal investment predictors of adolescent motivation orientation toward exercise. *Canadian Journal of Sport Sciences* 1990;15:185–192.

Tinsley BJ, Holtgrave DR, Reise SP, Erdley C, Cupp RG. Developmental status, gender, age, and self-reported decision-making influences on students' risky and preventive health behaviors. *Health Education Quarterly* 1995;22:3244–259.

Treiber FA, Baranowski T, Braden DS, Strong WB, Levy M, Knox W. Social support for exercise: relationship to physical activity in young adults. *Preventive Medicine* 1991;20:737–750.

Troiano RP, Flegal KM, Kaczmarski RJ, Campbell SM, Johnson CL. Overweight prevalence and trends for children and adolescents. The National Health and Nutrition Examination Surveys, 1963 to 1991. *Archives. Pediatriatrics and Adolescent Medicine* 1995;149:1085–1091.

Trost SG, Pate RR, Dowda M, Saunders R, Ward DS, Felton G. Gender differences in physical activity and determinants of physical activity in rural fifth grade children. *Journal of School Health* 1996;66:145–150.

U.S. Department of Agriculture, U.S. Department of Health and Human Services. Nutrition and your health: dietary guidelines for Americans. 4th ed. Washington, DC: U.S. Department of Agriculture, 1995. *Home and Garden Bulletin No. 232.*

U.S. Department of Health and Human Services. *Healthy people 2000: national health promotion and disease prevention objectives.* Washington, DC: U.S. Department of Health and Human Services, Public Health Service, 1990. DHHS Publication No. (PHS)91–50212.

U.S. Department of Health and Human Services. *1992 National Survey of Worksite Health Promotion Activities.* Washington, DC: Office of Disease Prevention and Health Promotion, Winter and Spring 1993.

U.S. Department of Transportation. *Final report: the National Bicycling and Walking Study: transportation choices for a changing America.* Washington, DC: U.S. Department of Transportation, Federal Highway Administration, 1994. Publication No. FHWA–PD–94–023.

U.S. Department of Transportation, Zehnpfenning G. *Measures to overcome impediments to bicycling and walking: the National Bicycling and Walking Study, case study No. 4.* Washington, DC: U.S. Department of Transportation, Federal Highway Administration, 1993. Publication No. FHWA–PD–93–031.

U.S. Preventive Services Task Force. *Guide to clinical preventive services.* Baltimore: Williams and Wilkins, 1989.

U.S. Preventive Services Task Force. *Guide to clinical preventive services.* 2nd ed. Baltimore: Williams and Wilkins, 1996.

Walter HJ. Primary prevention of chronic disease among children: the school-based Know Your Body intervention trials. *Health Education Quarterly* 1989;16:201–214.

Weber J, Wertheim EH. Relationships of self-monitoring, special attention, body fat percent, and self-motivation to attendance at a community gymnasium. *Journal of Sport and Exercise Psychology* 1989;11:105–114.

Wechsler H, Levine S, Idelson RK, Schor EL, Coakley E. The physician's role in health promotion revisited—a survey of primary care practitioners. *New England Journal of Medicine* 1996;334:996–998.

Weiss CH. *Research evaluation; methods for assessing program effectiveness.* Englewood Cliffs, NJ: Prentice-Hall, Inc., 1972.

Wells KB, Lewis CE, Leake B, Schleiter MK, Brook RH. The practices of general and subspecialty internists in counseling about smoking and exercise. *American Journal of Public Health* 1986;76:1009–1013.

Wells KB, Lewis CE, Leake B, Ware JE Jr. Do physicians preach what they practice? A study of physicians' health habits and counseling practices. *Journal of the American Medical Association* 1984;252:2846–2848.

Wilbur CS. The Johnson and Johnson program. *Preventive Medicine* 1983;12:672–681.

Williams CL, Carter BJ, Eng A. The Know Your Body program: a developmental approach to health education and disease prevention. *Preventive Medicine* 1980; 9:371–383.

Wilson MG, Crossman L, Davis D, McCarthy. Pychosocial and organizational characteristics of fitness program participants. *American Journal of Health Promotion* 1994: 8;422-424.

Wing RR. Changing diet and exercise behaviors in individuals at risk for weight gain. *Obesity Research* 1995; 3(Suppl 2):277–282.

Winkleby MA. The future of community-based cardiovascular disease intervention studies. *American Journal of Public Health* 1994;84:1369–1372.

Yordy GA, Lent RW. Predicting aerobic exercise participation: social cognitive, reasoned action, and planned behavior models. *Journal of Sport and Exercise Psychology* 1993;15:363–374.

Young DR, Haskell WL, Taylor CB, Fortmann SP. Effect of community health education on physical activity knowledge, attitudes, and behavior: the Stanford Five-City Project. *American Journal of Epidemiology* (in press).

Zakarian JM, Hovell MF, Hofstetter CR, Sallis JF, Keating KJ. Correlates of vigorous exercise in a predominantly low SES and minority high school population. *Preventive Medicine* 1994;23:314–321.

# LIST OF TABLES AND FIGURES

261

## Chapter 5: Patterns and Trends in Physical Activity

## Chapter 6: Understanding and Promoting Physical Activity

# INDEX

## A

Causality, 144–145
Centers for Disease Control and Prevention
(CDC), 5
Behavioral Risk Factor Surveillance System
(BRFSS), 175, 205
exercise recommendations, 23, 28, 33, 148
*Guidelines for School and Community Health
Programs to Promote Physical Activity
Among Youths*, 237, 244
School Health Policies and Programs Study,
236–237
Youth Risk Behavior Survey, 175, 176, 189,
193–199, 205
Cerebrovascular disorders, 7, 47, 45, 102–103,
104–107, 110
Child and Adolescent Trial for Cardiovascular
Health (CATCH) study, 239, 244
Children and physical activity, 75
assessment procedures, 29
behavioral research, 234–243
bone mass development, 131, 132
cardiovascular factors, 75, 91, 102
environmental factors, 73–74
goals, 28, 43
hypertension, 87
injuries, 142
minimum health standard, 17–18, 19
no regular activity, 4
obesity, 43, 47, 133, 134
obesity interventions, 248
regular, vigorous activity, 191
school-based interventions, 6
school program interventions, 236–243
Cholesterol, 19, 23, 47, 91, 102, 110–111
Church programs, 245
Cognition, 135, 141, 142
College Alumni Study, 36
Colon cancer, 4, 5, 7, 113–117, 146, 149
Colorectal cancer, 113
Communications interventions, 230–231
Community-based programs, 6, 227–229, 245–246

Community behavioral approaches, 227–229
Coronary artery
perfusion pressure increase, 64
vasodilation of, 64
Coronary artery bypass, 45
Coronary circulation, 63–64
Coronary disease, 16, 23, 28, 35, 37, 49, 47, 133,
140, 144–147, 149
inverse association with physical activity, 91
physical activity and, 4, 5, 7, 87, 90–91
population-based studies, 92–101
Coronary plaque, 110, 111, 112
Crime, 246–247

# D

Dehydration, 75, 143
Dementia, 136
Depression, 8, 135, 136, 140, 150
Detraining, 21, 61, 72
Diabetes mellitus, 4–6, 28, 35, 37, 43, 90, 125,
133, 144–149, 232
Diabetic retinopathy, 128
Diastolic blood pressure. *See under* Blood pressure
Diet, 5, 12–13, 116, 127, 128, 134, 232–233
*Dietary Guidelines for Americans*, 5, 28, 244
Disability. *See* Physically handicapped
Disuse atrophy, 72–73
Dyslipoproteinemia, 133

# E

Eating disorders, 136
Edema, 133
Educational factors
no physical activity and, 177, 178, 196
regular sustained physical activity, 183
regular, vigorous physical activity, 183, 187
strengthening activity, 191
stretching activity, 191

Eisenhower, President Dwight D., 17, 18
Elderly persons
  behavioral intervention programs for, 233
  cardiovascular response to exercise, 75–76
  cold stress in, 74
  community-based programs for, 245–246
  falling, 7, 132
  health-related quality of life, 142
  maximal oxygen uptake in, 32, 70
  osteoporosis, 130–133
  physical activity interventions for, 233
  physical assessment procedures for, 30
  psychomotor performance of, 35
  resistance training and, 44
Electrocardiographic changes, 111
Emotional functioning, 141
Emphysema, 140
End-diastolic volume. *See under* Blood pressure
Endocrine factors, 66, 67, 70
Endocrine glands, 5, 7
  hormonal responses to exercise, 66
  *See related* Hormones
Endometrial cancer, 7, 114, 120, 149
Endorphins, 141
Endurance training, 4, 18, 19, 21, 61, 63, 65
  capillary increase by, 69
  health benefits of, 7, 43
  health-related quality of life, 142
  insulin sensitivity and, 127
  ischemia and, 112
  lactate threshold and, 67
  metabolic adaptations, 69–70
  muscle fibers in, 67
  obesity and, 135
  osteoporosis and, 150
Enkephalins, 141
Environmental exposure, 19, 73–74
  air pollution, 74
  cold climate disorders, 74
  hot and humid conditions, 63, 73, 143

Epicondylitis, 143
Equilibrium, 35, 44
Ergometer tests. *See under* Exercise tests
Erythropoietin, 68, 74
Estradiol-progesterone, 68
Estrogen, 130, 131
Estrogen replacement therapy, 132
Exercise, 20, 21, 140. *See also* Physical activity;
  Physical activity, specific; Physical fitness;
  Physical fitness programs
Exercise physiology
  research, 18–20
  responses to, 61
  textbooks on, 61
Exercise tests
  accelerometers, 32
  bicycle ergometry, 62–63, 64, 66, 74–75
  maximal, 86, 87, 90
  motion sensors, 31–32
  for muscle fitness, 34–35
  pedometers, 31
  stabilometers, 32
  submaximal, 86, 87, 89
  treadmill, 32, 34, 122
Exercise training
  American College of Sports Medicine
    recommendations, 22
  benefits, 7
  bone adaptations, 67, 69
  cardiovascular diseases and, 45
  definition of, 20
  diabetes mellitus and, 128
  frequency of, 61
  interval vs. continuous, 19
  and lipoprotein, HDL, 43
  muscle, skeletal, adaptations, 67, 69
  triglycerides and, 111
  ventricular fibrillation, 112

Heat stroke, 74
Hematocrit, 43
Hematuria, 143
Hemoconcentration, 74
Hemoglobinuria, 143
High blood pressure *See* Hypertension
Hill's causality criteria, 144–145
Hip fracture, 130, 132
Hispanics
 bicycling activities by, 203
 child behavioral intervention program, 232
 diabetes mellitus and occupational physical
  activity, 126
 high school physical education enrollment and,
  205
 no regular activity by, 177, 195
 physical activity trends in, 8
 regular, sustained activity by, 183
 regular, vigorous activity by, 183, 187, 183,
  196–197
 sports team participation by, 200
 strengthening activities by, 191, 193, 198,
 stretching activities by, 191, 194, 201
 walking activities by, 203
Home care programs, 46
Hyaline cartilage, 130
Hydrogen ions (H+) concentration, 64
Hygiene, 11–18
Hyperglycemia, 127
Hyperinsulinism, 72
Hyperplasia, 69
Hypertension, 4–5, 7, 23, 47, 43, 63, 66, 71,
  126–127, 133
 obesity and, 133
 physical activity and, 103, 110, 144–145, 149
 population studies of, 108–109
Hyperthermia, 143
Hypertrophy, 69, 71, 76, 103
Hypoglycemia, 127–128, 143
Hypotension, 63, 74

# I

Immobilization, 71–72, 130
Immune system, responses to exercise, 7, 67
Immunoglobins, 67
Immunosuppression, 143
Inactivity. *See* Physical inactivity
Indian Health Service, 232
Industrywide Network for Social, Urban, and
  Rural Efforts (INSURE) project, 227
Infection control and exercise, 67
Injuries, 5
 exercise-related, 8, 44, 69, 150, 248
 joint, 129
 musculoskeletal, 142–143
 sports-related, 7
Insulin, 44, 67, 68, 72, 125–129
Intermodal Surface Transportation Efficiency Act,
  247
International Consensus Conference
 of Physical Activity Guidelines for Adolescents
  (1993), 28
 on Physical Activity, Physical Fitness, and
  Health (1988), 22
Interpersonal relationships, 46
 behavioral sciences theories, 213,
 social support role in activity, 214, 243
Intervention studies, adolescent, 8, 236
 accessibility, 236
 church programs for, 245
 determinants, modifiable, 243
 factors influencing, 243
 health care settings, 242
 outdoor activities, 243
 parental involvement, 243
 school-community programs, 242, 245
 school programs, 236–243, 236–243
 self-efficacy, 242, 248
 societal barriers, 246–247
 societal resources, 247

# O

Obesity, 7, 43, 133–135, 150, 248
  abdominal, 35, 128–129
  adult physical activity interventions, 232–234
  behavioral intervention programs, 232–233
  in adolescents, 102
  in children, 102
  childhood intervention, 244
  trends in, 47, 46
Occupational medicine, 15
Occupational physical activity, 113, 116, 175, 189.
  *See also* Worksite physical fitness programs

Olympic Games, 12, 15
Osteoarthritis, 7, 129–130, 133, 149–150
Osteoporosis, 7, 23, 43, 69, 130–133, 150.
  *See related* Bone density
Otitis externa, 143
Ovarian cancer, 7, 114, 116–118, 149
Overtraining, 21, 140
Overweight, 133. *See also* Obesity
Oxidative capacity, of muscle fibers, 65, 67
Oxidative energy system, 65, 66
Oxygen
  arterial-mixed venous, 62, 63, 70
  ATP production within mitochondria, 66
  body's use of, 61
  delivery, 74
  extraction, blood flow, 63
  myocardial demand/use, 63, 64
Oxygen consumption ($\dot{V}O_2$), 18, 31, 32, 34, 66, 70, 74, 110
Oxygen uptake. *See* Maximal oxygen uptake

# P

Pain threshold, 130
Paleolithic rhythm, 11
Pawtucket Heart Health Program (PHHP), 229
Pediatricians, physical activity counseling by, 244

Peripheral vascular disease, 45
Personality disorders, 136
Phosphocreatine (PCr), 65
Physical activity, 21
  of adolescents. *See* Adolescents and physical activity
  of adults. *See* Adults and physical activity
  adverse effects of, 142–144
  approaches to, 46–47
  of children. *See* Children and physical activity
  definition of, 20
  dosage, 146–148
  duration of, 44, 147, 148
  evolution of recommendations, 22–28
  frequency of, 44
  intensity of, 29–33, 35–36, 44
  measures of, 211–215
  no regular, 15–16, 23, 50, 46–48, 177–189, 188, 195, 248
  regular, intermittent, 11, 148
  regular, sustained, 4, 6, 23, 37, 49, 43, 110, 146–147, 182–183, 244
  regular, vigorous, 4, 6, 11, 23, 37, 50, 110, 127–128, 146–147, 182–187, 188, 244
  research considerations, 47, 150
  social environmental approaches to, 244–245
  surveys of, 175, 177
Physical activity, specific
  aerobics, 200, 205
  baseball, 129, 143, 200, 205
  basketball, 143, 200, 205
  bicycling, 4, 143, 144, 187, 200, 203
  boxing, 143
  carpentry, 140
  dancing, 14, 143, 144, 148, 187, 200, 205,
  football, 129, 143, 200, 205
  Frisbee, 197–198, 205
  gardening, 8, 140, 144, 147, 187
  golfing, 140
  hockey, 140, 148
  horseback riding, 14

Neither the U.S. Public Health Service nor the U.S. Department of Health and Human Services endorses any particular organization or its activities, products or services.

The United States Preventive Services Task Force Report: the **Guide to Clinical Preventive Services, 2nd edition** is likely to be the most influential book on the practice of medicine for this decade. The International Medical Publishing printing of the **USPSTF: Guide to Clinical Preventive Services, 2nd edition** includes all of the final revisions to the text completed in 1996. To provide your copy of the **Guide** a long and productive life, International Medical Publishing has sewn the binding and laminated the cover. Detachable prevention guideline table cards can be found behind the index.

The **Clinician's Handbook of Preventive Services** from the U.S. Public Health Service is the "How to" book for applying clinical guidelines. Published in 1994, the **Handbook** is the centerpiece of the "Putting Prevention into Practice Program" and is the perfect companion for the **Guide**. Each chapter details how the various recommended examinations, screening tests and counseling can be performed in practice.

| title | price | quantity | total |
|---|---|---|---|
| Guide to Clinical Preventive Services, 2nd ed. | $24.00 | _____ | _____ |
| Clinician's Handbook of Preventive Services | $17.00 | _____ | _____ |
| Physical Activity and Health: A Report of the Surgeon General | $17.00 | _____ | _____ |
| Shipping and Handling* | $3.00 | | _____ |
| Total | | | _____ |

Include Shipping address with your order. Purchase Orders accepted. For VISA or Mastercharge please include expiration date. Mail your order to:

International Medical Publishing, Inc.
13017 Wisteria Drive, #313
Germantown, MD 20874

*please remit $3.00 S&H per book.

The United States Preventive Services Task Force Report: the **Guide to Clinical Preventive Services, 2nd edition** is likely to be the most influential book on the practice of medicine for this decade. The International Medical Publishing printing of the **USPSTF: Guide to Clinical Preventive Services, 2nd edition** includes all of the final revisions to the text completed in 1996. To provide your copy of the **Guide** a long and productive life, International Medical Publishing has sewn the binding and laminated the cover. Detachable prevention guideline table cards can be found behind the index.

The **Clinician's Handbook of Preventive Services** from the U.S. Public Health Service is the "How to" book for applying clinical guidelines. Published in 1994, the **Handbook** is the centerpiece of the "Putting Prevention into Practice Program" and is the perfect companion for the **Guide**. Each chapter details how the various recommended examinations, screening tests and counseling can be performed in practice.

| title | price | quantity | total |
|---|---|---|---|
| Guide to Clinical Preventive Services, 2nd ed. | $24.00 | _____ | _____ |
| Clinician's Handbook of Preventive Services | $17.00 | _____ | _____ |
| Physical Activity and Health: A Report of the Surgeon General | $17.00 | _____ | _____ |
| Shipping and Handling* | $3.00 | | _____ |
| Total | | | _____ |

Include Shipping address with your order. Purchase Orders accepted. For VISA or Mastercharge please include expiration date. Mail your order to:

International Medical Publishing, Inc.
13017 Wisteria Drive, #313
Germantown, MD 20874

*please remit $3.00 S&H per book.